Mental Health Policy and Practice across Europe

The future direction of mental health care

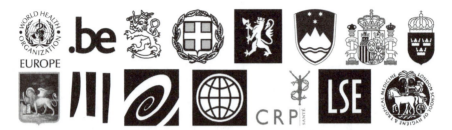

Mental Health Policy and Practice across Europe

The future direction of mental health care

Edited by

**Martin Knapp, David McDaid,
Elias Mossialos and
Graham Thornicroft**

 Open University Press

Open University Press
McGraw-Hill Education
McGraw-Hill House
Shoppenhangers Road
Maidenhead
Berkshire
England
SL6 2QL
email: enquiries@openup.co.uk
world wide web: www.openup.co.uk
and Two Penn Plaza, New York, NY 10121–2289, USA

Mental health policy and practice across Europe

First published 2007

Reprinted 2007

A catalogue record of this book is available from the British Library
ISBN-10 0 335 21467 3 (pb)   0 335 21468 1 (hb)
ISBN-13 978 0 335 21467 9 (pb)   978 0 335 21468 6 (hb)

Library of Congress Cataloging-in-Publication Data
CIP data applied for

Typset by RefineCatch Limited, Bungay, Suffolk
Printed in the UK by Bell & Bain Ltd, Glasgow

European Observatory on Health Systems and Policies Series

The European Observatory on Health Systems and Policies is a unique project that builds on the commitment of all its partners to improving health systems:

- World Health Organization Regional Office for Europe
- Government of Belgium
- Government of Finland
- Government of Greece
- Government of Norway
- Government of Slovenia
- Government of Spain
- Government of Sweden
- Veneto Region of Italy
- European Investment Bank
- Open Society Institute
- World Bank
- CRP-Santé Luxembourg
- London School of Economics and Political Science
- London School of Hygiene & Tropical Medicine

The series

The volumes in this series focus on key issues for health policy-making in Europe. Each study explores the conceptual background, outcomes and lessons learned about the development of more equitable, more efficient and more effective health systems in Europe. With this focus, the series seeks to contribute to the evolution of a more evidence-based approach to policy formulation in the health sector.

These studies will be important to all those involved in formulating or evaluating national health policies and, in particular, will be of use to health policy-makers and advisers, who are under increasing pressure to rationalize the structure and funding of their health system. Academics and students in the field of health policy will also find this series valuable in seeking to understand better the complex choices that confront the health systems of Europe.

The Observatory supports and promotes evidence-based health policy-making through comprehensive and rigorous analysis of the dynamics of health care systems in Europe.

Series Editors

Josep Figueras is the Director of the European Observatory on Health Systems and Policies, and Head of the European Centre for Health Policy, World Health Organization Regional Office for Europe.

Martin McKee is Head of Research Policy and Head of the London Hub of the European Observatory on Health Systems and Policies. He is Professor of European Public Health at the London School of Hygiene & Tropical Medicine as well as a co-director of the School's European Centre on Health of Societies in Transition.

Elias Mossialos is the Co-director of the European Observatory on Health Systems and Policies. He is Brian Abel-Smith Professor in Health Policy, Department of Social Policy, London School of Economics and Political Science and Director of LSE Health.

Richard B. Saltman is Associate Head of Research Policy and Head of the Atlanta Hub of the European Observatory on Health Systems and Policies. He is Professor of Health Policy and Management at the Rollins School of Public Health, Emory University in Atlanta, Georgia.

European Observatory on Health Systems and Policies Series

Series Editors: Josep Figueras, Martin McKee, Elias Mossialos and Richard B. Saltman

Published titles

Primary care in the driver's seat
Richard B. Saltman, Ana Rico and Wienke Boerma (eds)

Human resources for health in Europe
Carl-Ardy Dubois, Martin McKee and Ellen Nolte (eds)

Health policy and European Union enlargement
Martin McKee, Laura MacLehose and Ellen Nolte (eds)

Regulating entrepreneurial behaviour in European health care systems
Richard B. Saltman, Reinhard Busse and Elias Mossialos (eds)

Social health insurance systems in western Europe
Richard B. Saltman, Reinhard Busse and Josep Figueras (eds)

Health care in central Asia
Martin McKee, Judith Healy and Jane Falkingham (eds)

Hospitals in a changing Europe
Martin McKee and Judith Healy (eds)

Funding health care: options for Europe
Elias Mossialos, Anna Dixon, Josep Figueras and Joe Kutzin (eds)

Regulating pharmaceuticals in Europe: striving for efficiency, equity and quality
Elias Mossialos, Monique Mrazek and Tom Walley (eds)

Purchasing to improve health systems performance
Joseph Figueras, Ray Robinson and Elke Jakubowski (eds)

Forthcoming titles

Decentralization in Health Care
Richard B. Saltman, Vaida Bankauskaite and Karsten Vrangbæk (eds)

Contents

List of tables

List of figures

List of boxes

List of contributors

Francesco Amaddeo is Associate Professor of Psychiatry at the Department of Medicine and Public Health, Section of Psychiatry and Clinical Psychology, University of Verona, Italy.

Peter Anderson is a consultant in public health, with an honorary appointment with the Department of Primary Care, University of Oxford.

Robert Anderson is the Coordinator of the Living Conditions programme at the European Foundation for the Improvement of Living and Working Conditions, Dublin.

Thomas Becker is Professor of Psychiatry at the Department of Psychiatry II, University of Ulm, Germany.

Kathryn Berzins is a Research Associate at the Department of Public Health and Health Policy, University of Glasgow.

Peter Bower is Senior Research Fellow at the National Primary Care Research and Development Centre, School of Medicine, University of Manchester.

Traolach Brugha is Professor of Psychiatry and Honorary Consultant Psychiatrist, University of Leicester, Section of Social and Epidemiological Psychiatry, Department of Psychiatry and Brandon Mental Health Unit, Leicester General Hospital.

Lorenzo Burti is Associate Professor of Psychiatry at the Department of Medicine and Public Health, Section of Psychiatry and Clinical Psychology, University of Verona, Italy.

Claire Curran is a health outcomes associate at Lilly and a Ph.D. student at the London School of Economics and Political Science. She was a Research Officer in the Personal Social Services Research Unit at the LSE during the writing of this book.

Paul Cutler is the co-founder and a trustee of UK international mental health charity InterAction. Formerly he was the Deputy Director of the UK charity, the Hamlet Trust.

Natalie Drew is a technical officer of the Mental Health Policy and Service Development team in the Department of Mental Health and Substance Abuse at the World Health Organization.

Angelo Fioritti is Psychiatrist and Medical Director of the Azienda ASL di Rimini, Italy.

Michelle Funk coordinates the work of the Mental Health Policy and Service Development team in the Department of Mental Health and Substance Abuse at the World Health Organization.

Simon Gilbody is Senior Lecturer in Mental Health Services Research at the University of York and the editor of the Cochrane Depression and Anxiety Group.

David Goldberg (Sir) is Emeritus Professor, Health Services Research Department, Institute of Psychiatry, King's College London.

Robert Hayward is a psychologist who has been working as an NGO development consultant for over 15 years. He is the co-founder and Director of the UK international mental health charity, InterAction.

Eva Jané-Llopis is Technical Officer, Mental Health Promotion and Mental Disorder Prevention, WHO Regional Office for Europe, and was previously at the Department of Clinical Psychology, Radboud University of Nijmegen, the Netherlands.

Rachel Jenkins is Director of the WHO Collaborating Centre, and Head of Section on Mental Health Policy, The Institute of Psychiatry, King's College London.

Heinz Katschnig is Professor of Psychiatry and Chairman of the Department of Psychiatry, Medical University of Vienna, and Director of the Ludwig Boltzmann Institute for Social Psychiatry, Vienna, Austria.

Rob Keukens is Mental Health Consultant at the Global Initiative on Psychiatry and Senior Lecturer at HAN University, Nijmegen, the Netherlands.

Susan Kirkwood is a family member and was Treasurer and then Vice-President of EUFAMI (The European Federation of Associations of Families of People with Mental Illness) from to 1998 to 2004.

Martin Knapp is Professor of Social Policy and Director of the Personal Social Services Research Unit at the London School of Economics and Political Science, and Professor of Health Economics and Director of the Centre for the Economics of Mental Health at the Institute of Psychiatry, King's College London.

Viviane Kovess-Masféty is Professor and Director of the Fondation MGEN pour la santé publique, Paris.

Ville Lehtinen is Professor, National Research and Development Centre for Welfare and Health (STAKES), Mental Health R&D Group, Turku, Finland.

Jo Lucas is a freelance consultant in mental health, social work, NGOs and community development, mostly in Central and Eastern Europe and is Director of Kastanja Consulting.

Lorenza Magliano is Associate Professor at the Department of Psychiatry, University of Naples, Italy.

David McDaid is a Research Fellow in Health Policy and Health Economics at the Personal Social Services Research Unit, LSE Health and Social Care at the London School of Economics and Political Science, and at the European Observatory on Health Systems and Policies.

Elias Mossialos is Brian Abel-Smith Professor of Health Policy, and Director of LSE Health at the London School of Economics and Political Science, and Co-director of the European Observatory on Health Systems and Policies.

Camilla Parker is Mental Health and Human Rights Consultant for the Open Society Mental Health Initiative.

Dainius Puras is Associate Professor of Public Mental Health and Child Adolescent Psychiatry at the Faculty of Medicine, Vilnius University, Lithuania.

Diana Rose is Coordinator of SURE, the Service User Research Enterprise, based at the Institute of Psychiatry, King's College London.

Nikolas Rose is Professor of Sociology and Director of the BIOS Centre for the study of Bioscience, Biomedicine, Biotechnology and Society at the London School of Economics and Political Science.

Benedetto Saraceno is the Director of the Department of Mental Health and Substance Abuse at the World Health Organization.

Liz Sayce is Director of Policy and Communication at the Disability Rights Commission in Britain.

Edward Shorter is Hannah Professor in the History of Medicine in the Faculty of Medicine of the University of Toronto.

Michele Tansella is Professor of Psychiatry at the Department of Medicine and Public Health, Section of Psychiatry and Clinical Psychology, University of Verona, Italy.

Graham Thornicroft is Professor of Community Psychiatry and Head of the Health Services Research Department at the Institute of Psychiatry, King's College London, and is a Consultant Psychiatrist at the South London and Maudsley NHS Trust.

Toma Tomov is Professor of Community Psychiatry at the Department of Psychiatry at the Sofia Medical School and Director of the Bulgarian Institute for Human Relations at the New Bulgarian University, Sofia, Bulgaria.

Robert Van Voren is a Consultant at the Global Initiative on Psychiatry, Hilversum.

Charles Watters is Director of the European Centre for the Study of Migration and Social Care, and Senior Lecturer in Mental Health at the University of Kent.

Richard Wynne is a Director of the Work Research Centre, Dublin and a part-time lecturer at University College Dublin.

Series editors' introduction

European national policy-makers broadly agree on the core objectives that their health care systems should pursue. The list is strikingly straightforward: universal access for all citizens, effective care for better health outcomes, efficient use of resources, high-quality services and responsiveness to patient concerns. It is a formula that resonates across the political spectrum and which, in various, sometimes inventive, configurations, has played a role in most recent European national election campaigns.

Yet this clear consensus can only be observed at the abstract policy level. Once decision-makers seek to translate their objectives into the nuts and bolts of health system organization, common principles rapidly devolve into divergent, occasionally contradictory, approaches. This is, of course, not a new phenomenon in the health sector. Different nations, with different histories, cultures and political experiences, have long since constructed quite different institutional arrangements for funding and delivering health care services.

The diversity of health system configurations that has developed in response to broadly common objectives leads quite naturally to questions about the advantages and disadvantages inherent in different arrangements, and which approach is 'better' or even 'best' given a particular context and set of policy priorities. These concerns have intensified over the last decade as policy-makers have sought to improve health system performance through what has become a Europe-wide wave of health system reforms. The search for comparative advantage has triggered – in health policy as in clinical medicine – increased attention to its knowledge base, and to the possibility of overcoming at least part of existing institutional divergence through more evidence-based health policy-making.

The volumes published in the European Observatory on Health Systems and Policies series are intended to provide precisely this kind of cross-national health policy analysis. Drawing on an extensive network of experts and policy-makers working in a variety of academic and administrative capacities, these studies seek to synthesize the available evidence on key health sector topics using a systematic methodology. Each volume explores the conceptual background, outcomes and lessons learned about the development of more equitable, more efficient and more effective health care systems in Europe. With this focus, the series seeks to contribute to the evolution of a more evidence-based approach to policy formulation in the health sector. While remaining sensitive to cultural, social and normative differences among countries, the studies explore a range of policy alternatives available for future decision-making. By examining closely both the advantages and disadvantages of different policy approaches, these volumes fulfil central mandates of the Observatory: to serve as a bridge between pure academic research and the needs of policy-makers, and to stimulate the development of strategic responses suited to the real political world in which health sector reform must be implemented.

The European Observatory on Health Systems and Policies is a partnership that brings together three international agencies, seven national governments, a region of Italy, three research institutions and an international non-governmental organization. The partners are as follows: the World Health Organization Regional Office for Europe, which provides the Observatory secretariat; the governments of Belgium, Finland, Greece, Norway, Slovenia, Spain and Sweden; the Veneto Region; the European Investment Bank; the Open Society Institute; the World Bank; CRP-Santé Luxembourg; the London School of Economics and Political Science and the London School of Hygiene & Tropical Medicine.

In addition to the analytical and cross-national comparative studies published in this Open University Press series, the Observatory produces Health Systems in Transition (HiTs) profiles for a wide range of countries, the journal *EuroHealth* and the policy bulletin *EuroObserver*. Further information about Observatory publications and activities can be found on its website, www.euro.who.int/observatory.

Josep Figueras, Martin McKee, Elias Mossialos and Richard B. Saltman

Foreword

Mental health may be the most neglected public health issue. In much of Europe it remains a taboo to discuss the challenges that mental health raises for governments, societies, and particularly for people with mental health problems themselves. Stigma, prejudice and discrimination are widespread and deeply rooted and, if not addressed, can prevent any progress towards positive change. There are also significant legal and policy-related barriers to the full inclusion of people with mental health problems into society, and to date there has been little effort to address them. Since many governments fail to see the treatment of people with mental health problems as an issue of human rights, there is little political momentum for reform.

Mental Health Policy and Practice across Europe is an important step toward bringing the issue of mental health to the forefront of the public policy debate. In examining historical context, social factors, the legal and human rights perspective, community-based service provision and the role of people with mental health problems as advocates, it serves as a reference for those working to transform mental health policy and lays out a blueprint for moving forward. The editors have done a remarkable job in gathering eminent figures in the European mental health community to author the chapters, and in pulling together this wide array of subjects into a cohesive whole. While highlighting the challenges faced by those who are working in the field of mental health advocacy, this book also reminds us that there are many examples of good practice across Europe – both east and west – and that we have much to learn from each other.

For the past ten years I have had the privilege of working for the Open Society

Institute on promoting the rights of people with mental health problems and intellectual disabilities throughout central and eastern Europe and the former Soviet Union. Our work is focused on providing technical and financial support to organizations that provide community-based alternatives to institutionalization, as well as promoting the social inclusion of people with mental health problems and intellectual disabilities through advocating for policy changes and public awareness campaigns. Through my work with the Open Society Mental Health Initiative, I have had the opportunity to collaborate with many of the contributors to this book. Their commitment to developing mental health policies that promote the rights of people with mental health problems is demonstrated by the pockets of good practice in the region in which we work.

It says much that the Open Society Institute has been the only donor to address on a sustained basis the issue of mental health across central and eastern Europe and the former Soviet Union. Mental health issues remain a low priority among international donors as well as policy-makers. A poignant example of this is that new residential institutions for people with mental health problems and intellectual disabilities are still being built in the new central and eastern European member states of the European Union, despite the fact that some of their governments have stated their intent, over time, to close such institutions. In the former Soviet Union, the transition from state-dominated societies has created conditions that spell untold suffering for people with mental health problems and intellectual disabilities. Pervasive fiscal crises and cuts to government health and social welfare budgets have resulted in the further deterioration of conditions for people in long-term institutions and increased the isolation of those kept at home.

There is a great need for advocacy in mental health from a variety of angles, including the crucial work to address issues of social exclusion. In addition to promoting quality health care and social support, mental health policies must protect the human rights of people with mental health problems in terms of access to education, housing, employment, and leisure and cultural activities. Policies that support the development of community-based alternatives to institutional care are also essential to ensuring the full and equal participation of people with mental health problems in society. In many parts of Europe, however, community-based alternatives remain severely underdeveloped. To move forward, as a first step, governments must recognize the rights of people with mental health problems by elaborating policies that comply with international human rights standards and implementing financing mechanisms that make the shift of resources from institution to community realistic and possible. Perhaps most importantly, people who use mental health services and their families must have a voice in the planning, implementation and review of new policies.

Judith Klein
Director, Mental Health Initiative, Open Society Institute

Foreword by the Minister of Health and Care Services of Norway

It is an important time for the development of mental health policy and practice across Europe. There has never been so much visibility or recognition of the need to tackle mental health problems and promote good mental health. Now it is time to act. Across Europe, many people can expect to experience a mental health problem during their lifetime; many more of us will be affected by mental health problems experienced by family, friends and work colleagues. As this important volume demonstrates, in contrast to most physical health problems, the consequences of poor mental health are broad and persistent. They can, for instance, have an impact on the quality of family and other relationships, reduce the chances of employment, lead to social exclusion and to increased contact with the criminal justice system.

Another important issue, which sets mental health problems apart from many other health issues, is the need in specific circumstances to restrict individual liberty and/or use compulsory treatment. The importance of protecting and respecting human rights so that such powers are not abused cannot be stressed enough. The economic costs to society of poor mental health are also high, and as this book indicates, they are not restricted to the health and social care systems alone; the highest of costs are often due to the lost employment opportunities for both people with mental health problems and sometimes also family members who provide care and support.

Mental ill health is often associated with widespread stigma, ignorance and discrimination, impacting on all aspects of life. Several chapters of this book discuss the need to tackle stigma and improve public awareness in all our countries. Such stigma can be deeply ingrained. It can influence public attitudes, not only about people with mental health problems, but also about whether or not mental health should be seen as a priority issue for public investment.

One very visible experience in Norway can perhaps provide some insight. In 1998, our then Prime Minister, Kjell Magne Bondevik, made public the fact that he had to take three weeks off work because of depression. Mental health became a headline issue in the media and was generally received in a positive and sympathetic way by the general public. Undoubtedly this disclosure acted as a catalyst for both an improved public understanding of mental health problems and also the need for action to improve mental health across many sectors, including in the workplace, school and local community as well as in the health care system.

Throughout this book there is an emphasis on a holistic multi-sectoral, multi-dimensional and evidence-based approach to mental health policy and practice. While it is argued that there is a growing and increasingly robust evidence base on effective interventions, too often there remain gaps in service provision. Our ten-year National Programme for Mental Health, adopted in 1998, called for major investment, expansion and reorganization of services. Empowering service users and family members to participate in all levels of decision-making has been core to this programme. Services should be developed in an appropriate way to meet the needs of these stakeholders. Other key objectives have been to improve public awareness of mental health issues through education programmes; strengthen community-based prevention and early intervention services; expand specialized mental health services for adults, adolescents and children; improve the mental health workforce; improve the accessibility of accommodation and housing for clients of mental health services; and stimulate education and research.

This book rightly puts an emphasis not just on good treatment and rehabilitation but also on the promotion of good mental well-being. In Norway, actions to promote the mental well-being of the population can also be seen, for instance through initiatives such as the national programme for health-promoting workplaces or through the network for health-promoting schools.

In Helsinki, in January 2005, Ministers of Health from all across Europe, together with the World Health Organization, the European Union and the Council of Europe, endorsed a *Declaration and Action Plan* for mental health. In 2006, the European Union also published a Green Paper and launched a public consultation on its future strategy for mental health. Many actions have already been taken in Norway and in other countries. In our Government Programme from October 2005 we prioritize support and services for children and adolescents with mental health and drug problems. There is a growing acknowledgement all over Europe that we must put mental health higher on the agenda.

This book provides a valuable insight into many of the most pressing policy challenges which confront Europe's mental health systems today. It can also be of great assistance in understanding the differing contexts for system reform and will help to bolster efforts to turn recent fine intentions and potential actions into concrete policy and practice across Europe.

Sylvia Brustad
Minister of Health and Care Services, Norway

Acknowledgements

This volume is part of a series of books produced by the European Observatory on Health Systems and Policies. We are very grateful to the authors who wrote the chapters and later amended them following several rounds of rigorous discussions and comments from colleagues and peer-reviewing by external referees.

We particularly appreciate the detailed and very constructive comments of the chief reviewers, Norman Sartorius and Richard Warner. We would also like to thank Pierre Alexandre, Dan Chisholm, Christine Godfrey, David Goldberg, Marijke Gijswijt-Hofstra, Walter Holland, Clemens Huitink, Judith Klein, Judy Laing, Oliver Lewis, Joanna Murray, Steve Platt, Luis Salvador and Kristian Wahlbeck for comments on particular chapters. We would also like to acknowledge helpful information received from Roxana Radulescu and Jarno Habicht and thank Ingrid Zechmeister and Vidar Halsteinli for providing the case study material in Chapter 4.

The Observatory is especially grateful to the Norwegian Directorate for Health and Social Affairs for hosting the Authors' Workshop on 12–13 September 2003. Special thanks are extended to Bjorn Inge Larsen, Director General of the Norwegian Directorate for Health and Social Affairs and to Christine Furuholmen and Olav Valen Slättebrekk, principal coordinators of the workshop, as well as Brit Torill Gutbier and Berit Kolberg Rossiné for their central roles in its organization.

In addition to all the authors at the Workshop who provided detailed feedback on each other's chapters, special thanks are extended to Arlid Gjertsen, Reinhold Killian, Thorleif Ruud and Arman Vardanyan for useful comments.

Three policy briefs based on material from the book were prepared for the WHO European Ministerial Conference on Mental Health that took place in Helsinki in 2005 and we are grateful to our colleagues at the WHO Regional Office for Europe and the government of Finland for helping to facilitate this process.

We would particularly like to thank and acknowledge the work of Anna Maresso, who edited successive versions of the chapters, finalized the manuscript and contributed to project management and coordination. The editors were supported, sustained and gently cajoled throughout the whole process of commissioning, reviewing and editing by her characteristic efficiency.

Finally, while this book has benefited enormously from the contributions of numerous collaborators, responsibility for any errors remains with the editors.

The editors
May 2006

chapter One

Mental health policy and practice across Europe: an overview

Martin Knapp, David McDaid, Elias Mossialos and Graham Thornicroft

Morbidity, need and consequences

Recent years have seen mental health rise significantly up global and European health policy agendas. *The World Health Report 2001* was devoted entirely to mental health (World Health Organization 2001). The World Bank has emphasized better mental health as part of its strategy to improve disadvantaged economies (World Bank 2002). All 52 member states of the WHO European Region, as well as the European Union (EU) and Council of Europe, endorsed a *Declaration* and *Action Plan* on mental health in 2005 (World Health Organization 2005a, 2005b). The EU published its Green Paper on mental health later that same year, following on from other reports related to the state of mental health in Europe and EU actions related to mental health promotion and depression (Commission of the European Communities 2004; G. Henderson *et al.* 2004; Jané-Llopis and Anderson 2005).

International interest of this intensity is long overdue. One in four people experience a significant episode of mental illness during their lifetime, but the 'treatment gap' between the need for, and receipt of, appropriate services remains wide (Kohn *et al.* 2003). Suicide is one of the top ten leading causes of premature death in Europe, contributing an additional 2 per cent to the overall burden of illness (World Health Organization 2005c). The rate of suicide is much higher for men than women and, after traffic accidents, is the principal cause of mortality among 15–35-year-old males in the region. Mental health problems account for approximately 20 per cent of the total disability burden of ill health across Europe (World Health Organization 2004), but receive much lower proportions of total health expenditure (see Chapter 4), often below 5 per cent. Indeed, disability burden calculations of this kind could be underestimates as they overlook the broad impact that mental health problems can have on many aspects of life including physical health, family relationships, social networks, employment status, earnings and broader economic status. Moreover, they do not pick up the impacts on other family members, which are sometimes substantial (see Chapter 16). The stigma still very commonly associated with mental health problems can lead to discrimination, and may help to explain an apparent reluctance by some policy-makers to invest in mental health (see Chapter 13).

Despite growing policy attention, as well as advances in recognition and treatment, there are concerns that the situation in some parts of Europe could get worse before it gets better. Rapid economic and social change in central and eastern Europe has been accompanied by a decline in population mental health, with increasing rates of alcohol problems, violence and suicide (see Chapters 11 and 17). The mental health needs of people displaced through conflict, persecution or economic migration pose further challenges (see Chapter 15). The changing demography of Europe will clearly generate growth in age-related needs over the next few decades. Generally speaking, although the age-specific prevalence of most mental disorders would not be expected to rise (see Kessler *et al.* 2005), economic and social instability in some countries may bring their own inexorable pressures.

There is a strong relationship between poor mental health and social deprivation, with the causal influences working in both directions (Social Exclusion Unit 2004; see Chapter 3). For example, individuals living in areas of high unemployment are at increased risk of developing mental health problems, while deep-rooted stigma, profound ignorance and widely practised discrimination greatly limit education and employment opportunities for mental health service users, often dragging them down into poverty (Thornicroft 2006a). People with chronic mental health problems are at greater risk than the general population of becoming homeless. Contacts with the criminal justice system tend to be quite high for people with psychoses (whether as perpetrators or – all too often – as victims). The long-term impacts on children of people with mental health problems can also be significant: they may suffer from neglect and their schooling may be disrupted, curtailing their own long-term prospects.

Not surprisingly, the economic costs of mental health problems are very high: a few years ago they were conservatively estimated as amounting to between 3 and 4 per cent of gross national product (GNP) for the former EU–15 (Gabriel and Liimatainen 2000). The costs are also widely spread, and indeed the largest economic impacts usually arise outside the health sector (Knapp *et al.* 2004). Productivity losses can be especially large, stemming from short- and long-term absenteeism, reduced performance at the workplace (so-called 'presenteeism'), early retirement, other work cutbacks, reduced opportunities for career development, days 'out of role' for people not in paid work, and reduced lifetime productivity due to premature mortality. Productivity-related costs appear to be on the increase in many European countries (McDaid *et al.* 2005). Other potentially large, non-health costs may fall to social care, housing and criminal justice agencies (see Chapter 4), and of course, to families and service users themselves (see Chapters 14 and 16). Many of those economic impacts persist long into adulthood (Scott *et al.* 2001; Healey *et al.* 2004).

This is a long catalogue of needs, consequences and challenges. Perhaps more than any other health issue, mental health requires a concerted, coordinated, multi-sectoral approach to policy framing and implementation. Of course, Europe comprises a highly heterogeneous collection of countries, and that variety is reflected in the needs of people with mental health problems, their material and social circumstances, their access to treatment and support, and their quality of life. Logically, it should also lead to heterogeneity in policy responses.

Throughout this book we will therefore be searching for commonalities of need, experience, response and outcome, as well as trying to understand the reasons for differences and what they imply for the design and implementation of policy. Of course, we cannot cover every issue affecting mental health policy or practice across a collection of more than 50 countries which demonstrate diversity along so many dimensions. We have, for example, given less attention to mental health problems in childhood, adolescence and older age (and the policy responses to them) than we have to what are sometimes called 'working-age adults' (although the term in itself makes a number of assumptions worthy of debate). We have given more attention to the organization and configuration of services than to the details of the precise treatments they deliver – writing a psychiatry, psychology or nursing textbook was not our aim. There is little in this book on the aetiology of illness, or on the rapidly developing field of enquiry that seeks to unravel the interplay of genes and environment. Doubtless, there are other omissions that will disappoint some readers, but what the book aims to do is to identify, analyse and discuss many of the core and most pressing policy challenges confronting Europe's mental health system 'architects' today. In the remainder of this chapter we introduce those challenges.

Policy responses

Given the many and damaging consequences of poor mental health, one might have expected that promoting good mental well-being and intervening to tackle the consequences of illness would be major priorities for policy-makers. But both the development of national policies and the level of funding for mental health services or initiatives have been disappointing across almost the length and breadth of Europe. Consequently, mental health promotion continues to receive little attention in most countries (see Chapter 8), and treatment strategies are somewhat unevenly and inconsistently implemented (see Chapters 5, 6 and 9). Moreover, some therapeutic initiatives seem to overlook the broad functional and societal ramifications of a diverse group of disorders that includes chronic psychological malaise, destabilizing and disabling phobias and episodes of acute psychosis.

Institution-focused services continue to dominate much of the European mental health landscape and community-based support systems are patchy in availability and quality. Fundamental abuses of human rights continue to occur, perhaps most visibly within the institutions of central and eastern Europe, but certainly not confined to those settings or those parts of the continent (see Chapters 3, 13 and 17). Empowering service users – involving them in decisions and generally broadening the range of choice – is still a long way off in most countries (Mental Disability Advocacy Center 2005a; see Chapter 14).

Having a national policy on mental health is widely seen as fundamental to the task of raising awareness and securing resources, which, in turn, are necessary to deliver effective, equitable and affordable treatments (World Health Organization 2005a, 2005b). A national policy can obviously provide the framework within which to coordinate actions across the multiple agencies and sectors that one would hope would be in place to respond to the multiple needs of people with mental health problems. Developing and strengthening policy for mental health across Europe, therefore, remains a key concern, and most countries now have national or regional mental health policies in place. Some have a long pedigree (see Chapter 2), some are revisited and revised quite regularly, while others are rather dated and clearly in need of reform. Quite a few look out of touch with today's social norms, aspirations and mores. Some national policy frameworks fail to extend beyond the confines of the health system, failing to emphasize the need for concerted attention from the contiguous fields of housing, education, social care, criminal justice and employment (see Chapter 12). Clear statements on rights, enshrined in legislation, are still rare (see Chapter 13). Remarkably, in view of the high suicide rates in many countries, there also appear to be few national strategies for suicide prevention (Beautrais 2005). And even when policies are laid out, they may not actually be implemented (see Chapter 17).

There is a continuing need to take action to address human rights violations, stigma, discrimination and social exclusion more broadly. Few other health problems are characterized by such disadvantages. Violations of rights have been reported across Europe, but are most visible in the psychiatric institutions, dispensaries and social care homes that remain the mainstay of mental health systems in parts of central and eastern Europe. In some countries, individuals admitted to institutional settings still have a very low probability of returning to the community. There have also been well documented accounts by human rights groups and the Council of Europe of individuals being kept in 'caged beds' or being subjected to electro-convulsive therapy without anaesthesia or muscle relaxants in contravention of international guidelines (see Chapter 13).

Legislative instruments have obvious roles to play. There are already human rights instruments drawn up by the United Nations, the Council of Europe and the EU which are intended to protect people with mental health problems, the principles of which should underpin the development of national legislation. However, any such legislation can only be effective if implemented and monitored, with adequate sanctions to effect change. Legislation can ensure, for example, that compulsory treatment or detention is used as a last resort, and can build in safeguards such as access to an independent periodic review for people involuntarily treated or admitted to services.

Funding

In broad terms, there is a simple link between funding, the employment of staff and other resources, their combination to deliver services, treatments and support, and the achievement of individual, familial and societal mental health goals. In reality, of course, the links themselves are far from simple, but getting the right funding base established must accompany the development of a robust policy framework.

The levels and routes of mental health service financing vary somewhat from country to country, and indeed within countries, in response to a plethora of political, economic, cultural and other influences. Some funding routes can create incentives to better practice, while others erect barriers to the achievement of better individual-level and other outcomes (see Chapter 4). What is abundantly clear is that as the countries of Europe move away from mental health systems dominated by 'asylum management' to systems focused on 'community management', so too must the balance of funding shift from almost exclusive reliance on health systems to a more mixed economy of resources. As community models develop, services and supports from outside the health system will be called upon to help people to access appropriate housing, leisure facilities, associations, employment and all of those 'ordinary' ingredients that together greatly influence quality of life. Bureaucracy, immutable budgetary boundaries, official indifference, professional ignorance, pervasive stigma and sometimes simply the desperate scarcity of resources can stack up to deny people with mental health problems the liberties, opportunities and achievements enjoyed by others.

One of the major challenges across Europe, therefore, and unfortunately a challenge that has still to be taken up by many governments, is to create the incentives for the appropriate resources to be mobilized and, where necessary, moved between agencies and services so that people can access the support they need across relevant life domains. In countries such as the United Kingdom, where access to social care services is selective and means-tested, while access to health care is universal and free at the point of delivery, there are clearly ideological as well as practical difficulties to be overcome. In countries such as Austria, which has moved to a financing system based upon diagnostic-related groups, the problems are of a different kind, relating to the under-funding of mental health services. In countries where service users are expected to make substantial out-of-pocket contributions to the costs of their treatment, a major barrier will be affordability, particularly given that so many service users have to survive on very low incomes. In parts of eastern Europe the resource challenge is that governments do not, or cannot, prioritize mental health services, leaving the systems of support mired in outmoded practices dominated by institutions.

Institutions and communities

We emphasized earlier the heterogeneity of mental health policies and practices in Europe. Nowhere is this more evident than in the respect of institutional care: consigned to history in a few west European countries – where the gaze of policy attention is now more likely to be turning (albeit gradually) to social inclusion, destigmatization and empowerment – elsewhere it is still the primary focus of official action and still eating up the lion's share of total dedicated mental health expenditure.

The old asylums were promoted on a number of grounds. It was widely assumed that grouping people together in large numbers, with (hopefully) benign if (largely) unqualified staff, was the most effective way to contain and perhaps even to 'cure' people with mental health problems. Economies of scale were attractive. The preference of family members was often to have their 'disturbed' relatives accommodated in secluded settings, away from social embarrassment and harm (but also often then forgotten). Those asylums were undoubtedly also used as instruments of social control, not generally in the appalling way that psychiatric services were abused in the former Soviet system (see Chapter 17), but simply as an expedient, cheap and unobtrusive way of managing 'imbeciles', 'lunatics', promiscuous young women and other social 'deviants'.

The impetus to close the asylums came from equivalent, if diametrically opposite, arguments (see Chapter 10). It gradually came to be recognized that community-based services were more effective in promoting quality of life for the majority of people (Thornicroft and Tansella 2004), and also that they were not necessarily more expensive (Knapp et al. 1997). The views of individual service users were now sought, listened to and (increasingly, if slowly) acted upon, while the views of families and of wider society were mellowing – moving away from the need to hide 'peculiar' people away. Communities may be less hostile today, although one should be careful not to exaggerate the extent of any change. Similarly, the social control rationalization for asylums has been somewhat eroded, if not exactly swept away, by a slowly rising tide of support for human rights.

There is now quite wide acknowledgement that a 'balanced care' approach is required, where front-line services are based in the community but hospitals and other congregate care settings play important roles as specialist providers (Thornicroft and Tansella 2004). Where they are required, hospital stays should be as brief as possible, and should be offered in 'normalized' integrated facilities rather than in specialized, isolated locations. All but a few countries of the EU-25, for example, have seen the steady rundown of psychiatric hospital bed numbers over the last 30 or more years, although the decline generally has been slower in the newer member states (McDaid and Thornicroft 2005). Outside the EU, this shift away from institutional care generally has been slower, and there is often the added complication of a long tradition of using long-stay social care homes (*internats*). Perverse financial incentives sometimes link funding directly to bed occupancy, giving little encouragement or flexibility to local decision-makers to develop community-based alternatives.

New challenges may be looming. Some countries which have successfully closed most of their psychiatric hospitals may be moving into a phase of what some commentators have termed 'reinstitutionalization', where the kinds of individuals once accommodated in the old hospitals are now quite likely to find themselves in prisons, secure forensic units or care homes (Priebe *et al.* 2005).

Social inclusion and empowerment

Accompanying the move away from hospital-centred services across much of the European continent, particularly in higher-income countries, has been a gradual 'reconceptualization' of need, with more emphasis on human rights and social inclusion. As we have already stressed, a huge challenge for many people with mental health problems is stigma, which can lead to social marginalization, neglect and disadvantage. Even mental health professionals who themselves have used mental health services may experience discrimination from employers, colleagues and educators (Rooke-Matthews and Lindow 1998). A well received report from the Social Exclusion Unit (2004: 4) in England argued that there are:

> Five main reasons why mental health problems too often lead to and reinforce social exclusion: stigma and discrimination . . . low expectations of what people with mental health problems can achieve . . . lack of clear responsibility for promoting vocational and social outcomes . . . lack [of] ongoing support to enable them to work . . . [and] barriers to engaging in the community.

These reasons were identified in the English context, but would have their equivalents elsewhere (see Chapter 3).

One illustrative domain can be considered. Because paid work is so central to an individual's economic well-being, as well as to their social status and integration, attention is today being paid by some governments to the employment opportunities and needs of people with mental health problems. The detailed *Action Plan* endorsed by health ministers in Helsinki in 2005 called specifically for efforts to 'create healthy workplaces by introducing measures such as exercise, changes to work patterns, sensible hours and healthy management styles', and also to 'include mental health in programmes dealing with occupational health and safety' (World Health Organization 2005b: 2). Whether these positive words get turned into widely implemented deeds remains to be seen, but there are some encouraging signs in a few countries (Berkels *et al.* 2004; Henderson *et al.* 2005). Initiatives have been taken in some states to reform social welfare benefit structures in order to encourage people to return to work (Teague 1999). Such initiatives will have an impact on people claiming disability benefits, among whom are an increasing number of people with mental health problems (Jarvisalo *et al.* 2005).

While such reforms may act as an incentive for individuals to seek employment, changes to the social welfare system alone will not be sufficient to promote long-term job acquisition and retention by people with mental health problems. Welfare reform needs to be part of a broader package of measures that includes enforcement of anti-discrimination legislation, participation in vocational rehabilitation or supported employment schemes, improvements to workplace support, flexible working arrangements and better access to effective treatments. Health professionals may hold low expectations of what mental health service users can achieve, and may do little to encourage their employment aspirations. The previously mentioned report on social exclusion in England found a lack of clear responsibility for promoting social and vocational outcomes, a lack of ongoing support to enable people to work, and structural barriers to engagement in the community (Social Exclusion Unit 2004). It called for more choice and empowerment of service users, as well as help to retain jobs, to return to employment after an episode of illness, and to achieve career progression. Helping individuals to obtain and retain employment in the open job market could help reduce stigma and discrimination by employers, although breaking into this vicious cycle is not straightforward (Bond 1998).

Linked to the promotion of social inclusion is empowerment. There is, for example, evidence that many service-user organizations (as well as other stakeholders) in the United Kingdom support the use of 'advanced directives', where an individual, when well, specifies how they wish to be treated if they become unwell (Atkinson *et al.* 2004; C. Henderson *et al.* 2004). Such advance directives were thought to be empowering and potentially destigmatizing, although it was recognized that many problems need to be overcome in their implementation. Support for advance directives has also been reported among Dutch patient groups (Varekamp 2004). Crisis cards can be empowering (Sutherby *et al.* 1999). Consumer-directed services, such as arrangements that allow individuals to hold the budgets with which they can purchase some of the services they need, take service user control onto another plane. However, most such arrangements currently tend to exclude health care, and there are also numerous potential complications to be ironed out concerning the roles of family members, how the funding can be used and the extent to which individuals are empowered to take risks (Ungerson 2004). In fact, uptake of such arrangements in England has been disappointingly slow (Fernandez *et al.* 2006).

Conclusion: continuing challenges

What then, are the key questions for policy-makers in Europe and what are the toughest challenges they face as they seek to develop strategies and service systems that are fit for purpose in the new millennium, rather than stuck in a bygone age of narrow views, stigmatizing attitudes and bottom-of-the-pile priorities?

Fighting discrimination

Stigma distinguishes mental health disorders from most other health problems and is the major reason for discrimination and social exclusion. Tackling this discrimination remains a key policy challenge (Thornicroft 2006b). In some parts of central and eastern Europe fundamental human rights abuses continue to be seen in the psychiatric institutions and social care homes that are the mainstay of mental health systems (Mental Disability Advocacy Center 2005b). But abuse manifests itself in many ways; even where community-based care is the dominant mode of delivery, neglect and isolation can be widespread. Fear of stigmatization reduces an individual's willingness to seek treatment (Corrigan and Calabrese 2005). There are no easy solutions for policy-makers, but long-term actions such as intervention in schools to raise awareness of mental health (Pinfold *et al.* 2003, 2005), and constructive engagement with the media (which can reinforce negative social attitudes by sensationalist and inaccurate portrayals of mental illness) appear to be effective if concerted and prolonged (Hickie 2004; Jorm *et al.* 2005).

Closing the institutions

Clearly one of the biggest challenges in a number of European countries is to move the balance of care away from the old institutions. The large, closed asylums may have had their uses, but they embody and indeed reinforce wholly negative attitudes – including stigmatizing attitudes – about mental illness. As discussed in Chapters 4 and 10, it is relatively easy to close an institution but far harder to replace it with community-based arrangements that offer better support and greater opportunity by delivering high quality services of the kind that people actually want to use. Entrenched views held by the general public and by many mental health professionals need to be countered, and real efforts made to get people out of these institutions.

Developing caring communities

A related set of questions for policy-makers, therefore, is how to foster better community-based systems of support and treatment. This has to mean more than just replacing asylum provision with the occasional outpatient appointment. Policy-makers must assess the needs that people have, and identify appropriate configurations of community services to meet them. Are specialist services required to address specialist needs such as those associated with prodomal signs of serious illness, or the eruption of crises, or the need to keep people in contact with services? Has the development and rapid growth in uptake of new pharmacotherapies helped, or is too much reliance placed on them (see Chapter 7; Knapp *et al.* 2005)?

Promoting broad quality of life

The central concern of any mental health care system should be how best to promote the quality of life of individuals and families affected by, or at risk of developing, mental illness. Quality of life is a nebulous concept, inherently subjective, culture-bound and notoriously hard to measure well. What is clear, however, is the frequency and regularity with which service users emphasize certain dimensions of quality of life such as access to employment and other valued social roles, removal of discriminatory barriers and better social integration. This implies a pressing need for mental health systems to look beyond 'merely' alleviating symptoms or reducing the probability of relapse, and instead to encourage services and therapies that are more holistic and more ambitious in their aims.

Developing an evidence-based decision-making approach

What therapies, services and support arrangements achieve the outcome improvements wanted by service users and their families? If there is more than one option, which is the most cost-effective? There exist validated tools for measuring well-being and adjudging outcomes (Thornicroft *et al.* 2006), and an evidence base on effectiveness and cost-effectiveness is certainly developing (see Chapters 4–9, for example). But the volume and quality of evaluative evidence could certainly be improved. Steps need to be taken to ensure that available information is what policy-makers actually want, that it reaches them in a form that they can understand and employ, and of course, that they take into consideration. More can also be done to improve channels of communication between policy-makers, 'front-line' workers, researchers and other stakeholders. It must be asked whether the evidence is robust enough to allow mental health services to compete with other claims on a country's scarce health or wider resources. And if the evidence base is there for better treatments and interventions, are the right skills available within the workforce, and can the people with those skills be recruited to deliver what is needed?

Choice and control

A lot of attention has been focused recently on the promotion of self-determination through the empowerment of service users (see Chapters 3 and 14), linked to the protection of their human rights (Chapter 13). Do mental health service users have the same rights and opportunities to exercise choice and assume control as are available to other members of society? For policy-makers, one major challenge is to balance the need to keep vulnerable people in touch with services against the danger of interfering too assertively in their lives. Another is to design policy and practice measures that balance the need to protect individuals and communities from harm (including self-harm) against the risk of denying people their right to freedom and self-determination.

Understanding the money

We have already alluded to the funding challenge. By their very nature, many mental health problems are multiple, complex and (mostly) chronic. For people with more severe problems the consequence is therefore often a need for support from a range of different services and agencies. Policy-makers need to understand the widely ranging costs associated with mental health problems and look to create the right funding environment and the right structure of incentives to ensure that resources from across different agencies are combined in the best ways to enhance quality of life. The case for investment in mental health is surely very strong. There is now substantial evidence that greater expenditure in many areas of mental health is not only justified on the grounds of symptom alleviation and quality of life promotion, but also because it represents a more efficient use of health (and other sector) resources, allowing individuals to achieve, maintain or regain valued social roles.

Joining up decision-making

Even if there is sufficient political commitment to invest in effective interventions to promote better mental health, implementation remains problematic. Multiple responsibilities and multiple costs can raise a number of barriers (Knapp *et al.* 2006). One danger is that well-meaning initiatives or reforms are seriously under-funded and under-coordinated. Some of these problems may be addressed by creating joint health, social care and housing budgets for mental health, or by reaching agreements that facilitate the movement of money between different national or local government budgets in order to help overcome some of the disincentive (or perverse incentive) problems that can distort or inhibit appropriate action.

Promoting promotion

It is obvious from many chapters in this book that much more could be done to support mental health promotion. Few governments have given much attention to policies that can promote population well-being and individual mental health. Are the promotion possibilities recognized and responded to? Are governments setting up the right public mental health initiatives? One obvious challenge is that the development and implementation of strategies for public mental health promotion require action across many different agencies and sectors, as well across the life course. Examples include parent training programmes and interventions for the early identification of mental health problems in schools, flexible practices and access to counselling and support in the workplace, and bereavement counselling and social activities to reduce isolation and the risk of depression in older age. In turn, these efforts need mental health decision-makers to engage with a range of stakeholders including teachers, social workers, employers associations, trade unions and local community groups, including faith-based organizations.

From containment to opportunity

The most general over-arching challenge is to continue to move Europe's mental health systems out of the age of containment and confinement and into an era of opportunity and choice. The Helsinki Declaration of 2005 was most certainly a welcome development, setting out a whole range of actions to which signatory countries gave their commitment. The supra-national signatories to the Declaration (the EU, the World Health Organization and the Council of Europe) will want to work with national governments to support implementation of the *Action Plan*. The opening is there to create new opportunities for people affected by mental health problems to be socially included, to move from structures seemingly obsessed with containment to policies focused on lifestyle opportunities.

References

Atkinson, J.M., Garner, M.C. and Gilmour, W.H (2004) Models of advance directives in mental health care: stakeholder views, *Social Psychiatry and Psychiatric Epidemiology*, 39(8): 673–80.

Beautrais, A. (2005) National strategies for the reduction and prevention of suicide, *Crisis*, 26(1): 1–3.

Berkels, H., Henderson, J., Henke, N., Kuhn, K., Lavikainen, J., Lehtinen, V., Ozamiz, A., Van den Heede, R. and Zenzinger, K. (2004) *Mental Health Promotion and Prevention Strategies for Coping with Anxiety, Depression and Stress Related Disorders in Europe (2001–2003)*. Research report 1001. Bremerhaven: Federal Institute for Occupational Safety and Health.

Bond, G.R. (1998) Principles of individual placement and support, *Psychiatric Rehabilitation Journal*, 22(11): 23.

Commission of the European Communities (2004) *The State of Mental Health in the European Union*. Luxembourg: Commission of the European Communities.

Corrigan, P.W. and Calabrese, J.D. (2005) Strategies for assessing and diminishing self-stigma, in P.W. Corrigan (ed.) *On the Stigma of Mental Illness: Practical Strategies for Research and Social Change*. Washington, DC: American Psychological Association.

Fernandez, J.L., Kendall, J., Davey, V. and Knapp, M. (2006) Direct payments in England: factors linked to variations in provision, *Journal of Social Policy*, 36(1): 1–25.

Gabriel, P. and Liimatainen, M.-R. (2000) *Mental Health in the Workplace*. Geneva: International Labour Organization.

Healey, A., Knapp, M. and Farrington, D. (2004) Adult labour market implications of antisocial behaviour in childhood and adolescence: findings from a UK longitudinal study, *Applied Economics*, 36(2): 93–105.

Henderson, C., Flood, C., Leese, M., Thornicroft, G., Sutherby, K. and Szmukler, G. (2004) Effect of joint crisis plans on use of compulsory treatment in psychiatry: single blind randomised controlled trial, *British Medical Journal*, 329: 136–8.

Henderson, G., Henderson, J., Lavikainen, J. and McDaid, D. (2004) *Actions Against Depression: Improving Mental Health and Well Being by Combating the Adverse Health, Social and Economic Consequences of Depression*. Luxembourg: Commission of the European Communities, Health and Consumer Protection Directorate General.

Henderson, M., Glozier, N. and Holland Elliot, K. (2005) Long term sickness absence, *British Medical Journal*, 330: 802–3.

Hickie, I. (2004) Can we reduce the burden of depression? The Australian experience with beyondblue: the national depression initiative, *Australian Psychiatry*, 12(Suppl): S38–46.

Jané-Llopis, E. and Anderson, P. (2005) *Mental Health Promotion and Mental Disorder Prevention: A Policy for Europe*. Nijmegen: Radboud University Nijmegen.

Jarvisalo, J., Andersson, B., Boedeker, W. and Houtman, I. (eds) (2005) *Mental Disorders as a Major Challenge in the Prevention of Work Disability: Experiences in Finland, Germany, the Netherlands and Sweden*. Helsinki: The Social Insurance Institution, Finland.

Jorm, A.F., Christensen, H. and Griffiths, K.M. (2005) The impact of beyondblue: the national depression initiative on the Australian public's recognition of depression and beliefs about treatments, *Australian and New Zealand Journal of Psychiatry*, 39(4): 248–54.

Kessler, R.C., Demler, O., Frank, R.G., Olfson, M., Pincus, H.A., Walters, E.E., Wang, P., Wells, K.B. and Zaslavsky, A.M. (2005) Prevalence and treatment of mental disorders, 1990 to 2003, *New England Journal of Medicine*, 352: 2515–23.

Knapp, M., Chisholm, D., Astin, J., Lelliott, P. and Audini, B. (1997) The cost consequences of changing the hospital-community balance: the mental health residential care study, *Psychological Medicine*, 27(3): 681–92.

Knapp, M., Mangalore, R. and Simon, J. (2004) The global costs of schizophrenia, *Schizophrenia Bulletin*, 30(2): 279–93.

Knapp, M., Kanavos, P., King, D. and Yesudian, H.M. (2005) Economic issues in access to medications: schizophrenia treatment in England, *International Journal of Law and Psychiatry*, 28(5): 514–31.

Knapp, M., Funk, M., Curran, C., Prince, M., Gibbs, M. and McDaid, D. (2006) Mental health in low- and middle-income countries: economic barriers to better practice and policy, *Health Policy and Planning*, 21(3): 157–70.

Kohn, R., Saxena, S., Levav, I. and Saraceno, B. (2003) The treatment gap in mental health care, *Bulletin of the World Health Organization*, 82: 858–66.

McDaid, D. and Thornicroft, G. (2005) *Balancing Institutional and Community Based Care*. Policy brief. Copenhagen: WHO on behalf of the European Observatory on Health Systems and Policies.

McDaid, D., Curran, C. and Knapp, M. (2005) Promoting mental well-being in the workplace: a European policy perspective, *International Review of Psychiatry*, 17(5): 365–73.

Mental Disability Advocacy Center (2005a) *The Right to Vote at Risk in Bulgaria*. Budapest: Mental Disability Advocacy Center.

Mental Disability Advocacy Center (2005b) *Russia's Guardianship System Challenged at the European Court of Human Rights*. Budapest: Mental Disability Advocacy Center.

Pinfold, V., Toulmin, H., Thornicroft, G., Huxley, P., Farmer, P. and Graham, T. (2003) Reducing psychiatric stigma and discrimination: evaluation of educational interventions in UK secondary schools, *British Journal of Psychiatry*, 182: 342–6.

Pinfold, V., Thornicroft, G., Huxley, P. and Farmer, P. (2005) Active ingredients in anti-stigma programmes in mental health, *International Review of Psychiatry*, 17(2): 123–31.

Priebe, S., Badesconyi, A., Fioritti, A., Hansson, L., Kilian, R., Torres-Gonzaels, F., Turner, T. and Wiersma, D. (2005) Reinstitutionalization in mental health care: comparison of data on service provision from six European countries, *British Medical Journal*, 330: 123–6.

Rooke-Matthews, S. and Lindow, V. (1998) *The Experiences of Mental Health Service Users as Mental Health Professionals*. Findings 488. York: Joseph Rowntree Foundation.

Scott, S., Knapp, M., Henderson, J. and Maughan, B. (2001) Financial cost of social exclusion: follow-up study of antisocial children into adulthood, *British Medical Journal*, 323: 191–4.

Social Exclusion Unit (2004) *Mental Health and Social Exclusion*. London: Office of the Deputy Prime Minister.

Sutherby, K., Szmukler, G.I., Halpern, A., Alexander, M., Thornicroft, G., Johnson, C. and Wright, S. (1999) A study of 'crisis cards' in a community psychiatric service, *Acta Psychiatrica Scandinavica*, 100(1): 56–61.

Teague, P. (1999) Reshaping employment regimes in Europe: policy shifts alongside boundary change, *Journal of Public Policy*, 19(1): 33–62.

Thornicroft, G. (2006a) *Shunned: Discrimination against People with Mental Illness*. Oxford: Oxford University Press.

Thornicroft, G. (2006b) *Actions Speak Louder: Tackling Discrimination against People with Mental Illness*. London: Mental Health Foundation.

Thornicroft, G. and Tansella, M. (2004) Components of a modern mental health service: a pragmatic balance of community and hospital care: overview of systematic evidence, *British Journal of Psychiatry*, 185: 283–90.

Thornicroft, G., Becker, T., Knapp, M., Knudsen, HC., Schene, AH., Tansella, M. and Váquez-Barquero, J.L. (2006) *International Outcome Measures in Mental Health: Quality of Life, Needs, Service Satisfaction, Costs and Impact on Carers*. London: Gaskell, Royal College of Psychiatrists.

Ungerson, C. (2004) Whose empowerment and independence? A cross-national perspective on cash for care schemes, *Ageing and Society*, 24: 189–212.

Varekamp, I. (2004) Ulysses directives in the Netherlands: opinions of psychiatrists and clients, *Health Policy*, 70(3): 291–301.

World Bank (2002) *World Development Report 2002: Building Institutions for Markets*. Washington, DC: World Bank.

World Health Organization (2001) *The World Health Report 2001. Mental Health: New Understanding, New Hope*. Geneva: World Health Organization.

World Health Organization (2004) *The World Health Report 2004. Changing History. Geneva: World Health Organization.*

World Health Organization (2005a) *Mental Health Declaration for Europe: Facing the Challenges, Building Solutions*. Copenhagen: World Health Organization.

World Health Organization (2005b) *Mental Health Action Plan for Europe: Facing the Challenges, Building Solutions*. Copenhagen: World Health Organization.

World Health Organization (2005c) Suicide prevention website, http://www.who.int/mental_health/prevention/suicide/suicideprevent/en/index.html.

chapter two

The historical development of mental health services in Europe

*Edward Shorter**

This chapter traces the evolution of mental health care from the early nineteenth century to the present in the countries that came to form the European Union (EU) – and in the candidates for membership in 2004. What are the overall themes of change? What patterns emerge among the various states? Given that in Europe and America neuropsychiatric illness represents 43 per cent of the total burden of disability (Thornicroft and Maingay 2002), these are important questions.

This huge undertaking reminds us that there are two ways of looking at systems of mental health care: the vertical and the horizontal. The vertical dimension refers to how well the system is integrated, in the sense of providing continuous care from the community to mental hospital and back to the community; or from the community to the psychiatry department of a general hospital and back. The horizontal dimension refers to how comprehensive the system is: whether, in addition to family doctors and psychiatrists, a health care team based in community centres includes psychologists, psychiatric nurses and social workers, and even nutritionists and occupational therapists. (One can conceive this horizontal dimension as a functional model of disability rather than an illness model. As Bob Grove (1994: 431) puts it, 'The doctor or psychiatrist becomes only one expert among many others in the management of a disability.') Both dimensions, vertical and horizontal, have their own patterns of change.

Why begin in the early nineteenth century? One could, in fact, begin much earlier (Porter 1987). It goes without saying that patients with psychiatric illnesses have always existed, and that society has always devised some means of coping with them. Yet in Europe prior to the early nineteenth century, these coping stratagems were non-medical in nature, involving the Church and local authorities. A mental health care system presupposes a multidisciplinary approach to psychiatric illness, and makes the assumptions that (a) admission to a psychiatric facility is therapeutic rather than custodial, and (b) that effective psychopharmaceuticals or convincing physical therapies exist for assistance in community care. Although today biopsychosocial models of care, which involve many disciplines, are in vogue, historically the triumph of the doctor over the priest in the treatment of mental illness entailed, essentially, the triumph of the medical model (Shorter 1997: 1–22).

The history of mental health care within the territories that became the EU may therefore be divided into three periods. Period I, dating from the early nineteenth century to the mid-twentieth, represents the epoch of institutional mental health care, as a district-level network of mental hospitals was constructed across Europe, and spas and private sanatoriums became the elective sites of care for 'nervous' illnesses among the middle and upper classes.

Period II, from the end of the Second World War to the 1970s, represents the beginning of systematic community mental health systems, in the form of extensive private-practice psychiatry, the advent of effective psychoactive medications, and the establishment of day care and outpatient clinics in most psychiatric hospitals. This period really represents the first wave of community-based care.

Period III, dating from the 'long-term programme' in 1970 of the WHO Regional Office for Europe to the present (Freeman *et al.* 1985: 5), represents a systematic expansion of vertical care, in the form of sectorization and deinstitutionalization, as well as horizontal care, in the form of the continent-wide expansion of the comprehensive community-care patterns that had begun after the Second World War.

Period I: the era of the asylum

The legacy of this initial period in the modern history of psychiatric care was the institutional impulse (Porter and Wright 2003). It represented a cultural, political and social reflex that made admission to a mental hospital the benchmark of quality mental health care. Undoubtedly, in a situation where community mental health care was non-existent for the majority of people, hospital admission did represent an appropriate treatment for major illness, all the more so in the absence of effective psychopharmaceuticals. Yet as a legacy to an era that possesses pharmacologic alternatives, the institutional reflex is inappropriate, chaining mental health care to giant structures of brick and mortar.

A bit of perspective is useful here, however. It has become fashionable to deplore the 'confinement' of psychiatric patients in mental hospitals and to demand community care. But one recalls that, in the context of the history of psychiatry, the early therapeutic asylums were a decided step forward in view of the often terrible conditions that these individuals encountered in the 'community'. In Denmark, for example, as late as 1840, the mentally ill were locked up in wooden cages in the villages or chained in stalls; 142 such cages were known to officials. As late as 1908 this kind of community care was customary in rural Sweden and Finland (Pandy 1908: 3n.). Under these circumstances, admission to a clean, orderly mental hospital was often welcome to the patients and their families.

Although Europe had known custodial asylums since the Middle Ages, a page in the history of psychiatry was turned with the advent of the first therapeutic asylums. Arguably, the first was formed in the 1780s in Florence under the aegis of Vincenzo Chiarugi, several others in Paris in the 1790s under Philippe Pinel, and then an increasing number in many other countries in the following years (Shorter 1997: 8–21). Yet the therapeutic aims of these early institutions were soon overwhelmed by the press of numbers. And from the viewpoint of mental health care systems, the crucial event in this first phase was the laying down of a district-level network of asylums, each with its own catchment area. This began in England with the County Asylums Act of 1808, in France with the Law of 1838, and in other countries at successively later dates (Pichot 1983: 17, 33–4; Jones 1993).

By the last third of the nineteenth century, an impressive array of district-level asylums was flung across western Europe. The table of contents of one of the standard asylum directories conveys the sheer amount of institutional care involved: the 1890 edition of Heinrich Laehr's directory of the German-speaking psychiatric world shows, solely in towns beginning with 'B', 19 public asylums and 14 private psychiatric clinics. That is just one letter of the alphabet, and omits the institutions for the mentally retarded, for alcoholics, for persons with epilepsy, and institutions mainly with 'open' doors – all of which are listed separately (Laehr 1891: vii–xi). Continent-wide, such institutions contained hundreds of thousands of beds. Yet these asylums tended to be self-contained little worlds, the patients admitted through judicial orders or a county health officer. Thus, in Europe during these years there was scarcely a trace of vertical integration of care. Patients discharged from asylums were *grosso modo* on their own, at best supervised by the district officer of health.

But before the First World War there were three exceptions to this rule, which were rudimentary yet pioneering. One was the practice of boarding out, or placing psychiatric inpatients in the homes of private individuals. This was routinely done in asylums across Europe. The homes were those of nearby villagers or the patient's own friends in his or her home town. Home care was begun in 1764 by the Engelken family, owners of a private psychiatric clinic in Rockwinkel near Bremen. It spread sooner or later to virtually every European country with the exceptions of the Iberian peninsula and England. Villages such as Dun-sur-Auron in France, Gheel in Belgium, and Uchtspringe in Germany became synonymous with family care, and an 1876 law made it possible for the General Board of Commissioners in Lunacy for Scotland to admit patients directly to home care without passing through the asylum (Pandy 1908: 524–72). In Scotland, around a fifth of all of the 'insane' were accommodated in 'boarding-out' arrangements (Letchworth 1889: 130). Thus, furloughing an asylum patient to a private residence did represent a kind of two-stage care system that foreshadows the more systematic integration that occurred after the Second World War.

The second exception to the predominance of the large asylums were the urban psychiatric clinics – first proposed by Wilhelm Griesinger (1868), professor of psychiatry in Berlin – that had by the turn of the century blossomed in a number of cities. Intended for acute cases, urban clinics usually had fewer than 100 beds and were suitable for short-stay patients, who would either recover or be transferred to a large asylum. Many university psychiatric hospitals also functioned as short-stay clinics in this sense (Sérieux 1903: 22–4, 31–3, 675–86). In practice, however, these urban boutique clinics were not always kept small: for example, around the year 1900 the one in Frankfurt had 300 beds.

The final exception was the existence of community organizations for post-discharge care, almost always organized by private charities and foundations. These were not to be found universally, yet existed in enough large cities to make a difference. In France, the first *Oeuvre de patronage pour les aliénés convalescents* was founded in Paris in 1843. In England, the Mental Aftercare Association was established in London in 1869 (Bennett 1991: 323). Among the 15 such foundations in existence in Germany by 1900, the first was founded in Wiesbaden in 1829, the others dating to the 1870s and 1880s (Sérieux 1903: 650). In Italy, a society to help reintegrate 'the poor insane' discharged from the (otherwise very) progressive asylum at Reggio-Emilia, was set up in 1874 (Sérieux 1903: 671–4).

In addition, although the state mental hospital remained the dominant public institution in the asylum era, it was not the only one. Relatively early, general hospitals began admitting mentally ill patients into psychiatry divisions. After the Second World War, the shift from asylum to general hospital was to take on positive, progressive overtones – the tip of the lance of 'de-asylumization', to coin a phrase. Yet this was not always so. In Hungary, for instance, the psychiatry 'annexes' of general hospitals were initially conceived as dumping grounds for chronic patients who presumably had no access to the psychiatric treatments and psychotherapy that the state asylums had on offer. Towards 1900, there were only four state asylums in Hungary (with 2300 patients), but 12 general hospital annexes with more than 100 patients apiece, in addition to numerous other smaller psychiatry wards in general hospitals, housing a total of over 5000 patients. In subsequent years, these general hospital units came to admit acute cases of all kinds, not just chronic patients dumped from the progressive asylums; and they also eventually acquired psychiatrists as directors (Pandy 1908: 439–40; Nyiro 1968: 77–8). Yet the Hungarian case is a reminder that the general hospital link in the vertical referral chain has not always been a forward-looking one.

Before the Second World War, the best example of integrated mental health care was found not in the public sector but in the private: the whole world of spa therapy and private sanatoriums for the middle classes and the wealthy (Shorter 1990). It is often forgotten that in the past, generally the well-to-do in Europe received their health care in private clinics, and above all in spas. It was a not so well-kept secret that the prime clientele for spa therapy (aside from the tuberculars in such dedicated settings as Davos) were the 'nervous' patients, a euphemism for psychiatry patients (Shorter 1997: 119–28). For example, the water-cure clinic in Boppard am Rhein, ostensibly a refuge for patients with aching joints seeking the healing waters, was in fact, primarily, a psychiatric facility. Admission statistics on 1185 patients between 1883 and 1888 show that only a fifth were somehow outside the psychiatric spectrum. Fifty-two per cent of the clinic's patients had 'neurosis' (neurasthenia, hysteria, hypochondria); 5 per cent had organic CNS conditions such as 'progressive paralysis', a contemporary term for neurosyphilis; 13 per cent were alcoholics, and 9 per cent were 'psychotic', meaning mainly melancholia and obsessive-compulsive disorders (Hoestermann 1889: 29–30). The Boppard am Rhein water-cure clinic captured the whole world of spa and sanatorium therapy in a microcosm.

There were essentially three kinds of such clinics in the mental health area: openly acknowledged private asylums for mental illness, hydrotherapy clinics such as Boppard am Rhein for 'nervous' illness, and general medical sanatoria for what sounded like organic conditions (but often were not), such as 'disturbances of nutrition', 'problems of metabolism', and 'weakness and fatigue'. Between 1880 and 1930 the private asylums in German-speaking Europe increased by 60 per cent, hydrotherapy services for nerves rose more than threefold, and general medical clinics (whose main clients had nervous conditions) increased over twenty-five fold (Shorter 1995: 291, Table 1). So in the mental health area, the growth was definitely on the euphemism-filled organicity side rather than the explicit psychiatric side.

Yet the point is that the spas and private sanatoriums represented both horizontally and vertically integrated mental health care – for the well-to-do, of course. It was vertically integrated, in the sense that the referral route functioned smoothly from family doctor or psychiatrist in the big city to the 'hydrotherapy' specialist in the spa. And back again: for as the patients were discharged they returned with referral notes about the successful treatment of their 'neurasthenia' to the family doctor, and all the participants waited for the entire cycle to begin again the following year. The system was also horizontally integrated, in that the spa or sanatorium offered a wide variety of physical and dietetic therapies, in addition to an extensive social programme. At bottom, this is not greatly different from the panoply of psychologists, occupational therapists, nutritionists, biofeedback specialists and so forth who greet the psychiatric patient today as part of the mental health care team. Indeed, the spas and sanatoriums would have offered splendid models for today's world of integrated care, had they not been reserved for a small fragment of the population.

As for the funding of mental health care, the Bismarckian health insurance law of 1883 – and its subsequent amendments – covered organic 'nervous' complaints and patients who consulted insurance fund physicians would not bear the expenses themselves. There were, however, two provisos. Firstly, the insurance stopped after 26 weeks, whereas many psychiatric illnesses tend to be chronic. Secondly, many community psychiatrists (*Nervenärzte*) had not signed contracts with the insurance funds, and demanded private compensation, thus making themselves unavailable to working patients and their families. (If Sigmund Freud, a typical community *Nervenarzt*, ever treated a single working-class patient, it is beyond our knowledge.) Costs of mental hospitalization were borne either by the insurance fund or, in the case of indigent patients, by the local community. After 1889, some somatization disorders, psychiatric in origin, were covered by the Reich Insurance Office (Eghigian 2000: 106). Aspects of this German system were widely copied in the Austro-Hungarian monarchy (and its successor states), Great Britain, the Netherlands, Norway,

Serbia, Romania and Yugoslavia. During the 1920s and 1930s, France and Sweden adopted similar legislation.[1] Certain kinds of spa and sanatorium therapy also were included after the First World War so the integration of mental health care into social insurance systems was well underway before the Second World War.

Period II: the rise of mental health systems

The key theme of the post-war years is the gradual inclusion of mental health within social insurance plans and the welfare state. In terms of mental hospitals, the 1950s and 1960s were eras of growth. All the countries in the then European Community, except the United Kingdom and Ireland, had a higher number of mental health beds in 1970 compared to 1950 (Mangen 1985: 21–2, Table 1.2). By 1971, a quarter of the mental hospitals in the WHO European Region had more than a thousand beds. 'Impersonal custodial regimes, lack of privacy and of . . . stimuli leads to apathy and the aggravation of symptoms' noted a WHO report (1975: 37). However, the great turnabout was soon in coming. The 1970s saw the beginning of deinstitutionalization: there is no country where the number of beds failed to decline between 1970 and 1979 (Mangen 1985: 21–2, Table 1.2).

This gathering deinstitutionalization took place under the aegis of the integration of psychiatric care, meaning the erasure of the firewall between asylum and the community. In 1948, the National Health Service (NHS) in the United Kingdom made the first move in this erasure by taking over responsibility for asylums from the local authorities. As Charles Webster noted, 'The NHS marked the end of a 25-year campaign to end separate administration of mental health services . . . 'Integration' was seen as the key to modernization and to the development of services freed from the taint of the Poor Law and lunacy code' (1991: 104). One bears in mind that the great 'bins', as the English mental hospitals were known, had already begun the process of opening up to the outside. As examples of isolated initiatives of this kind, the Maudsley Hospital in London began admitting psychiatric patients in 1923, and accepted male and female outpatients (on alternate days) while the Mental Treatment Act in 1930 had introduced voluntary treatment (Bennett 1991: 324–5).

It remained for the Mental Health Act of 1959 to enshrine deinstitutionalization in the United Kingdom, emphasizing community care. The Hospital Plan for England and Wales, promulgated by the Ministry of Health in 1961, called for a big decrease in asylum beds and a corresponding increase in psychiatry beds in general hospitals together with day hospitals and community services. As an American visitor commented in 1965 on the British mental hospitals he had visited, 'Personal liberty is actively promoted. Closed wards and locked doors appear to be at an irreducible minimum. Patients wear their own clothes, are encouraged to visit outside and to have visitors. Good relations with the surrounding community are fostered' (Furman 1965: 2). Thus, the British experience gives us the flavour of gathering reform.

By the mid-1960s five patterns of organizing local mental health services had evolved in western Europe, as identified by Sylvan Furman (1965: 4–5):

1 Mental-hospital dominated: the hospital looks after its own aftercare and may not involve the community. Graylingwell and Littlemore Hospitals in England corresponded to this model, as did most of the asylums in Italy until 1978.
2 Partnership between mental hospital and community health authority: York, England, represents a model of this arrangement (Furman 1965: 24–8).
3 The psychiatric division in a general hospital looks after a catchment area: examples are the Glostrup State Hospital in Denmark, a large psychiatric service adjacent to an 850-bed general hospital, and the psychiatry divisions of the general hospitals in Hungary (Furman 1965: 124–9; Tringer 1999).
4 Community care controlled by a public health authority: the Netherlands in the 1960s comes to mind at once as an example, with the large public health departments of Amsterdam and Rotterdam integrating the mental health care of the local populations covered by national health insurance (Furman 1965: 104–16). Stationary care remained mainly voluntary and religious, financed by the Poor Laws of the municipalities. At this point integration with mental hospitals, which were mostly in towns, had not been achieved.
5 Transitional systems, from large mental hospitals to community care centered in general hospitals: In the 1960s and 1970s Sweden conformed to this model, with the funding going to the large asylums and the start of sectorization (WHO 1978: 7).

In this second period, an attachment to spa therapy and to physical therapy for 'nervous' and mental disorders remained strong among the continental members of the EU as well as among those candidate states which had strong spa traditions. A 1985 guide to spa treatment in Romania, for example, listed either central nervous system (CNS) or 'asthenic neurosis' indications for the great majority of facilities that it mentioned (Teleki *et al.* 1985: 292–4). For the Sliac spa, situated in today's Slovakia, the prime indications were, 'Diseases of the nervous system and the spinal cord, neuralgia, neuritis, tabes dorsalis, neurasthenia, mental exhaustion, disorders of the visceral nervous system. Nervous symptoms in diseases of a gouty origin' (Simon 1954). Sliac, and many similar spas in the Czech Republic and Slovakia, still refer to a folk tradition of mental health spa therapy that goes back to the early nineteenth century.

In sum, this second period saw increasing horizontal and vertical integration of mental health care, accomplished under the militant banners of the welfare state and all-embracing social insurance programmes. The timid initiatives of the first period had now become state policy almost everywhere in the EU.

Period III: 1970s to the present

This period is characterized by the vertical extension of mental health care, as the smooth passage from the mental hospital to the community becomes the norm; and by the horizontal extension of care, as mental health teams based in non-hospital settings take the baton from isolated community psychiatrists and family doctors. Mental health care starts to become demedicalized, in the sense that numerous non-physician specialists begin to assume a role. It must be emphasized, though, that mental health care remains firmly within the province of medicine to the extent that it involves psychopharmacology and procedures such as electroconvulsive therapy (ECT). Community care, however praiseworthy as a goal, does not imply the exclusion of medicine.

To what extent are the achievements of community care a result of the advent of psychopharmacology? Treatment with medication is clearly replacing psychotherapy as the predominant treatment mode of psychiatry. In the United States, for example, the percentage of depressed outpatients treated with pharmacotherapy rose from 44.6 per cent in 1987 to 79.4 per cent in 1997 (Olfson *et al.* 2002). Do the gains of community care thus rest on a solid basis of psychopharmaceuticals? Not really. There clearly is some overlap, because the depot phenothiazines do facilitate the integration of patients with schizophrenia into community life. But the one is not a precondition of the other. For one thing, deinstitutionalization in the form of open-door policies and the like began before the advent of the antipsychotics in 1954. The emptying out of the asylums was not really caused by the prescription of chlorpromazine but by the upswing of social and community psychiatry from the 1940s onwards (Shorter 1997: 229–39). The growing provision of ECT in the early 1940s and later also played a cardinal role. Secondly, a certain underlying antipathy has divided the philosophical orientations of biological psychiatry from those of community care: the former seeing mental illness as arising in the neurochemistry of the brain and treatable through medication, and the latter seeing the origin of mental illness as somewhat inscrutable, and treatable, certainly, not solely through psychiatrists' prescriptions but through team efforts and the beneficent influences of community life. As one WHO consultant observed in 1977 (in remarks published in 1978), 'Psychiatric training and community mental health services [are] like ships that pass in the night with only the briefest awareness of each other's presence and without communication' (WHO 1978: 17).

Yet there is a sense in which psychopharmacology did encourage incipient mental health care reforms, and this was the advent of the depot antipsychotics. Squibb's fluphenazine decanoate (Ayd 1991: 75) debuted in 1973, dovetailing in Britain with the growing network of district-level care. Increased patient compliance meant better community care. As a World Rehabilitation Fund report commented in 1986, 'Easily accessible depo-neuroleptic clinics dispense these medications to patients living in the community and patients appear less resistant to medication maintenance' (Jansen 1986: 3).

What larger trends, if not psychopharmacology, are driving mental health care in Europe today? The search for a single index of progressive care has proven to be vexatious. Some writers suggest reductions in length of hospital stays as an index of forward-looking community care (Uffing *et al.* 1992). And indeed the 'institutionalism' that accompanies truly long stays is undesirable. However, David Healy and his associates have discovered, in the catchment area of a psychiatric hospital in North Wales, that the longer stays of the past were associated with lower suicide rates than the shorter stays of today (Healy *et al.* 2005). In general though, the shortening of the average length of stay in hospital does seem a reasonable proxy for the modernization of care (Rössler *et al.*

1994), as shorter stays usually mean more intensive attempts to provide therapy and return the patient to the community. However, average stay-duration data are not available for all countries.

This chapter proposes a ratio – the number of mental hospital beds as a percentage of all psychiatric beds – as a possible measure of the shift away from classical forms of care. Table 2.1 suggests certain trends over the past three decades among the old and newer EU member states on the basis of this measurement. These figures give some indication of the progression of care away from the asylum. To the extent that psychiatry beds are established in general hospitals, psychogeriatric settings, private sanatoriums and charitable psychiatric hospitals – among other sites of non-asylum residential care – mental health care is being 'de-asylumized'. (Of the three WHO surveys which reported statistics on psychiatric beds for these years, the 1972 survey by Anthony R. May is the least reliable [WHO 1979: 18]. Yet the bed data in even this questionable report should be more or less useful for the analysis of change over time within a given country. In any case, differences in data collection from country to country probably mean that one would not want to push fine cross-national comparisons too far.)

It must be emphasized that 'de-asylumizing' residential care does not necessarily imply deinstitutionalization, for we are measuring merely the presence of beds in other residential settings, not ambulatory care. Yet the shift away from the asylum is progressive in historical terms, and the numbers in Table 2.1 do give us a rough measure of this trend.

Essentially three patterns emerge from Table 2.1:

1 Countries where the asylum never predominated. These include Hungary and other east European countries where, as we have seen, non-asylum settings such as general hospitals provided residential care going back to the beginning of the twentieth century.
2 Countries where the ice began to break up very rapidly after the 1970s, in the form of a massive political and cultural assault upon the very notion of public mental hospital care. These include Italy – the best known case – where Law 180 in 1978, driven forward by ideological forces, abolished the asylum (Barbato 1998); Finland, where residential psychiatric care became largely shifted to community general hospitals;[2] and Denmark, where principles of community care took hold very rapidly after a 1976 law shifted responsibility for psychiatric hospitals from the state to the local government counties. In Denmark, the number of psychiatry beds dropped 43 per cent between 1980 and 1991 while the number of ambulatory psychiatric visits rose by 74 per cent (EOHSP 2001b: 15–16, 50). The experience of these three countries does not yet reveal whether the pessimism that the national mental health directors expressed in 1979 at a WHO meeting in Bielefeld about abolishing the asylum was justified: 'There [is] little confidence in the idea that an inpatient psychiatric service based only on a district general hospital could meet all the needs of a sector for inpatient psychiatric care' (WHO 1979: 9). Indeed, the Danish experience suggests that a precipitous dismantling of residential care can have adverse effects. Responding to a doubling of the suicide rate in Denmark between 1970 and 1987, in 1997 the Danish Psychiatric Society

Table 2.1 Beds in state psychiatric hospitals as a percentage of total psychiatric beds: EU states and candidate states, 1972–2001

	1972	1982	2001
EU-15			
Austria	96	94	90
Belgium	98	96	66
Denmark	89	80	26
Finland[1]	90	–	0
France	80	76	64
Germany[2]	–	92	63
Greece	98	99	49
Ireland	99	93	85
Italy[3]	–	96	0
Luxembourg	88	87	71
Netherlands	70	54	82
Portugal[4]	96	100	27
Spain	99	92	84
Sweden	75	58	–
UK	95	86	–
Candidate states (in 2001)			
Bulgaria[5]	39	–	49
Czech Republic[6]	49	44	86
Estonia	–	–	78
Hungary	15	15	24
Latvia	–	–	97
Lithuania	–	–	91
Malta	83	89	99
Poland	79	74	79
Romania	65	77	77
Slovakia	–	–	66
Slovenia	–	–	57

Sources: For 1972 and 1982 data: Freeman *et al.* (1985: 32–5, Tables 1–2); for 2001 data: WHO *Atlas* (2001), *passim.*
1 Finland omits other-psychiatric beds for 1982. 1982 public-psychiatric beds were 19,095, almost the same as 1972. The 2001 figure of '0' for 'psychiatric beds in mental hospitals' may be questionable, as another source indicates that 'the state . . . owns two psychiatric hospitals' (EOHSP 2001c: 26).
2 Data are for West Germany only for 1982. In 1982 the public-psychiatric percentage of total beds in East Germany was virtually the same as in West Germany. No data available for 1972. No information given in 1982 or 2001 on private psychiatric hospitals or other non-general hospital institutions. A 1990 law artificially shrank the denominator by ceasing to consider some beds in rehabilitation hospitals and health resorts as psychiatric beds (see Haug and Rössler 1999).
3 In Italy no breakdown on public psychiatric beds vs. other psychiatric beds in 1972 is available.
4 Portugal reported no other psychiatric beds for 1982 (as opposed to 420 in 1972).
5 Bulgaria failed in 1982 to report a large number of other-psychiatric beds that were evidently present.
6 Czechoslovakia in 1972, 1982.
NB: All 2001 figures calculated from the rates given in the source (N public psychiatric hospital beds per 10,000 population/N total psychiatric hospital beds/10,000 population); 1972 and 1982 figures calculated from absolute numbers of beds. No 2001 data are available for Sweden or United Kingdom. 'Other-psychiatric' beds, aside from public mental hospitals, will include psychiatry wards in general hospitals, psychogeriatric institutions, charitable psychiatric hospitals and private psychiatric hospitals, among other institutions.

urgently requested the government to pump up the number of psychiatry beds (Munk-Jorgensen 1999).

3 Countries where the shift from public hospital to community care has been slower, yet part of a steady process. These include the United Kingdom and virtually all of the remaining EU-15 countries. The changes in West Germany, for example, following the publication in 1975 of a psychiatric reform report, have been impressive: the number of general hospital psychiatric units rose from 21 in 1971 to 165 in 2001 (Bauer *et al.* 2001). By 1992, the number of ambulatory psychosocial services had risen to 250; and in the 1990s, the supply of private medical psychotherapists increased by 215 per cent. Yet comprehensive services, based in the community, are still said to be missing in Germany (EOHSP 2000b: 61, 71–2).

In the United Kingdom, the achievements of community psychiatry have been quite spectacular. Even though advocates continue to complain of a lack of resources, the extension of community care in Greater London, for example, would be the envy of mental health workers in Poland or Slovakia. As a recent study of the Primary Care Trusts in Greater London demonstrated, in two-thirds of them psychiatric liaison services with emergency departments of general hospitals are provided by a psychiatrist; many local government boroughs have emergency duty teams and crisis intervention teams, 'assertive outreach teams' and 'community mental health teams', not to speak of 'drop-in services' and 'employment schemes' (Greater London Authority 2003: 85).

Results in such previously deprived areas as Portugal have been dramatic, as psychiatric care in that country, following the enactment of a 1963 law, was shifted from six large mental hospitals to 18 new mental health care centres. In 1984 all mental health care was integrated into a single directorate (Caldas de Almeida 1991). There remains the interesting exception of the Netherlands, which is distinctive among EU nations because its asylum share has recently risen due a large increase in psychogeriatric beds and lack of funding for community services.[3] Community psychiatry has yet to make a dent in residential care in Austria, despite some promising experiments in social psychiatry around Vienna (Marksteiner and Danzinger 1985; WHO 1987: 169; Haug and Rössler 1999). In psychiatry, as in most areas of medicine in Austria, there is high use of inpatient care. Although the hospital investment plan of 1999 is intended to strengthen outpatient mental health services, Austria remains the EU nation where the least has been done in this area. This holds true despite a 450 per cent increase in the number of psychotherapists – who tend to be private-practice psychologists – in the years 1991–2001 (EOHSP 2001a: 52–3, 68, 99).

The winds of change have been slower in the countries of eastern Europe, where reformers must still fight against massive bureaucracies predisposed to asylum care. Indeed, with the abolition of other types of psychiatric beds, the proportion of beds in state psychiatric hospitals in eastern Europe has actually risen. At a joint WHO–European Commission meeting in 1999, the consensus on eastern Europe was that 'In many cases reform initiatives originated from the non-governmental field, with governments either being largely indifferent or even hostile'. In the Czech Republic, for instance, changes had been 'mainly the result of work by enthusiastic persons, often working on a volunteer basis'. The spirit of official psychiatry was thought still to permeate the asylums (WHO/EC 1999: 6).

As a last observation on eastern Europe: the measure used in Table 2.1 – the percentage of total psychiatry beds in state asylums – does not capture important changes in ambulatory care, for example, the spread of community psychiatry in Poland (Puzynski and Moskalewicz 2001).

The inadequacy of existing cross-national data

Cross-national studies in the provision of mental health services are of the utmost importance. The successful harmonization of care requires accurate information on the status quo, as well as some respect for the different historical traditions from which this status quo has evolved. Yet the main cross-national source of data is currently the WHO *Atlas* (2001).[4] And though one is mindful of the difficulties under which WHO epidemiologists labour, the results leave an often incomplete image of the real picture.

The main problem is that the WHO data give little information about what one might think of as the politics of care, such as national attitudes towards such often politicized issues as the legitimacy of ECT, the preferred style of psychotherapy (whether cognitive-behavioural or psychodynamic) and the desirability of any form of institutional care. So crude are the WHO measures of morbidity that the suicide rate is made to serve as 'a surrogate indicator of the overall level of mental health' (EC/WHO 2001: 15). It may well be that suicide was the only statistical parameter available to the WHO epidemiologists. Yet suicide is not a proxy for overall 'mental health'; many victims, for example, do not have a diagnosable psychiatric illness.[5]

National contexts are also important. The WHO monograph on Italy contains no hint of the national Italian antipathy towards ECT, of the distaste for psychiatric institutionalization of any kind – the monograph indicates without explanation that '0' psychiatric beds are available in Italy – or of the lingering Italian fondness for Freudian psychoanalysis (WHO 2001: 333–4). These national preferences make Italy dramatically different from Germany, the United Kingdom or the Czech Republic, for example, yet the artless reader would remain unaware of these important national variations. New EU states searching for an established model of care to adopt would end up with strikingly different results were they to adopt an Italian model instead of an English one.

What is required, in other words, are cross-national data that raise our awareness of less tangible elements in a system of care than the number of beds or the number of psychiatric nurses (van Os and Neeleman 1994). It is desirable to standardize the modes of treatment as well as the rough structures within which treatment is encased – and to harmonize treatment on the basis of state-of-the-art scientific data about evidence-based psychiatry, rather than on the basis of past fads and fancies.[6]

A lack of historical continuity

In retrospect, it is puzzling that the momentum of history has had so little heft. Normally, one expects that patterns laid down in the eighteenth or nineteenth centuries will continue to resonate in some form even into the twenty-first. Yet in mental health care this seems not to be the case. With the exception of such singularities as the thriving of home boarding in Belgium, an inheritance of the colony of Gheel (EOHSP 2000a: 48–9), few of the regularities of the nineteenth century have survived into the twenty-first.

- The uniformity of the former Austro-Hungarian Empire has dissolved on the threshold of the twenty-first century. Austria continues to have high rates of asylum care with little provision for community mental health. Hungary shows the opposite pattern.
- Today, many east European countries have a large surplus of clinical beds, many of them unneeded and an inheritance of the Soviet emphasis on 'more is better'. 'What countries from the eastern parts of Europe have in common', comments one observer, 'is not so much ancient history and traditions as their shared recent past. Essentially, the political division of postwar Europe interfered with the historical course that each respective country had been following earlier' (Tomov 2001: 22). Classically, some of these lands, such as Bohemia, offered well-ordered asylum care; others did not.
- Countries in which the private and voluntary sectors once excelled, such as Britain and the Netherlands, have now gone over to statist national health and social insurance services in which non-state players have little to say about mental health. (The growing voice of psychiatric consumers might be seen as a qualification to this statement, yet voluntary charitable organizations, as such, have receded in importance.)
- Countries that once constituted Europe's rearguard in mental health care, such as Portugal, are now in the vanguard – as a result of political realignments.

Truly, the momentum of the past seems today to count for little. The reason, of course, has to do with the vast political discontinuities introduced after the Second World War, as Europe became divided into a Soviet camp in the East and a welfare state camp in the West (a camp more recently embracing Spain and Portugal). Both effaced traditional patterns, ensuring that the history of mental health care would be, essentially, a history of the past 50 years.

From history to policy

This historical analysis closes with a present-day observation. A WHO report noted that 'The concept of what constitutes mental illness varies amongst cultures based on local beliefs and practices' (WHO 2002: 28). In other words, policy-makers need to craft programmes based on the national illness representations of the population; otherwise the services will be shunned.

If we wish to integrate mental health services into primary care, it is important to get around these fears. 'There still appears to be a division between so-called "physical" and "mental" health' write Üstün and Jenkins, who believe that people worldwide find organicity more appealing because it is 'concrete', mental health issues less so because they are more 'abstract' (1998: 483). But this is unlikely to be the real reason for the preference for organic-sounding settings and diagnoses. Much of the population of central and eastern Europe still fears the notion of psychiatric illness, preferring to think of mental afflictions as affections of the 'nerves'. They prefer, in other words, the 'N' word to the 'P' word. The population of the United Kingdom and western Europe is scarcely more enlightened, although several generations of exposure to the concept of mental health have, in fact, borne some fruit. In western Europe today, for example, ECT therapy, though a useful treatment for major depression, is not widely used because patients fear it. The first- and second-line treatments for major depression in these countries remain psychopharmaceuticals. ECT is refused. The issue, therefore, is to deliver care that is congruent with patients' representations of illness.

How can representationally congruent care in the area of psychiatry and mental health be achieved? Here some lessons from history may serve us well. Before the Second World War, as we have seen, much of the population of Europe sought care in spas and private sanatoriums for 'nervous' complaints, symptoms that would now be regarded as psychiatric in nature. The care they received was primarily physical treatments plus milieu therapy, a mixture of applications of water and electricity, plus the environmental benefits flowing from a relaxed spa environment that calmed and reassured on a twenty-four hour a day basis. Even today, the folk doctrine of nerves, together with a belief in the meliorative influence of spa and sanatorium treatment, have survived as an attenuated echo in the medical folklore of these regions. Doubters need merely consult the *Deutscher Bäderkalender* (*German Spa Guide*), where, under the indications 'conditions of general weakness and re-convalescence, vegetative dystonias, fatigue states, and premature aging', the editors have noted: 'all of the health-baths and spas are suitable' (*Deutscher Bäderverband* 1988: 139).

In Europe as a whole, numerous groups in the population still believe in the curative nature of spa and sanatorium treatments. Until recently in Germany, generous social insurance plans made it possible for patients to spend up to a month in spas, receiving milieu therapy for a variety of complaints, many of which were 'nervous' in nature. That link between spas and nerves has always been indissoluble. This same belief lingers as an echo in east central and eastern Europe today, despite the levelling effects of 50 years of the Semashenko health system imposed in some of these countries by the Soviet Union.

Delivering representationally congruent mental health care to the eastern regions of Europe will involve building on these memories of trust in spas and sanatoriums, because the 'P' and 'M' words – psychiatry and mental health – are still shunned in a vast belt from the Oder-Neisse river to the Carpathian mountains. To the extent that there are alternative approaches to psychiatry in the new EU states, they lie in this area: a preference for veiling mental illness as an organic disease of the body. As a WHO report on Lithuania commented, 'One of the obstacles to a more rapid process of deinstitutionalisation is the high level of stigmatisation of mentally ill people among the general public' (WHO 2001: 343). Mental health sometimes needs to be smuggled in, and it may be most effectively delivered in settings that do not necessarily announce themselves as psychiatric clinics or community mental health services, but as centres for physical therapy with a focus upon the central nervous system.

Nor is this organic-sounding labelling necessarily a deceit: in North America, pain clinics that offer physical therapy also supply psychoactive medications and counselling. There is no reason why this highly effective package should be denied to Europeans.

Our current concepts of mental health rely heavily on the acknowledgement of psychogenicity: that the patient, in fact, has a mental disorder rather than a nervous one. In the absence of such acknowledgement, patients refuse to seek psychiatric treatment, and the facilities sit idle. After half a century of psychodynamic psychotherapy in North America and western Europe, the doctrine of psychogenicity has a certain following. Psychiatry and mental health care do not need to hide their lights. The situation elsewhere may be different, however. And in the absence of this kind of acknowledgement, policy-makers who wish to deliver representationally congruent care will seek to give the consumers what they want.

Notes

*   The author wishes to thank Professor Marijke Gijswijt-Hofstra for some helpful editorial suggestions.
1   The standard history of social insurance (Köhler *et al.* 1982) contains very little on mental health. A compact overview of the issue appears in Elster (1923: 932–42).
2   According to Ville Lehtinen, a mental health specialist in Finland, there are still about 6000 psychiatric beds in Finland, but almost all are in the psychiatry divisions of general hospitals rather than in state asylums. In a 1991 reform, several older asylums were simply declared to be psychiatric annexes of nearby general hospitals, an issue of definition rather than a fundamental change (personal communication). There are apparently still two state psychiatric hospitals in operation in Finland (see Table 2.1, note 1).
3   Psychogeriatric beds in the Netherlands have climbed from 8680 in 1980 to 26,332 in 1996, while asylum beds have scarcely declined and psychiatric beds in general hospitals have dropped by 19 per cent (Mangen 1985; Wiersma 1991: 198–9; Schene and Faber 2001: 76, Table 1).
4   A promising initiative was the conference in Germany in 2000 on the occasion of the 25th anniversary of the German *'Psychiatrie Enquete'* that helped launch reform in that country. Yet the comparative data presented there are limited to nine countries, and treatment issues are not covered (Becker and Vázquez-Barquero 2001).
5   See for example Power *et al.* 1997. It goes without saying that a majority of suicide victims do have a psychiatric illness; yet the minority without seems significant enough to impair the usefulness of the suicide rate as a cross-national indicator of 'mental health'. A sudden change in the suicide rate within a country, of course, raises questions about care.
6   It is recommended that WHO's in some ways exemplary gathering of cross-national mental health data be augmented by the work of an independent commission or information-gathering body that is more sensitive to context. Such a commission would consist of observers sensitive to cross-national differences in the context of care, rather than merely in such quantitative variables such as the number of

psychiatry beds. The context of care is determined by its community and institutional framework: by variables, in other words, measuring integration of care. It is also determined by the kind of care provided: biological treatments, the various kinds of psychotherapies, the availability of ECT and the number of physicians vs. non-physicians involved in care. The membership of such a commission would reach across the spectrum of biomedicine and social science, and its report would constitute an evidence-based goal to which to aspire.

References

Ayd, F. Jr. (1991) The early history of modern psychopharmacology, *Neuropsychopharmacology*, 5(2): 71–84.

Barbato, A. (1998) Psychiatry in transition: outcomes of mental health policy shift in Italy, *Australian and New Zealand Journal of Psychiatry*, 32(5): 673–9.

Bauer, M., Kunze, H., von Cranach, M., Fritze, J. and Becker, T. (2001) Psychiatric reform in Germany, *Acta Psychiatrica Scandinavica*, 104 (suppl. 410): 27–34.

Becker, T. and Vázquez-Barquero, J.L. (2001) The European perspective on psychiatric reform, *Acta Psychiatrica Scandinavica*, 104 (suppl. 410): 8–14.

Bennett, D. (1991) The drive towards the community, in G.E. Berrios and H. Freeman (eds) *150 years of British Psychiatry, 1841–1991*. London: Gaskell.

Caldas de Almeida, J. (1991) Portugal, in H. Freeman and J. Henderson (eds) *Evaluation of Comprehensive Care of the Mentally Ill*. London: Gaskell.

Deutscher Bäderverband (ed.) (1988) *Deutscher Bäderkalender (German Spa Guide)*. Deutscher Bäderverband e.V. Gütersloh, Flöttmann.

Eghigian, G. (2000) *Making Security Social: Disability, Insurance, and the Birth of the Social Entitlement State in Germany*. Ann Arbor, MI: University of Michigan.

Elster, L. (ed.) (1923) *Handwörterbuch der staatswissenschaften (Social and Political Science Encyclopedia)*. Jena: Fischer.

European Commission/World Health Organization Regional Office for Europe (EC/WHO) (2001) *Highlights on Health in Bulgaria*. Copenhagen: WHO Regional Office for Europe (E73818).

European Observatory on Health Systems and Policies (EOHSP) (2000a) *Health Care Systems in Transition: Belgium*. Copenhagen: European Observatory on Health Systems and Policies.

European Observatory on Health Systems and Policies (EOHSP) (2000b) *Health Care Systems in Transition: Germany*. Copenhagen: European Observatory on Health Systems and Policies.

European Observatory on Health Systems and Policies (EOHSP) (2001a) *Health Care Systems in Transition: Austria*. Copenhagen: European Observatory on Health Care Systems.

European Observatory on Health Systems and Policies (EOHSP) (2001b) *Health Care Systems in Transition: Denmark*. Copenhagen: European Observatory on Health Care Systems.

European Observatory on Health Systems and Policies (EOHSP) (2001c) *Health Care Systems in Transition: Finland*. Copenhagen: European Observatory on Health Care Systems.

Freeman, H.L., Freyers, T. and Henderson, J.H. (1985) *Mental Health Services in Europe: 10 years on*. Copenhagen: WHO Regional Office for Europe.

Furman, S.S. (1965) *Community Mental Health Services in Northern Europe: Great Britain, Netherlands, Denmark, and Sweden*. Bethesda: National Institute for Mental Health, PHS Pub. no. 1407.

Greater London Authority/Mayor of London (2003) *Availability of mental health services in London*. London: GLA.

Griesinger, W. (1868) Über irrenanstalten und deren weiterentwickelung in Deutschland (On mental hospitals and their further development in Germany). *Archiv für Psychiatrie und Nervenkrankheiten*, 1: 8–43.

Grove, B. (1994) Reform of mental health care in Europe: progress and change in the last decade, *British Journal of Psychiatry*, 165: 431–3.

Haug, H.-J. and Rössler, W. (1999) Deinstitutionalization of psychiatric patients in Central Europe, *European Archives of Psychiatry and Clinical Neuroscience*, 249(3): 115–22.

Healy, D., Harris, M., Michael, P., Cattell, D., Savage, M., Chalasani, P. and Hirst, D. (2005) Service utilization in 1896 and 1996: morbidity and mortality data from North Wales, *History of Psychiatry*, 16(61 Pt 1): 27–42.

Hoestermann, K.E. (1889) *Zur erinnerung an die feier des fünfzigjährigen bestehens der wasserheilanstalt marienberg zu Boppard am Rhein*. Boppard: Richter.

Jansen, M.A. (1986) *International Exchange of Experts and Information in Rehabilitation. Final Report: European Mental Health Policies and Practices: Rehabilitation of Persons with Chronic Mental Illness*. New York: World Rehabilitation Fund.

Jones, K. (1993) *Asylums and After: A Revised History of the Mental Health Services: From the Early 18th Century to the 1990s*. London: Athlone.

Köhler, P.A., Zacher, H.F. and Partington, M. (1982) *The Evolution of Social Insurance, 1881–1981: Studies of Germany, France, Great Britain, Austria and Switzerland*. London: Frances Pinter.

Laehr, H. (1891) *Die Heil – und pflegeanstalten für psychisch-kranke des deutschen sprachgebietes im J. 1890 (Asylums for the Acute and Chronic Care of the Mentally Ill in German-language areas*, 1890). Berlin: Reimer.

Lehtinen, V. Personal communication.

Letchworth, W. (1889) *The Insane in Foreign Countries*. New York: Putnam's.

Mangen, S.P. (1985) Psychiatric policies: developments and constraints, in S.P. Mangen (ed.) *Mental Health Care in the European Community*. London: Croom Helm.

Marksteiner, A. and Danzinger, R. (1985) *Gugging: versuch einer psychiatriefreform: 100 jahre niederösterreichisches landeskrankenhaus für psychiatrie und neurologie klosterneuburg (Gugging: A Project of Reform in Psychiatry: 100 Years of the Lower-Austrian Provincial Hospital for Psychiatry and Neurology in Klosterneuburg)*. Salzburg: AVM-Verlag.

May, A.R. (1976) *Mental Health Services in Europe: Review of Data Collected in Response to a WHO Questionnaire*. Geneva: WHO.

Munk-Jorgensen, P. (1999) Has deinstitutionalization gone too far? *European Archives of Psychiatry and Clinical Neuroscience*, 249(3): 136–43.

Nyiro, G. (1968) Hungary, in A. Kiev (ed.) *Psychiatry in the Communist World*. New York: Science House.

Olfson, M., Marcus, S., Druss, B., Elinson, L., Tanielian, T. and Pincus, H.A. (2002) National trends in the outpatient treatment of depression, *Journal of the American Medical Association*, 287(2): 203–9.

Pandy, K. (1908) *Die irrenfürsorge in Europa: eine vergleichende studie (The Care of the Mentally Ill in Europe: A Comparative Study)*. Berlin: Reimer.

Pichot, P. (1983) *A Century of Psychiatry*. Paris: DaCosta.

Porter, R. (1987) *Mind-forg'd Manacles: A History of Madness in England from the Restoration to the Regency*. Cambridge, MA: Harvard.

Porter, R. and Wright, D. (2003) *The confinement of the insane: international perspectives, 1800–1965*. Cambridge: Cambridge University Press.

Power, K., Davies, C., Swanson, V., Gordon, D. and Carter, H. (1997) Case-control study of GP attendance rates by suicide cases with or without a psychiatric history, *British Journal of General Practice*, 47(417): 211–15.

Puzynski, S. and Moskalewicz, J. (2001) Evolution of the mental health care system in Poland, *Acta Psychiatrica Scandinavica*, 104 (suppl. 410): 69–73.

Rössler, W., Salize, H.J., Biechele, U. and Riecher-Rössler, A. (1994) Stand und Entwicklung der psychiatrischen Versorgung (Condition and development of care in psychiatry), *Nervenarzt*, 65: 427–37.

Schene, A.H. and Faber, A.M.E. (2001) Mental health care reform in The Netherlands, *Acta Psychiatrica Scandinavica*, 104 (suppl. 410): 74–81.

Sérieux, P. (1903) *L'assistance des aliénés*. Paris: Imprimerie municipale; Préfecture du département de la Seine, Conseil Général.

Shorter, E. (1990) Private clinics in Central Europe, 1850–1933, *Social History of Medicine*, 3(2): 159–95.

Shorter, E. (1995) Ceti medi e consumi sanitari in Europa tra l'Otto e il Novecento (The middle classes and health consumption in Europe during the nineteenth century), in G. Aliberti (ed.) *L'Economia Domestica* (Secc. XIX–XX). Pisa: Istituti editoriali e Poligrafici Internazionali

Shorter, E. (1997) *A History of Psychiatry from the Era of the Asylum to the Age of Prozac.* New York: Wiley.

Simon, B. (ed.) (1954) *Spas and Climatic Health Resorts of Czechoslovakia.* London: Williams.

Teleki, N., Munteanu, L., Stoicescu, C., Teodoreanu, E. and Grigore, L. (1985) *Spa Treatment in Romania.* Bucharest: Sport-Turism Publishing House.

Thornicroft, G. and Maingay, S. (2002) The global response to mental illness, *British Medical Journal*, 325: 608–9.

Tomov, T. (2001) Mental health reforms in Eastern Europe, *Acta Psychiatrica Scandinavica*, 104 (suppl. 410): 21–6.

Tringer, L. (1999) Focus on psychiatry in Hungary, *British Journal of Psychiatry*, 174: 81–5.

Uffing, H.T, Ceha, M.M. and Saenger, G.H. (1992) The development of de-institutionalization in Europe, *Psychiatric Quarterly*, 63(3): 265–78.

Üstün, T.B. and Jenkins, R. (1998) Epilogue: the way forward – proposals for action, in R. Jenkins and T.B. Üstün (eds) *Preventing Mental Illness: Mental Health Promotion in Primary Care.* Chichester: Wiley.

van Os, J. and Neeleman, J. (1994) Caring for mentally ill people, *British Medical Journal*, 309: 1218–21.

Webster, C. (1991) Psychiatry and the early National Health Service: the role of the Mental Health Standing Advisory Committee, in G.E. Berrios and H. Freeman (eds) *150 Years of British Psychiatry, 1841–1991.* London: Gaskell.

Wiersma, D. (1991) The Netherlands, in H. Freeman and J. Henderson (eds) *Evaluation of Comprehensive Care of the Mentally Ill.* London: Gaskell.

World Health Organization, Department of Mental Health and Substance Dependence, Mental Health Determinants and Populations (WHO) (2001) *Atlas: Country Profiles on Mental Health Resources.* Geneva: WHO.

World Health Organization, Department of Mental Health and Substance Dependence, Mental Health Evidence and Research (WHO) (2002) *Prevention and Promotion in Mental Health.* Geneva: WHO.

World Health Organization/European Commission (WHO/EC) (1999) *Balancing Mental Health Promotion and Mental Health Care: A Joint World Health Organization (WHO)/ European Commission (EC) Meeting, Brussels, 22–24 April 1999.* Typescript. WHO, MNH/NAM/99.2, www5.who.int/mental_health/download.cfm?id=0000000043 (accessed 15 January 2003).

World Health Organization, Regional Office for Europe (WHO) (1975) *Health Services in Europe*, 2nd edn. Copenhagen: WHO Regional Office for Europe.

World Health Organization, Regional Office for Europe (WHO) (1978) *Constraints in Mental Health Services Development: Report on a Working Group, Cork, 28 June–1*

July 1977. Typescript. Copenhagen: WHO Regional Office for Europe, ICP/MNH 030 II.

World Health Organization, Regional Office for Europe (WHO) (1979) *Mental Health Policy Formulation in the WHO European Region: Report on a Meeting of National Mental Health Advisers, Bielefeld, 26–30 November 1979*. Typescript. Copenhagen: WHO Regional Office for Europe, ICP/MNH 054.

World Health Organization, Regional Office for Europe (WHO) (1987) *Mental Health Services in Pilot Study Areas: Report on a European Study*. Copenhagen: WHO Regional Office for Europe.

three

Tackling social exclusion across Europe

Liz Sayce and Claire Curran

Adults with long-term mental health problems are one of the most excluded groups in society. Although many want to work, fewer than a quarter actually do – the lowest employment rate for any of the main groups of disabled people ... Stigma and discrimination against people with mental health problems is pervasive throughout society ... Fewer than four in ten employers say they would recruit someone with a mental health problem. Many people fear disclosing their condition, even to family and friends.

(Social Exclusion Unit 2004: 3–4)

To date there has been no national or European initiative strong enough to make a significant system-wide impact on rates of exclusion faced by people with mental health problems or psychiatric disabilities.[1] There are significant opportunities to develop more effective interventions, based on Article 13 of the European Union (EU) Directive on Employment (2000) that requires governments to pass laws outlawing discrimination on grounds including disability. In late 2003, the then Commissioner for Employment and Social Affairs, Anna Diamantopoulou, additionally announced that a European Directive on disability discrimination would be developed – with potential coverage of education, transport and goods and services. In early 2006 this was still in abeyance.

This chapter challenges the effectiveness of purely educational initiatives, especially those based on the popular 'mental illness is an illness like any other' message, and explores more evidence-based approaches. It outlines evidence of social exclusion in Europe across four key domains: excess mortality, stigma, employment and human rights. The chapter also identifies promising interventions to reduce social exclusion that:

- address the power issues behind discrimination rather than relying on education alone;

- increase opportunities for contact between users/survivors of mental health services and other citizens;
- break the connections between mental ill health and both violence and incompetence;
- bring mainstream mental health inclusion into generic employment, educational and economic programmes.

What is social exclusion and what is its relationship with psychiatric disabilities?

Defining and conceptualizing social exclusion is not straightforward. It is perhaps helpful to provide a brief history of the concept's origin in order to explain its diverse meanings and usages. Modern usage emerged in France in the 1970s, where it referred specifically to the group of people administratively excluded by the state from the services provided under the social insurance system. '*Les exclus*' (the excluded) were disabled people, lone parents and the uninsured unemployed, especially young adults. Still in France, the term became more widely applied to specific groups of disaffected youths and isolated individuals living on large estates on the peripheries of large cities that experienced an increasing intensity of social problems. In France the concept is very closely linked to ideas of citizenship, rights, solidarity and the unity of the state (Burchardt *et al.* 2002).

Meanwhile in the United Kingdom, during the Conservative government of the 1980s, poverty fell off the policy agenda. It has been argued that in order to continue conversations at the European level that were essentially about poverty, the term 'social exclusion' was used so as not to offend the sensibilities of the Conservative government (Burchardt *et al.* 2002). In contrast to France, where social exclusion is intimately related to ideas of citizenship and rights, in the United Kingdom the concept was initially a proxy term for poverty, before being captured by the wider social policy agenda to include employment, housing, social networks, and political and social participation. When the term is used in the European context it refers more to the EU objective of achieving social and economic cohesion (Percy-Smith 2000). It is therefore perhaps helpful, if an oversimplification, to suggest that definitions of social exclusion fall broadly into two categories: those of rights and those of participation. A definition that falls into the latter category has emerged from the research carried out by the ESRC Centre for the Analysis of Social Exclusion at the London School of Economics and Political Science which suggests that 'an individual is socially excluded if he or she does not participate in key activities of the society in which he or she lives', with these key activities defined as consumption, production, policy engagement and social interaction (Burchardt *et al.* 1999).

The United Nations Development Programme has attempted to conceptualize social exclusion in terms that fit all countries regardless of their stage of economic and social development (Gore and Figueiredo 1997). These attempts resulted in the identification of the significance of enforceable civil and social rights; for example, adequate health care, basic education and material wellbeing. Social exclusion is therefore conceptualized as a lack of recognition of basic rights, or where that recognition exists, lack of access to the political and legal systems necessary to make those rights a reality. This approach can be pursued along the theme of discrimination and lack of enforceable rights (Burchardt *et al.* 2002). Although in some countries, for example the United Kingdom, this is not a common approach to social exclusion, it has been explored in some studies (Leslie 1997; Sayce 2000) and is the most appropriate concept for pursuing the issue of social exclusion in relation to individuals experiencing mental health problems. For that reason, this is the dominant concept of social exclusion employed in this chapter. An issue that is only briefly touched upon here but deserves highlighting is the idea of agency or power; that is, who is doing the excluding. This has clear ramifications for individuals with mental health problems who may find themselves unable to make decisions about their life and their medical treatment, as well as being vulnerable to more major abuses of basic human rights in many countries.

The next important question is: what is the relationship between social exclusion and individuals with mental health problems? According to a report by the United Kingdom government's Social Exclusion Unit (2004), people with mental health problems are at increased risk of becoming socially excluded, and similarly, people who experience social exclusion are at increased risk of experiencing a mental health problem. It is likely that causality works in both directions and compounds the experience. Empirical evidence from the United Kingdom shows an association between disadvantage, variously measured, and higher frequencies of common mental disorders. Prevalence rates were shown to be higher in social groups exhibiting less education, unemployment and lower income and material assets (Fryers *et al.* 2003). A review of the international evidence also supports the notion that material poverty is a risk factor for a negative outcome among people with mental health problems (Saraceno and Barbui 1997). Both the experience of (mental) health problems and of social exclusion are mediated by a range of factors, which can function both inter- and intra-generationally (Hobcraft 2002) and include: discrimination, unemployment, poverty, stress, lack of access to services and reduced social networks.

Exclusion from citizenship

This chapter addresses both social exclusion and the discrimination – distinguishing between human differences and treating some groups unfavourably as a result – that amplifies, compounds and results in social exclusion. People with psychiatric impairments are among the most excluded of all European citizens (see Sayce 2000; European Foundation for the Improvement of Living and Working Conditions 2003). Social exclusion is a particularly powerful descriptor of the experience of mental health service users/survivors. It has been defined in terms of:

> the inter-locking and mutually compounding problems of impairment, discrimination, diminished social role, lack of economic and social participation and disability. Among the factors at play are lack of status, joblessness, lack of opportunities to establish a family, small or non-existent social

networks, compounding race or other discriminations, repeated rejection and consequent restriction of hope and expectation.

(Sayce 2001: 122)

In this chapter we describe just four examples. A fifth example, on the situation faced by asylum seekers and refugees, is discussed in Chapter 15.

An equal chance of life itself?

Around the world, people with some types of mental health problem or learning disability are more likely to die prematurely even when compared with smokers. One factor in this disparity appears to be a pattern of unequal access to health promotion, prevention and treatment for both psychiatric and, particularly, somatic illnesses. Or, more formally, they are excluded from consuming (accessing) services that are available to others. Yet there is no significant attention to health improvement for these at-risk groups comparable, say, to smoking prevention/cessation programmes.

An international review (Harris and Barraclough 1998) of empirical evidence on the 'excess mortality' associated with learning disability and mental health problems found that – for natural causes (excluding suicide) – there is a significantly raised risk of premature mortality for groups including:

- People with 'mental retardation' (learning disability): the mortality rate from natural causes is 7.8 times higher than expected. By comparison, the mortality rate from natural causes among smokers is only 2.5 times higher than expected.
- People with schizophrenia – 1.4 times higher than the expected mortality rate (it is higher in some countries; for instance, it is 2.5 times in Britain) (Department of Health 1991).
- Other psychotic disorders – 2.4 times higher.

The type of diseases accounting for premature death include infectious, circulatory, endocrine, respiratory, coronary heart disease (CHD), digestive and genito-urinary illnesses. One study estimated that, for schizophrenia, these figures translate, on average, into lives shortened by ten years for men and nine years for women (Allebeck 1989). Another study looked into the reasons behind a higher mortality rate due to ischaemic heart disease in Western Australian psychiatric patients between 1980–98 (Lawrence *et al.* 2003). The conclusions were diverse but included lower revascularization procedure rates in the psychiatric population, particularly in those with psychoses. In Western Australia these revascularization processes tend to be elective procedures through private health insurance, with reduced access for those accessing the service through Medicare (the Australian public health insurance scheme). Only 13 per cent of people with psychosis had any private insurance compared with 32 per cent in the general population. Other factors that explained the higher mortality rates in the psychiatric population included more risky behaviours such as smoking, for which rates were 43 per cent in the psychiatric service user population compared with 24 per cent in the non-psychiatric population, with rates even higher among those with psychosis. Obesity was also higher in the psychiatric service user population for a range of reasons, including under-activity, lack of knowledge of dietary principles and side-effects of medications. There were also reduced admission rates in the psychiatric population compared to the non-psychiatric population and this was explained as being due to reduced effective communication of symptoms; increased social isolation; lack of perception of symptoms; and medical practitioner focus on psychiatric symptoms (Lawrence *et al.* 2003).

This lack of access to appropriate services and care is a commonly reported problem for people with mental health problems. Surveys of people with mental health problems, learning disabilities and their families (Read and Baker 1996; Singh 1997) have repeatedly shown a lack of equal access to health assessment and treatment – a factor likely to contribute to unequal health outcomes. Read and Baker (1996) found that of 500 people with mental health problems surveyed, 50 per cent reported unfair treatment on the part of general health services; for instance, being met with the assumption that any physical complaint could be explained away as a psychiatric symptom. Breast lumps went unexamined and valium was prescribed for palpitations that later turned out to be major heart disease. A study of long-stay psychiatric patients in northern Finland concluded that the 'notably higher' rates of mortality in this population were due in part to 'inadequately organized somatic care and the prevailing culture of "non-somatic" treatment in psychiatry' (Rasanen *et al.* 2003: 297). Another study following the closure of long-stay hospitals in Italy found that mortality rates were twice as high for individuals being cared for in the community compared with the general population, and that, in fact, this was an improvement on mortality rates in the long-stay hospitals (D'Avanzo *et al.* 2003). The authors suggest the reason for the high mortality rates is multi-causal, involving the high frequency of concurrent pathological conditions in the psychiatric service user population, as well as smoking and other lifestyle habits, a tendency to self-neglect, and quality of living conditions and care. A longitudinal study of excess mortality after discharge from long-term psychiatric care in Scotland suggests that access to health care may be more limited for this group, or that they might be treated differently from people who have not had a mental illness (Stark *et al.* 2003).

In Britain the Disability Rights Commission (DRC) is undertaking a formal investigation into physical health inequalities experienced by people with mental health and/or learning disabilities, with a particular focus on potential solutions through primary care. The Commission has produced a summary of available evidence (Nocon 2004) and an interim report. The final report describes new evidence from large data sets on disparities in health outcomes and service and treatment access for people with mental health problems compared to other citizens (Disability Rights Commission 2006).

Equal respect?

Common ideas about madness – the moral taint, the 'life not worth living', the notion that 'mad' people's views are invalid by definition – recur with alarming regularity in the media and wider culture (Wahl 1995, 2003; Sayce 2000; Sieff 2003). As Otto Wahl put it, there is probably no detective on prime time TV who has not had a mentally ill villain to apprehend (Wahl 1995). If the person is not portrayed as dangerous the other likely option is that they are seen as a 'poor unfortunate', unable to help themselves. Across children's media 'references to mental illnesses are typically used to disparage and ridicule' (Wahl 2003: 249), with mentally ill characters 'almost entirely devoid of admirable attributes' (Wilson *et al.* 2000: 440). Images of people with mental health problems contributing – working, raising children, being involved in their communities – are notable by their absence. There is some evidence that this distorted discourse impacts upon public attitudes and on discriminatory behaviour (Angermeyer and Matschinger 1996; Penn and Wykes 2003; Sieff 2003).

People with psychiatric impairments are seen through the lens of risk: that they might be violent or unable to cope. It has often been noted that a mental health service user can be compulsorily detained for a level of risk of violence which – if it were applied to young men who drink alcohol – would mean thousands of young men detained in advance of committing any crime (Sayce 1995). But the notion of risk to self can be equally pernicious. As one corporate senior manager put it after returning to work following mental ill health: 'They gave my junior most of my job, so I wouldn't be "stressed" – I think they actually thought they were being helpful. They didn't think to ask me how I might react to that. I did point out that a Disability Discrimination Act case from one of their senior managers might not put the company in too good a light' (Personal Communication).

Within the risk-dominated stereotypes, there is precious little attention given to the (very high) risk of social exclusion – and the associated risk to health. A concentration on risk in terms of violence and vulnerability leads to social exclusion, as people's autonomy is denied and the wider public's tendency to desire social distance is magnified. A mark of respect would be to stop subjecting mental health service users to a different set of assumptions and rules on risk than applies to other citizens. Without the choice to take risks, there can be no autonomy, no social participation and no achievement.

Attitude and awareness research in Europe shows a mixed picture. A European public opinion survey (in the 15 countries of the EU in 2003) found that people with mental health problems or learning disabilities were most likely to be perceived as not having 'the same chance of getting a job, training or promotion' as anyone else. Eighty-seven per cent thought they would have less chance than anyone else: higher than for physically disabled people (77 per cent), people over 50 (71 per cent) and people from ethnic minorities (62 per cent). Much lower proportions thought that young people or gay or lesbian people would have less chance (Eurobarometer 2003).

This may suggest strong public recognition of discrimination on grounds of psychiatric status. However, when asked whether discrimination against these groups in work, education, housing and services was always or usually wrong, in relation to 'mental disability' a significant proportion considered that it was not. The authors note that 'issues of discrimination and mental disability are more vulnerable than other examples to confusion in respondents' minds between selection, which is fair, and discrimination, which is unfair'. This may echo how women were perceived 40 years ago – when it was widely believed that women could not undertake many types of work, given the essential fact of mothering. The public may lack awareness of the possibility that far more people with mental health problems could work, with 'adjustments' and supports – just as in the 1960s many people could not yet imagine how the workplace, home and child care could be organized to increase opportunities for women.

The United Kingdom government's Social Exclusion Unit reported that 83 per cent of respondents to the consultation process for their report on mental health and social exclusion identified stigma as a key issue (Social Exclusion Unit 2004). Link *et al.* (1997) found that stigma and discrimination can affect people long after the symptoms of mental health problems have been resolved. Discrimination can lead to relapses in mental health problems and can intensify existing symptoms.

Discrimination can occur in many areas of day-to-day life but in relation to employment it can be particularly damaging. Read and Baker (1996) state that a third of people with mental health problems report having been dismissed or forced to resign from their job and almost four in ten felt they had been denied a job because of their previous psychiatric history. Another survey reports over two-thirds had been put off applying for jobs for fear of unfair treatment (Mind 2000).

An equal chance to contribute?

Employment-related discrimination translates into reduced opportunities to contribute (see also Chapter 12). The employment rate of people with 'moderate disability' in the EU was 43 per cent in 2003, and 22 per cent for 'severe disability'. There are considerable variations by country: rates for 'moderate disability' vary from 27 per cent in Ireland to 54 per cent in Germany, and for 'severe disability' from 13 per cent in Spain to 37 per cent in France (European Foundation for the Improvement of Living and Working Conditions 2003).

There are also significant variations by impairment type. People with mental health problems tend to have the lowest employment participation across Europe (European Foundation for the Improvement of Living and Working Conditions 2003). For instance in Britain, 21 per cent of people with long-term mental health problems are working, as compared to 51 per cent of disabled people generally (Disability Rights Commission 2005). Even where disabled people – including those with mental health problems – are working there are differentials between disabled and non-disabled people's wages. Earnings for disabled people in Germany are 35 per cent less than non-disabled, 20 per cent less in Ireland and 6 per cent less in Sweden. Moreover, 9 per cent of disabled people of working age in Europe have no income from either employment or benefits: they make up 1.4 per cent of the total European working age population (European Foundation for the Improvement of Living and Working Conditions 2003).

In the EU about 500,000 disabled people (particularly those with mental health problems or learning disabilities) are based in separate 'sheltered work', where remuneration is often very low, far below the accepted minimum wage. There is generally a low rate of exit to open employment. In Belgium, France, Spain, Ireland and Scotland less than 3 per cent go on to open employment each year (European Foundation for the Improvement of Living and Working Conditions 2003).

Exclusion can begin in childhood. Only 59 per cent of European disabled children are in mainstream schools. In some countries, including Spain, Greece, Ireland and Portugal, children with disability-related needs (including mental health problems) do not go beyond primary school because there is no infrastructure to support their education. Young people with mental health problems are disproportionately likely to leave school without qualifications, to be excluded from school, to be underestimated and to hold low aspirations about their own futures (Rutter and Smith 1995; Gray 2002).

The European Foundation for the Improvement of Living and Working Conditions (2003) proposed a target of 50 per cent employment of people with moderate impairments and 30 per cent for people with severe impairments, by 2010. Some countries have gone further. The British DRC and Trades Union Congress in 2004 called for a target of 60 per cent employment of disabled people of working age, by around 2014 (Disability Rights Commission 2004).

Employment can confer a range of benefits beyond the obvious financial one. In addition, work can provide structure to the day, increase self-esteem and increase the number of people in an individual's social network. Surveys have reported up to 90 per cent of those with severe mental health problems expressing a desire to work (Perkins and Rinaldi 2002) and yet, as already reported, those with mental health problems have among the lowest employment rates of any group. Returning to the issue of the financial benefit associated with employment, the majority of countries in Europe provide social protection in the form of financial assistance to those unable to work. While the prevention of poverty should be a key policy aim for any country intending to reduce social exclusion, this 'compensation' tradition emerges from the individual model of disability and can produce unexpected disincentives to work, i.e. incentives not to work, among those who have the desire and the ability to do so (van Oorschot and Hvinden 2000). Often individuals with mental health problems receive sickness or incapacity payments rather than unemployment payments, as these are worth more. However, this then classifies the individual as economically inactive, rather than unemployed, which has repercussions in terms of access to advice about jobs; in some cases it limits eligibility to back-to-work programmes. More importantly, in many countries applying for and receiving benefits is a difficult process that can take many months to set up. These various factors can lead to a 'benefit trap'. This is the process by which an individual is at risk of becoming financially vulnerable if they take paid work, compared with remaining on benefits. While countries in Europe are beginning to tackle this disincentive to work it is essential that policies are formulated that do not increase the risk of increasing poverty levels among those with mental health problems and that support those people, particularly those with fluctuating conditions, who are not able to sustain continuous paid employment.

Human rights?

At the extreme, people with mental health problems are subjected to major human rights abuses (see also Chapter 13). For example, in Hungary in 1997:

> Closed from public view in institutions with no human rights oversight or advocacy available to them, people are vulnerable to the most serious human rights violations prohibited by international law. Major restrictions on individual liberty are routinely delegated to the administrative discretion of ward staff without due process of law.
>
> Some people are placed in cages as a form of physical restraint and permanent detention. Cages are constructed of a metal frame supporting a cloth or wire mesh over a bed. People can sit up or roll over in the cage but they cannot stand up. Some individuals are placed in cages for weeks or months for behavioural control. Other individuals are kept permanently in cages because of lack of staff to supervise them. With such limited movement, people in cages are subject to dangerous, and potentially life threatening pressure ulcers (bedsores).
>
> (Mental Disability Rights International 1997: xvii, xxii)

In Hungary, one indication of 'exclusion' from society was that some long-stay institutions serving people with learning or psychiatric impairments from Budapest were located 'near the enemy' – near the Austrian border (EASPPD 2002). By 2002 pioneering service providers and non-governmental organizations were using every tactic to bring services back into Budapest and other local communities – against a backdrop of NIMBY (not in my back yard) campaigns, in which local residents protested against the resettlement plans.

Mental Disability Rights International (1997) has reported serious human rights abuses in countries in eastern Europe, including Bulgaria and the Kosovan region of Serbia and Montenegro. However, human rights abuses do not only occur in central and eastern Europe. In 2000 an investigation into North Lakeland NHS Trust in Northern England found that elderly patients with dementia had been made to eat while tied to commodes, fed on inadequate liquid diets and left outdoors in winter with inadequate clothing. The investigation, conducted some five years after initial reports of abuse, found 'whole system failure' (Commission for Health Improvement 2000).

As well as these major abuses of human rights, some individuals with mental health problems are also denied the right to appropriate treatment, or treatment in an appropriate setting. Priebe *et al.* (2005) report on the apparent 're-institutionalization' occurring in mental health care across Europe following the closure of the long-stay psychiatric hospitals during the 1980s. Characteristics of re-institutionalization include rising numbers of forensic beds, involuntary hospital admissions and places in supported housing (often in the absence of flexible support enabling people to live independently). Between 1990 and 2002 all of the six European countries in the study (England, Germany, Italy, the Netherlands, Spain, and Sweden) reported an increase in the number of forensic beds and places in supported housing. Involuntary admissions rose in England, the Netherlands and Germany but fell slightly in Italy, Spain and Sweden. The general prison population has risen in all six countries. Priebe *et al.* suggest one reason for the increasing size of the prison population is the growing tendency towards 'risk containment' in twenty-first-century European society. In this sense, the rise in prison numbers and in compulsory institutionalization of people with mental health problems are part of one risk-averse trend. Although a citizenship approach requires equal rights and responsibilities for people with mental health problems – including taking responsibility for crime whenever someone is mentally competent – it seems that investment in incarceration is taking the place of investment in support for participation in social networks and civic opportunities.

Setting priorities

A key question is: what practical, policy and legislative changes need to be introduced in order to eliminate this unfair experience of social exclusion by people with mental health problems? As dimensions of social exclusion are broad and 'interactive', responses must also be diverse and multi-agency. The recent policy recommendations from the United Kingdom's Social Exclusion Unit (2004) included a 27-point action plan for major government departments: health, work and pensions, finance, education and employment. At the international level, the World Health Organization's (WHO) European Ministerial Conference on Mental Health in Helsinki in January 2005 prioritized tackling stigma, discrimination and inequality, and the empowerment and support of people with mental health problems, as well as stating social participation and action against discrimination as major action points (WHO 2005). The *European Declaration on Mental Health* and its *Action Plan* for Europe was endorsed by the 52 member states of the WHO European region.

Both the *Action Plan* for Europe and the United Kingdom's *Action Plan* address a range of issues including discrimination, poverty alleviation, access to appropriate services and support, and finding and sustaining employment. Housing, education and inter-agency cooperation also feature prominently in the *Action Plan*. However, while such documents may state that they are targeting stigma and discrimination it is possible to question how high a priority this actually is, and how it is best achieved. As this chapter addresses social exclusion from the perspective of a lack of basic or enforceable rights due to discrimination, the following sections focus on why this should be the major priority, and discuss practical methods of achieving it.

Improving the bottom line and human rights

It might seem intuitively sensible to begin the challenging task of overturning exclusion by improving the 'bottom line' of life and human rights. There are opportunities: as European Commissioner for Employment and Social Affairs Anna Diamontopoulou put it, 'the European Union was born from the ashes of the holocaust' (speech to the Italian Presidency Conference, Milan, 2003). The determination to avoid a repetition of past abuses is reflected at EU level in the annual human rights report that included, for the first time in 2003, a chapter on the rights of disabled people.

This determination is evident culturally as well as politically. As part of the European Year of Disabled People 2003, an Austrian disability organization developed a project to commemorate resistance to the Nazi so-called 'euthanasia' programmes. At Schloss Hartheim in Upper Austria 70,000 people with psychiatric or learning disabilities, criminals, prostitutes and orphans were murdered and/or used for experiments. A few people spoke out courageously against this, including architect Herbert Eichholzer, sculptor Walter Ritter and painter Anna Neumann. In 1943 Eichholzer was killed for his resistance activities and Neumann imprisoned. In 2003, *Klump* wooden toys, designed by Eichholzer and Ritter and painted by Neumann, were made again, this time by people with learning disabilities, thereby giving a powerful symbolic message on the importance of resistance.

However, where inclusion activities have focused only on improving the rights of the least powerful – for instance, challenging coercive mental health laws – progress has generally been slow, and has certainly not extended beyond the institutions in which people are incarcerated. A society is more likely to stop treating classes of people inhumanely when that group comes to be seen as equals. Then a new spotlight may be thrown on laws and practices that degrade them. As Nelson Mandela put it in relation to prisons, 'prison conditions would not change until the country changed' (Mandela 1995). As long as the public perception is that mental health service users are 'psychos' there will be little public outcry. The challenge is to go beyond objecting to gross abuses – important as that is – and push forward, for the positive benefits of participation.

Evidence also tells us that because discrimination is a persistent phenomenon, attempts to counter it in one area merely mean it pops up again in another guise, like a many-headed hydra (Link and Phelan 2001). Initiatives need to be multi-faceted and multi-level.

Reducing discrimination and exclusion

Link and Phelan (2001: 367) argue that 'stigma' (discrimination),[2] 'is entirely dependent on social, economic and political power'. This has huge implications for determining which approaches and types of programme are most likely to create change. They argue that it is not enough to label and disparage another group for them to become 'stigmatized': psychiatric service users may label some clinicians 'pill pushers' and treat them differently from other clinicians. This does not make these clinicians a stigmatized group, because patients 'simply do not possess the social, cultural, economic and political power to make their cognitions about staff have serious discriminatory consequences'.

Anti-discrimination work must either change the deeply-held attitudes and beliefs of powerful groups that lead to labelling, stereotyping, setting apart, devaluing and discriminating; or it must limit the power of such groups (Link and Phelan 2001); or both (Sayce 2003).

The problem with much anti-stigma work in Europe is that it has not addressed power. The World Psychiatric Association anti-stigma and discrimination initiative includes many examples of educational initiatives on its website (www.wpanet.org). In Belgium there has been a programme to inform people about 'the causes and consequences of mental illness', using evening lectures, tours of mental health services and introductions to group therapy, music therapy and sports therapy. In Slovenia there have been sessions for service users, professionals, relatives and schoolchildren. These programmes may be helpful – the Slovenian programme, for instance, resulted in increased confidence among professionals – but they rely on the assumption that education and information are enough to challenge discrimination. There is no evidence that just providing information on the causes and consequences of mental illness is enough to change attitudes, let alone behaviour.

It is more helpful to use power as part of the initiative. In the United Kingdom, the first European country to pass a disability discrimination law, the Disability Discrimination Act (DDA) 1995 outlaws discrimination against people with psychiatric disabilities. It has been used to achieve justice and set some legal precedents. One example is Ms Brazier, who had a diagnosis of psychosis, and in 2003 took a case against North Devon Homes who were seeking to evict her following complaints by neighbours about her behaviour. The court found that her disability was the cause of much of her conduct and that to evict her would be to discriminate against her under the DDA. This discrimination could not be 'justified' because, although the neighbours experienced discomfort, there had at no point been a danger to anyone's health or safety (*North Devon Homes Ltd* vs. *Brazier 2003*, EWHC 57). Other housing cases have been less helpful to tenants with mental health problems.

The existence of the law – the iron fist behind the velvet glove – means advice, with an explicit or implicit threat of law, is often enough to achieve change. In another example, Mr Watkiss's offer of a senior job with a construction company was withdrawn after his diagnosis of schizophrenia came to light. He challenged the company under the DDA in 2001 (see Box 3.1). The company settled, admitting unlawful discrimination and providing substantial compensation (*Watkiss* vs. *John Laing Employment Tribunal 1999*, proceedings for discrimination under the DDA 1995; case number 6002547).

However, British law is imperfect, particularly in relation to people with mental health problems, because of the way legal definitions are framed and interpreted. Under the DDA, people with mental health problems had a success rate at employment tribunals of 18 per cent – lower than those with hearing impairments (29 per cent) and diabetes (39 per cent) (Disability Rights Commission 2003). The first problem with the law is that the definition of disability is harder for people with psychiatric impairments to meet: it relies on a list of 'day-to-day activities' that are biased towards the physical, not the emotional and cognitive (Equal Opportunities Review 2000).

It has also proved easier for employers to 'justify' discrimination against people with psychiatric impairments on (usually spurious) health and safety grounds. This reflects the depth of prejudice in our societies. People seeking work in health or social care have been viewed as being too high a risk to clients, on the grounds of their diagnosis (bi-polar disorder, bulimia); or too high a risk to themselves, because the employer thinks the job (for example, probation

Box 3.1 A personal testimonial of work discrimination

Mr Watkiss writes (speech to Mind Conference 2001):

I received a curt letter from the personnel director stating that 'my standard of health did not measure up to the job, and therefore the offer was being withdrawn'. A more intelligent, sober and kindly reaction would have been to enquire a little further: perhaps to have contacted me to find out more about this illness that the one sentence in the medical report revealed. To have contacted, perhaps, my doctor or psychiatrist or my then employer to find out a little more, and having done all this, then make a decision.

My argument was that its [the company] action had been contrary to the requirements of the DDA – which say that it is illegal to treat, in this case a candidate for interview, less favourably than another solely on the grounds of disability. I argued that its reaction was based on ignorance and prejudice and was discriminatory. I applied for damages on the basis of loss of earnings and injury to feelings. And I won!

My solicitor described it as a landmark decision . . . I hope it will mean that more people with mental illness apply for work and are successful in getting it . . . I would like to think that my case took a swipe at social prejudice as well as questioning the equation that mental illness equals incapacity.

officer, for someone with a history of depression) will be 'too stressful'. Often such risk assessments are based on stereotypes, not on a genuinely individual assessment of whether the person can do the particular job, with adjustments (for example, extra support) if needed, as required by the DDA.

The British DRC has analysed the case law and recommended specific legal reform to government, including changes to the list of 'day-to-day activities' (Disability Rights Commission 2003). Evidence indicates that discrimination frequently occurs on the basis of unnecessary questions during recruitment such as 'have you ever experienced mental illness?'. Therefore, the DRC proposes that questions about disability should only be permitted during recruitment (before job offer) in highly specified circumstances. In 2005 the United Kingdom government did make it easier for people with mental health problems to secure their rights by removing the requirement that people with mental health problems – but not other types of disability – had to show their condition was 'clinically well recognized'. Since 2004 direct discrimination can no longer be justified, which should prove helpful to litigants in future.

By the end of 2003, under the EU Directive on Employment, Article 13, countries (and new EU countries prior to membership) had to have passed legislation debarring employment discrimination on grounds including disability; and to set up institutions to ensure enforcement. Research conducted for the EU suggests that by 2003 there were 21 institutions in 15 countries devoted to enforcing anti-discrimination provisions, with some countries having more than one such body, to deal with distinct issues such as race, gender and disability (www.eumc.eu.int).

It appears that EU and peer pressure is speeding up progress in legislating against discrimination (even beyond EU countries). For instance, the Norwegian Parliament set up a Commission, gathered evidence from Europe and beyond, and adopted anti-discrimination provisions in the labour market (under Paragraph 55 of its 2001 legislation on the work environment, which amended Acts No 313 and 311 in the Collection of Laws – Labour Code). This followed lobbying based on the European Directive on Employment and the influence of pre-existing Swedish legislation. Slovakia adopted a new employment act which came into force in 2004 and which provided measures to encourage the active involvement of disabled persons in the workplace (under Act No. 5 on Employment Services).

European countries have the potential to avoid the pitfalls in British law when developing their legislation. Furthermore, in the USA and Britain there is extensive material on what 'reasonable adjustments' can mean in the workplace for people with mental health problems, from off-line support to additional supervision or flexible hours (Employers Forum on Disability 1998). In Germany and Russia, there are strong incentives for employers to recruit and retain disabled people – and fines for non-compliance that are ploughed back into implementation programmes.

Systemic legal powers are likely to have an even greater impact than individual redress. In Britain the DRC can conduct formal investigations into whole sectors or organizations that appear to be discriminating – and make recommendations for systemic change, backed by the force of law. The government has also legislated to introduce a public sector duty, requiring that public sector organizations proactively promote equality of opportunity – rather than tackling discrimination only after the event. This came into force in December 2006 under the Disability Discrimination Act 2005. It will be crucial to evaluate the impact of the range of legal and policy measures and spread good practice across Europe.

Intervening in the different stages of discrimination

Link and Phelan (2001) argue that stigma has four components:

- distinguishing between and labelling human differences;
- linking the labelled persons to undesirable characteristics;
- separating 'them' (the labelled persons) from 'us'; culminating in
- status loss and discrimination that lead to unequal outcomes or life chances.

Sayce (2003) analyses evidence for potential interventions in each of these stages to achieve reduced discrimination. Here, two particularly salient lessons from evidence are further developed.

Linking the person to undesirable characteristics

To replace 'undesirable' with 'desirable' characteristics requires, first, attending to very specific stereotypes and identities. Promoting the very general message that discrimination against any human being is wrong has not dislodged myths about mental health service users. In Britain in the late 1990s, when public attitudes towards 'disabled people' were becoming more accepting through campaigns and increased participation, social distance towards those with mental health problems actually increased (Department of Health 2003).

Media Consulta, a Berlin-based PR company working on a 2003 EU public information campaign in employment ('Down with discrimination') found it challenging to devise images and messages that 'worked' across race, gender, disability, age, sexual orientation and religion/belief. They settled for an image of robots in the office – to caricature the horrors of a European workplace without diversity. While this was a clever resolution of a tricky brief, it would be very surprising if it reduced prejudice towards mental health services users and all the other sub-groups whom the new laws are designed to protect (migrant workers, travellers, older people, gays and lesbians).

Secondly, when considering messages centred on a 'desirable' characteristic – to replace the negative stereotype – it is essential to test whether the proposed characteristic actually is viewed as desirable, by people with psychiatric impairments and by the intended audience. It is all too easy to replace one stereotype with another.

Evidence suggests that one type of message that can 'work' is one that disrupts the link between mental ill health and violence (Penn and Martin 1998; Penn *et al.* 1999; Read and Law 1999). This matches the finding that the association between dangerousness and mental illness is 'the core' of stigma (Link *et al.* 1999). People who associate mental illness with violence are most likely to hold discriminatory attitudes (Link *et al.* 1987) and where educational interventions break the link with violence, discriminatory attitudes wane.

Another promising message focuses on the contribution of mental health service users – as employees and community leaders. The New Zealand Like Minds campaign profiled people with mental health problems working and succeeding, including a well-known New Zealand rugby player, as well as more ordinary citizens. This emphasis may have been a factor in the campaign's success in measurably improving public attitudes (Ministry of Health 2003). It appears to have helped replace the stereotype of helplessness and/or dangerousness with images of people with something to offer. This campaign tackles the view – perhaps as pernicious as the assumption of violence – that people with mental health problems are incompetent. More evaluations of such campaigns are needed.

Beyond these areas, evidence for the effectiveness of particular messages is much less clear-cut. It is troubling that many anti-stigma campaigns worldwide are using – or even relying on – messages for which there is no clear evidence base. One of the commonest is the message that 'mental illness is an illness like any other' (or is a brain disease). In fact, recent evidence from Germany suggests that these messages result in outcomes that are the opposite of those intended: the more that people recognize biology as a cause of mental health problems –

in this particular case, schizophrenia – the more social distance they desire between themselves and the affected individual (Angermeyer and Matschinger 2005).

It is unsurprising that people afflicted by discrimination want to benefit from the more benign attitudes towards people with, say, coronary heart disease than to those with schizophrenia (Lai *et al.* 2001). This can lead to the naïve view that emphasizing illness terminology – and explaining aetiology in disease terms – will transfer the acceptance of physical illness directly across to the mental health sphere. There are a number of problems with this assumption, the first being that the disease conception does not disrupt the link between mental illness and violence. In popular culture, 'sickness' can sometimes co-exist too readily with the idea of 'evil' – as 'sick monster' newspaper headlines in some countries attest. A second problem is that the disease conception also fails to disrupt the link between mental illness and incompetence; in fact, it may re-enforce it. Physical impairments can be linked to assumed incompetence, as with the 'Does he take sugar?' comment often addressed to the companion of a wheelchair user (rather than to the wheelchair user her/himself). We would not respond to that patronizing attitude by explaining the facts of the accident that broke the disabled person's spine. The cause is simply irrelevant. The effective challenge is a demonstration of competence and/or assertion of how the person wishes to be treated. In the same way, we should not assume that explaining the causes of schizophrenia will moderate discriminatory attitudes. Why should it?

If people with physical illnesses can be subjected to pity and stigma, when the diseased organ is the brain itself – the site of the personality, or mind – the whole person's credibility and capability is thrown into question. Add to that the fear of mental illness as a metaphor for wider disorder and lack of control (Sontag 1978) and it seems clear that simply stating that 'madness' is a brain disease is unlikely to 'use up' the metaphor, in Sontag's terms – to remove its sting.

A third problem associated with the brain disease/illness model is the removal from the individual of the burden of responsibility for his or her condition and the behaviour flowing from it; if it is an illness, it is not a person's fault. This can be cited as a positive outcome, and indeed research in the United States does show a link between biological understandings of mental illness and reduced blame of the individual (Phelan *et al.* 2002). However, now Angermeyer and Matschinger (2005) have replicated this study in Europe, results opposite to those achieved in America have been reported. American citizens are considerably more likely than Europeans to see individuals as responsible for poverty (Wilson 1997) – and for 'their own fate' more broadly. While Angermeyer and Matschinger (p. 331) report that 'parallel to an increase in the public's tendency to endorse biological causes, an increase in the desire for social distance from people with schizophrenia was found'. The report authors suggest that in Germany, the more the survey respondents endorsed biological factors as a cause, the more lacking in self-control, unpredictable and dangerous they believed individuals with schizophrenia to be. This, in turn, was associated with a higher degree of fear, which resulted in a stronger desire for social distance. Read and Harre (2001) found a similar result: when a sample of the public understood the 'brain disease' message they became more, not less, likely to believe the person was incapable and not responsible: a poor unfortunate, rather than an equal citizen. If a person is not responsible for their behaviour then they cannot control it and are even more dangerous. As Read and Harre put it, the brain disease messages are related to negative attitudes, including perceptions that 'mental patients are dangerous, anti-social and unpredictable, with reluctance to become romantically involved with them . . . It is recommended that de-stigmatization programmes consider abandoning efforts to promulgate illness-based explanations and focus instead on increasing contact with, and exposure to, users of mental health services' (Read and Harre 2001: 223).

Some British evidence suggests that the public is more accepting when they think a mental health problem stems from understandable causes – like bereavement or unemployment – than when it is biologically caused or not understandable at all (Sayce 2000). However, this can mean they see a gulf between acceptable, understandable distress and being 'mental': the acceptability of understandable distress does not 'rub off' on views of madness, so may not 'work' as an anti-discrimination strategy.

If biological understandings reduce individual blame, then blame is replaced by what can be seen as more positive attitudes and behaviours – such as pity, sympathy or willingness to help (Phelan *et al.* 2002). This begs a fundamental question: are pity and a desire to help the positive responses that challenge discrimination? As one American consumer put it: 'People used to be called crazy and lunatic. A lot of hatred was directed at them. NAMI [National Alliance for the Mentally Ill] stepped in and said no, don't hate them, they're sick. Pity them. Now we're stuck with a lot of pity. I wish someone had had more foresight and substituted something different for the hatred' (cited in Sayce 2000: 207).

Being 'ill' means one can be subjected to what Corrigan *et al.* (2001) called the stigma of benevolence. People are then seen as innocent and childlike. Importantly, this is linked to the desire for social distance, just as the fear of violence is. Illness also means one is excused from social roles which may be exactly what the individual does not want. Phelan *et al.* (2002) argue that biological and genetic explanations are 'a double-edged sword'. While they are associated with reduced blame, they are also linked to pessimism about recovery and, in the case of genetic causation, to fear of spread of the genetic taint and to 'stickiness' of the mentally ill label even if the person has been symptom-free for years.

Hinshaw and Cicchetti (2000) note that historically, biological/disease models of mental illness have been as much associated with punitive societal responses as have models of demonic possession; in either case, the person receives an authoritarian response to the perceived 'disorder' of brain or spirits. It appears that there are no grounds to privilege biological understandings, from the point of view of reducing discrimination; but equally no grounds for privileging social causation, since this can mean some (understandable) conditions are accepted while others are rejected (Sayce 2000).

Finally, from a cross-cultural perspective, there is no consensus on which explanatory model is most helpful for individuals' self-perception and no evidence that the western medical model is more helpful in anti-discriminatory terms than others. Haj-Yahia (1999) found that in a traditional Arab society, although religious views of mental illness were growing, rejection of people with mental health problems was not necessarily linked to this. Lefley (1990) notes that different world views should be seen as strengths, to be worked with, not homogenized into a common, global understanding of mental ill health as 'disease'.

Several authors have discussed possible reasons for the frequent use of the brain illness/disease model in anti-discriminatory work. Rose (1998) notes that in the 1950s and 1960s the notion of 'an illness like any other' was central to the community psychiatry movement, which sought to reduce coercion in favour of care, strip madness of its terrors and make mental health services a branch of ordinary medicine. There is thus profound professional investment in the 'illness like any other' model, which may help explain its assumed usefulness in the absence of empirical evidence. Pharmaceutical companies may have vested interests in the illness conception, as it opens up markets for the sale of bio-medical solutions. Relatives of mental health service users can find comfort in the 'brain disease' model as the emphasis on nature rather than nurture absolves them of behavioural responsibility. However, there is no evidence that any particular model of what madness/mental illness is, or what causes it, is any more useful than any other model in anti-discrimination work. Far too much confidence has been placed in the brain disease model, which may compound rather than challenge the stereotypes of dangerousness and, particularly, incompetence.

The assumption that public understanding of the 'illness' model is positive is so deep-rooted that it sometimes emerges in research studies as an assumed (not demonstrated) positive outcome. For instance, the Royal College of Psychiatrists cited as a success of their Defeat Depression campaign an increase in the proportion of the public believing that depression was 'a medical condition like any other illnesses' (Royal College of Psychiatrists 1995). Stuart and Arboleda Florez (2001) use knowledge that schizophrenia is a biological illness as one of several indicators of accurate public knowledge, in order to assess links between accurate knowledge and stigma. This type of research does not enable us to ascertain whether belief in an illness model is linked, positively or negatively, with important outcomes from the service user's point of view, such as social distance. It is necessary both for research and for evidence-based practice to discard the assumption that biological understandings reduce discrimination. Causation is not the key to countering discrimination.

More promising are messages that ignore causation, focusing rather on contribution and equal citizenship, breaking the links with violence and incompetence. The disability rights model – which draws attention to disabling barriers and to people's rights to participate, with adjustments where needed – seems much more likely to effect changes in attitude and behaviour than the chimera that as scientific understanding of causation percolates through society, so discrimination will ebb away. Evidence to support or contradict this approach is limited. However, the New Zealand government's Like Minds project appears to have had some success in reducing discriminatory attitudes, especially desire for social distance, while there is some evidence that conventional programmes raising awareness of biological causation may not effectively reduce stigma (Angermeyer and Matschinger 2005). More research is needed in this area to provide policy-makers with evidence for how best to reduce discriminatory attitudes and behaviours.

Separating 'them' (the labelled persons) from 'us'

The most consistent research finding on reducing discrimination or stigma is that attitudes improve as a result of contact or familiarization with a person/people with experience of mental health problems (Angermeyer and Matschinger 1997; Read and Law 1999; Meise *et al.* 2000). Opposition to mental health facilities disappears once the facilities open and neighbours 'see service users as people' (Repper *et al.* 1997). Contact appears to reduce fear of the 'other' and to increase empathy. Contact affects attitudes whether or not the contact is voluntary (Link and Cullen 1986; Desforges *et al.* 1991; Corrigan *et al.* 2001). Contact can be retrospective or prospective – in other words, engineering contact as an anti-discrimination intervention promises to be effective (Couture and Penn 2003).

In the New Zealand Like Minds campaign, government employees receiving training said it was the personal experience that moved them from a concern about how people with mental illness might behave, to looking at their own behaviour: what they could say or do when someone was mentally unwell.

Research into what types of contact have most impact on which attitudes and behaviours is not yet conclusive (Alexander and Link 2003). Wider research into the impact of contact in relation to groups facing discrimination (e.g. ethnic and religious minorities) shows that key factors are that people should be brought together under conditions of equal status, in situations where stereotypes are likely to be disconfirmed, where there is inter-group cooperation, where participants can get to know each other and where wider social norms support equality (Hewstone 2003). There is some evidence in the mental health field that supports these conclusions, particularly on equal status (Corrigan and Penn 1999) and cooperative activity (Desforges *et al.* 1991). Where people with psychiatric impairments have ongoing significant roles as employees, bosses or teachers, or are trainers with status, this is likely to impact positively on the attitudes of those around them. There are provisos: the impact will not occur if the person hides their psychiatric status, or if non-disabled people see them as so different from their stereotypes that they do not generalize from this individual, and instead see him or her as an 'exception' (Hewstone 2003).

Compared to contact, specific information has less research backing as an effective changer of attitude. Wolff *et al.* (1996) found in one study that attitudes changed as a result of a community intervention, in which neighbours were given information and met service users, even though knowledge did not increase at all. Link *et al.* (1999) note that at a time in the United States when public awareness about mental illness had grown, the desire for social distance remained strong. Knowledge does not seem to be either a necessary or a sufficient condition for attitude change.

Inclusion itself is a powerful way of changing non-disabled people's beliefs (see Box 3.2). Recent British research finds that the group with the highest DDA awareness and the most inclusive attitudes about disability are people who 'know someone who is disabled at work' (Disability Rights Commission 2002). Inclusive schools also influence non-disabled children to hold more accepting attitudes towards disabled children (Gray 2002).

Thus, a key challenge is to make it safer for disabled people to assert the right to

Box 3.2 Strategies for greater inclusion

- Evidence shows contact between people with mental health problems and other citizens has the most positive effects on attitudes and behaviour.
- Contact should involve equal status.
- Inclusion in employment and education in itself changes attitudes and behaviour.
- Educational messages that contradict stereotypes of violence and incompetence, and emphasize contribution, are also effective.
- Messages focused on the cause of mental health problems – for instance 'an illness like any other' – are at best unproven and may add to discrimination.

participate. It is encouraging that a recent American survey of professionals and managers with mental health problems (from across industries and sectors) found that the vast majority (87 per cent) had disclosed at work; and most (61 per cent) had no regrets. One of the factors significantly associated with disclosure was awareness of the Americans with Disabilities Act. Anti-discrimination law can encourage confidence, and at best deliver greater safety to disclose (Ellison *et al.* 2003). Increasing the proportion of European disabled people who know their rights is crucial. Eurobarometer (2003) found that only just over a third of Europeans would know their rights if they experienced discrimination.

Policy directions

A report from the European Foundation for the Improvement of Living and Working Conditions (2003: 26, 56), commenting on European labour markets and income, concluded that 'different studies find that people with mental illness are those with most problems in comparison with other types of illness and disability . . . Information campaigns have tried to de-stigmatise mental illness, but there is still a strong stigma attached to it'.

Stigma is clearly a key factor in unequal life chances generally and should be accorded much greater attention in mainstream work to reduce exclusion (Link and Phelan 2001). The exclusion of people with psychiatric impairments is unfortunately often mirrored in a second exclusion – from the arena of policy-making on inclusion of disabled people:

> Based on seven years of work, I find that two distinct groups of persons with disabilities, those with intellectual and those with psychiatric disabilities, are systematically more marginalized and isolated than other groups of disabled people . . . Modern disability policy creates a motion from exclusion towards inclusion. It is high time that the most vulnerable groups amongst

disabled people, including persons with psychiatric disabilities, will be included in this world-wide development. To achieve this it is a responsibility we must all share.[3]

To be excluded even from the 'disability inclusion' agenda is problematic, since this agenda is itself marginalized from broader social and economic policy. Disability discussions tend to focus on the issue of rights, which attracts consensus but often fails to generate active policies that improve conditions for people (European Foundation for the Improvement of Living and Working Conditions 2003).

In the next phase of EU policy development the key issue is mainstreaming. This means mental health policy analysts and advocates should be building the mainstream rationale for inclusion – not arguing only from the basis of distinct policy and rights.

To give an example, Burchardt (2000) notes that in Britain disabled people make up half of those who are out of work and want to work; and a third of those ready to start in a fortnight. Would any reasonable employer, especially in times of low unemployment, screen out half of all potential recruits? Would any government aiming to increase employment participation leave so many (disabled) people out of its policy equation? As Burchardt puts it, 'anti-poverty strategies will need to take into account the needs of disabled people as a central part of the programme, not just as a special case with a token budget' (p. 65). Social exclusion of disabled people needs to come out of the ghetto of 'disability policy' or even 'disability rights policy'; and mental health policy-makers need to join in.

In Europe, mental health problems account for 25 per cent of new disability benefits cases, and this share is rising (European Foundation for the Improvement of Living and Working Conditions 2003). Mainstream policy-makers are seeking solutions. If disability policy-makers and advocates can offer cost-effective ways of increasing social participation, including for people with mental health problems, there is a chance they will be heard (see Box 3.3).

Box 3.3   Policy directions for greater inclusion

- Policy-makers need to focus on inclusion, not mental health services alone.
- They should support multi-level, multi-faceted anti-discrimination initiatives.
- They should view the inclusion of mental health service users through the mainstream lens of policies on education, employment or economic regeneration, and devise mainstream solutions.
- Mental health policy-makers and advocates need to work with others in disability and wider networks to bring mental health policy into wider agendas.

Conclusion

Evidence is growing on the social exclusion of people with mental health problems in Europe and what works to overcome it. People with mental health problems face discrimination and exclusion in all facets of life, including health, personal respect and opportunities to contribute to their communities, as well as in terms of equal human rights. The days of well-intentioned ad hoc programmes to 'inform people about mental illness' to reduce stigma should be over. What is needed are anti-discrimination initiatives based on multi-faceted, multi-level programmes that centrally address power imbalances, that mainstream mental health service users' rights and interests into general economic and social policy and that also disrupt the highly specific stereotypes that have dogged mental health service users for centuries. In particular, the notion that mental health service users should be subject to a different set of assumptions and rules about risk than other citizens – because they are viewed as 'dangerous' and/or 'incompetent' – should be actively challenged. A positive focus on participation seems to be a key element in formulating effective anti-discrimination strategies. Evidence shows that contact between people with mental health problems and other citizens, particularly through inclusion in employment and education, has the most positive effects on attitudes and behaviour.

Although this work is highly complex by its very nature, there is evidence about 'what works' and major opportunities in Europe, with the passage of the European Directive on Employment (Article 13) and a new commitment to a disability Directive beyond employment. Europe's first disability discrimination law, passed in the United Kingdom, has had important successes for people with psychiatric impairments and other member states are developing similar legislation in response to the EU Directive. If resulting policies include mental health dimensions from the outset and are monitored and continuously reformed, with lessons learnt internationally, the momentum could bring tangible benefits in terms of reduced discrimination faced by people with mental health problems across Europe.

Finally, power relationships cannot be changed unless the work to change them itself models the new power relations (see Chapter 14). Policy-makers, advocates and service users need to access wider networks and maintain a presence within wider policy agendas. More importantly, disabled people must lead the process, with allies contributing as appropriate. Link and Phelan (2001) note that a key issue in stigmatization is 'whose cognitions prevail'. In this context, it is the cognitions of users and survivors of mental health services that must prevail.

Notes

1   We use the term disability in terms of a social model of disability. People are disabled by the barriers and attitudes they encounter, and solutions depend on stripping away discrimination. The alternative model is the so-called medical model in which individuals are financially compensated for the limitations in functioning that they experience which prevents full participation in society (Van Oorschot and Hvinden 2000).

2 We use the term discrimination to describe the overall process termed 'stigma' by Link and Phelan. For discussion of the respective merits of these concepts, see Link and Phelan (2001) and Sayce (2003).
3 Dr Bengt Lindqvist, United Nations Special Rapporteur on Disability. Speech to a World Health Organization meeting on Mental Health and Human Rights, Geneva, April 2001.

References

Alexander, L.A. and Link, B.G. (2003) The impact of contact on stigmatising attitudes towards people with mental illness, *Journal of Mental Health*, 12(3): 271–90.

Allebeck, P. (1989) Schizophrenia: a life-shortening disease, *Psychiatric Bulletin*, 15(1): 81–9.

Angermeyer, M.C. and Matschinger, H. (1996) The effects of violent attacks by schizophrenic persons on the attitude of the public towards the mentally ill, *Social Science & Medicine*, 43(12): 1721–8.

Angermeyer, M.C. and Matschinger, H. (1997) Social distance towards the mentally ill: results of representative surveys in the Federal Republic of Germany, *Psychological Medicine*, 27(1): 131–41.

Angermeyer, M.C. and Matschinger, H. (2005) Causal beliefs and attitudes to people with schizophrenia: trend analysis based on data from two population surveys in Germany, *British Journal of Psychiatry*, 186: 331–4.

Burchardt, T. (2000) *Enduring Economic Exclusion: Disabled People, Income and Work*. York: Joseph Rowntree Foundation.

Burchardt, T., Le Grand, J. and Piachaud, D. (1999) Social exclusion in Britain 1991–1995, *Social Policy and Administration*, 33(3): 227–44.

Burchardt, T., Le Grand, J. and Piachaud, D. (2002) Introduction to understanding social exclusion, in J. Hills, J. Le Grand and D. Piachaud (eds) *Understanding Social Exclusion*. Oxford: Oxford University Press.

Commission for Health Improvement (2000) *Investigation into the North Lakeland NHS Trust: Report to the Secretary of State for Health*. London: Commission for Health Improvement.

Corrigan, P.W. and Penn, D.L. (1999) Lessons from social psychology on discrediting psychiatric stigma, *American Psychologist*, 54(9): 765–6.

Corrigan, P.W., Edwards, A.B., Green, A., Diwan, S.L. and Penn, D.L. (2001) Prejudice, social distance and familiarity with mental illness, *Schizophrenia Bulletin*, 27(2): 219–5.

Couture, S.M. and Penn, D.L. (2003) Interpersonal contact and the stigma of mental illness: a review of the literature, *Journal of Mental Health*, 12(3): 291–306.

D'Avanzo, B., La Vecchia, C. and Negri, E. (2003) Mortality in long-stay patients from psychiatric hospitals in Italy: results from the Qualyop Project, *Social Psychiatry and Psychiatric Epidemiology*, 38(7): 385–9.

Desforges, D.M., Lord, C.G., Ramsay, S.L., Mason, J.A., Van Leeuwen, M.D., West, S.C. and Lepper, M.R. (1991) Effects of structured co-operative contact on changing negative attitudes towards stigmatised groups, *Journal of Personality and Social Psychology*, 60(4): 531–44.

Department of Health (1991) *Health of the Nation*. London: Department of Health.

Department of Health (2003) *Attitudes to Mental Illness 2003*. London: Department of Health.

Disability Rights Commission (2002) *Public Attitudes Survey*. Conducted by BMRB for the Disability Rights Commission. London: Disability Rights Commission.

Disability Rights Commission (2003) *Disability Equality: Making it Happen. A Review of the Disability Discrimination Act 1995*. London: Disability Rights Commission.

Disability Rights Commission (2004) *Strategic Plan 2004–2007*. London: Disability Rights Commission.

Disability Rights Commission (2005) *Disability Briefing*. London: Disability Rights Commission.

Disability Rights Commission (2006) *Equal Treatment: Closing the Gap. Results of a Formal Investigation into Health Inequalities Experienced by People with Learning Disabilities and/or Mental Health Problems*. London: Disability Rights Commission.

EASPPD (2002) *Report to European Association of Service Providers of People with Disabilities*, www.easpd.org.

Ellison, M.L., Russinova, Z., Macdonald-Wilson, K.L. and Lyass, A. (2003) Patterns and correlates of workplace disclosure among professionals and managers with psychiatric conditions, *Journal of Vocational Rehabilitation*, 18(1): 3–13.

Employers Forum on Disability (1998) *Practical Guide to Employment Adjustments for People with Mental Health Problems*. London: Employers Forum on Disability.

Equal Opportunities Review (2000) The DDA after four years: part 1 – the meaning of disability, *Equal Opportunities Review*, 94: 12–19.

Eurobarometer (2003) *Discrimination in Europe. For Diversity, Against Discrimination*. Brussels: European Commission.

European Foundation for the Improvement of Living and Working Conditions (2003) *Illness, Disability and Social Inclusion*. Brussels: European Foundation for the Improvement of Living and Working Conditions.

Fryers, T., Melzer, D. and Jenkins, R. (2003) Social inequalities and the common mental disorders: a systematic review of the evidence, *Social Psychiatry and Psychiatric Epidemiology*, 38(5): 229–37.

Gore, C. and Figueiredo, J.B. (eds) (1997) *Social Exclusion and Anti-Poverty Policy*. Geneva: International Institute of Labour Studies.

Gray, P. (2002) *Disability Discrimination in Education. A Review Undertaken on Behalf of the Disability Rights Commission*. London: Disability Rights Commission.

Haj-Yahia, M.M. (1999) Attitudes towards mentally ill people and willingness to employ them in Arab society, *International Sociology*, 14(2): 173–93.

Harris, E.C. and Barraclough, B. (1998) Excess mortality of mental disorder, *British Journal of Psychiatry*, 173: 11–53.

Hewstone, M. (2003) Intergroup contact: panacea for prejudice? *The Psychologist*, 16(7): 352–5.

Hinshaw, S.R. and Cicchetti, D. (2000) Stigma and mental disorder: conceptions of illness, public attitudes, personal disclosure and social policy, *Development and Psychopathology*, 12(4): 555–98.

Hobcraft, J. (2002) Social exclusion and the generations, in J. Hills, D. Le Grand and D. Piachaud (eds) *Understanding Social Exclusion*. Oxford: Oxford University Press.

Lai, Y.M., Hong, C.P. and Chee, C.Y. (2001) Stigma of mental illness, *Singapore Medical Journal*, 42(3): 111–14.

Lawrence, D.M., Holman, C.D., Jablensky, A.V. and Hobbs, M.S. (2003) Death rate from ischeamic heart disease in Western Australian psychiatric patients 1980–1998. *British Journal of Psychiatry*, 182: 31–6.

Lefley, H.P. (1990) Culture and chronic mental illness, *Hospital and Community Psychiatry*, 41(3): 277–85.

Leslie, D. (1997) *Unemployment, Ethnic Minorities and Discrimination*. Florence: European University Institute.

Link, B.G. and Cullen, F.T. (1986) Contact with people with mental illnesses and perceptions of how dangerous they are, *Journal of Health and Social Behaviour*, 27(4): 289–302.

Link, B.G. and Phelan, J.C. (2001) On the nature and consequences of stigma, *Annual Review of Sociology*, 27(1): 363–85.

Link, B.G., Cullen, F.T., Franck, J. and Wozniak, J.F. (1987) The social rejection of mental patients: understanding why labels matter, *American Journal of Sociology*, 92(6): 1461–500.

Link, B.G., Struening, E.L., Rahav, M., Phelan, J.C. and Nuttbrock, L. (1997) On stigma and its consequences: evidence from a longitudinal study of men with dual diagnoses of mental illness and substance abuse, *Journal of Health and Social Behavior*, 38(2): 177–90.

Link, B.G., Phelan, J.C., Bresnahan, M., Stuene, A. and Pescosolido, B.A. (1999) Public conceptions of mental illness: labels, causes, dangerousness and social distance, *American Journal of Public Health*, 89(9): 1328–33.

Mandela, N.R. (1995) *Long Walk to Freedom*. London: Abacus.

Meise, U., Sulzenbacher, H., Kemmler, G., Schmid, R., Roessler, W. and Guenther, V. (2000) 'Not dangerous but still frightening' – a school programme against stigmatisation of schizophrenia, *Psychiatric Praxis*, 27(7): 340–6.

Mental Disability Rights International (1997) *Human Rights and Mental Health, Hungary*. Washington, DC: MDRI.

Mind (2000) *Mindout for Mental Health, Working Minds: Making Mental Health your Business*. London: Mind.

Ministry of Health (2003) *Like Minds, Like Mine. National Plan 2003–2005*. Wellington, New Zealand: Ministry of Health.

Nocon, A. (2004) *Equal Treatment: Closing the Gap. Background Evidence for the DRC's Formal Investigation into Health Inequalities Experienced by People with Learning Disabilities or Mental Health Problems*. Stratford-on-Avon: Disability Rights Commission.

Penn, D.L. and Martin, J. (1998) The stigma of severe mental illness: some potential solution for a recalcitrant problem, *Psychiatric Quarterly*, 69(3): 235–47.

Penn, D.L. and Wykes, T. (2003) Stigma, discrimination and mental illness, *Journal of Mental Health*, 12(3): 203–8.

Penn, D.L., Kommana, S., Mansfield, M. and Link, B.G. (1999) Dispelling the stigma of schizophrenia II: the impact of information on dangerousness, *Schizophrenia Bulletin*, 25(3): 437–46.

Percy-Smith, J. (2000) Introduction: the contours of social exclusion, in P. Smith (ed.) *Policy Responses to Social Exclusion: Towards Inclusion?* Buckingham: Open University Press.

Perkins, R. and Rinaldi, M. (2002) Unemployment rates among people with long-term mental health problems: a decade of rising unemployment, *Psychiatric Bulletin*, 26(8): 295–8.

Phelan, J., Cruz-Rojas, R. and Reiff, M. (2002) Genes and stigma: the connection between perceived genetic etiology and attitudes and beliefs about mental illness, *Psychiatric Rehabilitation Skills*, 6(2): 159–85.

Priebe, S., Badesconyi, A., Fioritti, A., Hansson, L., Kilian, R., Torres-Gonzales, F., Turner, T. and Wiersma, D. (2005) Reinstitutionalization in mental health care: comparison of data on service provision from six European countries, *British Medical Journal*, 330(7483): 123–6.

Rasanen, S., Hakko, H., Viilo, K., Meyer-Rochow, V.B. and Moring, J. (2003) Excess mortality among long-stay psychiatric patients in Northern Finland, *Social Psychiatry and Psychiatric Epidemiology*, 38(6): 297–304.

Read, J. and Baker, S. (1996) *Not Just Sticks and Stones: A Survey of the Stigma,Taboos and Discrimination Experienced by People with Mental Health Problems*. London: Mind.

Read, J. and Harre, N. (2001) The role of biological and genetic causal beliefs in the stigmatization of 'mental patients', *Journal of Mental Health*, 10(2): 223–35.

Read, J. and Law, A. (1999) The relationships of causal beliefs and contact with users of mental health services to attitudes to the 'mentally ill', *International Journal of Social Psychiatry*, 45(3): 216–29.

Repper, J., Sayce, L., Strong, S., Wilmot, J. and Haines, M. (1997) *Tall Stories from the Back yard. A Survey of Nimby Opposition to Community Mental Health Facilities Experienced by key Service Providers in England and Wales.* London: Mind.

Rose, N. (1998) Governing risky individuals: the role of psychiatry in new regimes of control, *Psychiatry, Psychology and Law*, 5(2): 177–95.

Royal College of Psychiatrists (1995) *Results of Second MORI Poll on Attitudes Towards Depression.* London: Royal College of Psychiatrists.

Rutter, M. and Smith, D.J. (1995) *Psychological Disorder in Young People.* Chichester: Wiley.

Saraceno, B. and Barbui, C. (1997) Poverty and mental illness, *Canadian Journal of Psychiatry*, 42(3): 285–90.

Sayce, L. (1995) Response to violence: a framework for fair treatment, in J. Crighton (ed.) *Psychiatric Patient Violence.* London: Duckworth.

Sayce, L. (2000) *From Psychiatric Patient to Citizen: Overcoming Discrimination and Social Exclusion.* London: Macmillan.

Sayce, L. (2001) Social inclusion and mental health, editorial, *Psychiatric Bulletin*, 25(4): 121–3.

Sayce, L. (2003) Beyond good intentions: making anti-discrimination strategies work, *Disability and Society*, 18(5): 625–42.

Sieff, M. (2003) Media frames of mental illnesses: the potential impact of negative frames, *Journal of Mental Health*, 12(3): 259–70.

Singh, P. (1997) *Prescriptions for Change: a Mencap Report on the Role of GPs and Carers in the Provision of Primary Care for People with Learning Disabilities.* London: Mencap.

Social Exclusion Unit (2004) *Mental Health and Social Exclusion.* London: Office of the Deputy Prime Minister.

Sontag, S. (1978) *Illness as Metaphor.* New York: Doubleday.

Stark, C., MacLeod, M., Hall, D., O'Brien, F. and Pelosi, A. (2003) Mortality after discharge from long-term psychiatric care in Scotland, 1977–94: a retrospective cohort study, *BioMed Central Public Health*, 3(September): 30.

Stuart, H. and Arboleda Florez, J. (2001) Community attitudes towards people with schizophrenia, *Canadian Journal of Psychiatry*, 46(3): 245–52.

Van Oorschot, W. and Hvinden, B. (2000) Introduction: towards convergence? Disability policies in Europe, *European Journal of Social Security*, 2(4): 293–302.

Wahl, O.F. (1995) *Media Madness: Public Images of Mental Illness.* Piscataway, NJ: Rutgers University Press.

Wahl, O.F. (2003) Depictions of mental illnesses in children's media, *Journal of Mental Health*, 12(3): 249–58.

Wilson, C., Nairn, R., Coverdale, J. and Panapa, A. (2000) How mental illness is portrayed in children's television, *British Journal of Psychiatry*, 176: 440–3.

Wilson, J. (1997) *When Work Disappears: the World of the New Urban Poor.* New York: Vintage.

Wolff, G., Pathare, S., Craig, T. and Leff, J. (1996) Public education for community care, *British Journal of Psychiatry*, 168(4): 440–3.

World Health Organization (2005) *Mental Health Declaration for Europe: Facing the Challenges, Building Solutions.* WHO European Ministerial Conference on Mental Health. Helsinki, January 2005.

chapter four

Financing and funding mental health care services

Martin Knapp and David McDaid

The centrality of funds and resources

Although prevalence rates for the majority of psychiatric disorders vary little across Europe, different health systems identify different levels of need, devote different levels of funding to meet those needs and choose different ways to deliver services. These variations in need, funding and response arise for many reasons, including demographic pressures, socioeconomic contexts, macro-economic capabilities, societal attitudes, cultural and religious orientation, and – of course – the political commitment and policy priorities that flow from them. In turn, these factors tend to influence the routes and details of mental health services financing and resourcing. Despite these inter-country economic differences, there is a common core of resource challenges to be faced. The aim of this chapter is to discuss those challenges.

Mental health interventions include actions and services for the promotion of mental well-being, prevention of mental health problems, treatment of symptoms and their sequelae, rehabilitation and support. Good quality services that are also well coordinated and well targeted will have significant impacts on the mental health and general well-being of individuals and populations. Those services will be delivered by skilled staff with access to appropriate information and support, evidence-based medications, psychological therapies and psychosocial interventions in specialist and other settings. That is the ideal: the key to a successful mental health system is obviously access to good physical and human capital resources. The reality is usually rather different: pervasive limitations on resources restrict access and constrain health improvements.

The structure of this chapter is as follows. We first introduce a conceptual framework that links resources and outcomes and helps to stylize the complex interplay between funding and provision. Many people with mental health problems have multiple needs, often eliciting multiple responses from health care and other bodies, adding necessary complexity to these frameworks. We set them out in the following sections. We then pull out some key topics for more focused attention, starting with financing arrangements and mental health budgets, then looking at the efficient and equitable targeting of resources, and finally discussing resource challenges for mental health in Europe and how to overcome them.

Production of welfare

Descriptions of the resources available to a mental health system tend to focus primarily on those used in providing treatment of identified symptoms or needs. In fact, resources might be deployed in various ways:

- promotion of well-being and prevention of symptoms;
- screening for, and assessment of, needs;
- purchasing or providing treatment for identified needs;
- maintenance of, or rehabilitation back into, 'mainstream' activities and lifestyles;
- coordination of treatment and rehabilitation services (brokerage);
- monitoring of service quality and service users' outcomes;
- regulation of procedures, services, choices and opportunities; and
- research and development.

What then do we mean by resources? How are they linked to outcomes?

We can start with a simple framework which represents the links between budgets, the resource inputs they purchase or fund, the services produced by those inputs, and the health and quality of life outcomes that hopefully will result for service users, their families and relevant others. These are among the most pertinent links in any mental health system and the framework therefore helps us identify many of the issues faced by decision-makers.

The framework is illustrated schematically in a highly simplified form in Figure 4.1 and shows the connections between a number of entities:

- The *resource inputs* used in promoting good mental health or in assessing, supporting, treating or monitoring people with mental health problems. These are mainly staff, physical capital, medications and other consumables.
- The *costs* of these resource inputs expressed in monetary terms.
- The service volumes and qualities (perhaps weighted in some way for user characteristics, including casemix) produced from combinations of the resource inputs, which we can call the *intermediate outputs*.
- The *final outcomes* from prevention and care, principally outcomes for individual service users and others gauged in terms of symptom alleviation, improved functioning and quality of life, improved family well-being and perhaps some wider social consequences.
- The *non-resource inputs*, which do not have a readily identified cost (since they are not directly marketed) but which exert influences on user outcomes and also mediate the influences of the resource inputs. Examples would be the

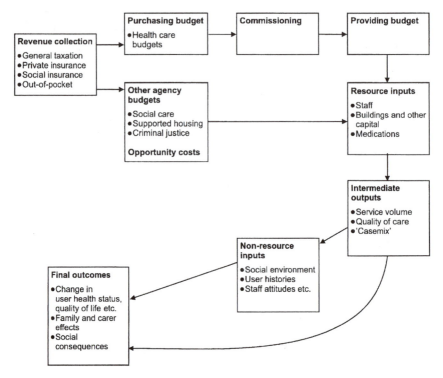

Figure 4.1 The production of welfare framework, revenue collection and commissioning

    social milieu of a care setting, service users' personal histories (especially their previous treatment experiences) and staff attitudes.
- The *commissioning* links between costs (or budgets) and the intermediate (service) outputs.
- *Revenue collection*, 'the process by which the health system receives money from households and organizations or companies, as well as from donors' (World Health Organization 2000: 95).

    What the schematic diagram represents, therefore, is the assumed or evidenced connections between what goes in (the funds and the resource inputs they purchase) and what comes out (the outputs of services and particularly the outcomes for service users and families), made possible by the treatment and support processes and the broader economic and societal contexts. This representation has been called the *production of welfare framework* (Knapp 1984, 1995) because of its analogies with production processes in mainstream economics but with its primary concern being the promotion of well-being (quality of life). The framework shows how financing and resources are linked to many of the key features of a mental health system. It thus provides a starting point for discussing the resource barriers to better mental health care in Europe and a platform for discussing how they might be overcome (see below). The framework also provides a conceptual structure for cost-effectiveness evaluations of different policies or interventions and for discussions of equity (again, see below).

The success of a mental health system in improving the health and quality of life of the population will depend on the mix, volume and deployment of resource inputs and the services they deliver, which in turn are dependent on the finances made available. And, of course, we know that different countries choose different levels and mixes of resource inputs. To give an example, we can see very different patterns of employment of professional staff across Europe. According to the (2005a) WHO *Atlas* on mental health, northern European countries generally employ more mental health staff than eastern or southern European countries. Denmark, Finland, Iceland, Ireland, Luxembourg, the Netherlands, Norway, Sweden and the United Kingdom, with San Marino being the southern exception, have more than 100 mental health personnel (including social workers) per 100,000 population. Within this group of countries, Finland has the highest figure at 436 personnel per 100,000 of population. Of the 52 countries in the European Region, Bulgaria, with 41.5 personnel per 100,000, is the median. This is just one illustration of variations in approach; others will be considered later.

Multiple needs, multiple resources

It is quite common for someone with a mental health problem to have needs for support across multiple life domains. For instance, someone who experiences recurrent bouts of psychosis may need not only health care but assistance or support in finding and/or retaining paid employment. If they are not working they are likely to need some alternative source of income and may qualify for financial support from government or a social insurance fund. They may have relationship or family difficulties, in more extreme cases even leading to the involvement of social care agencies. If the consequences of their illness are especially debilitating, or if they have dislocated normal family relations, they may need help in finding appropriate housing, or family members may themselves need services or financial support. For some people with behavioural problems, desperation or victimization might lead to higher than average contact with the criminal justice system.

Some symptoms of mental illness have a tendency to generate multiple needs because they are chronically disabling for the person concerned, distressing for the family and widely misunderstood by the community. Regardless of circumstances, where or from whom an individual gets their support, treatment might almost be a lottery in some countries. Some people may be supported by health services, some by social care services, some by their employers, some by religious and charitable groups, some solely by family members, and some – unfortunately – by no one at all: across the world, many needs still go unrecognized or ignored (World Mental Health Survey Consortium 2004).

In well-developed and well-resourced health systems, the multiple needs of individuals and populations are likely to be identified, assessed and addressed by a range of agencies. Similarly, dedicated promotion and prevention strategies may be in place in a number of settings such as schools or workplaces (see

Chapter 8). One of the organizational challenges in this complex 'de facto mental health system' (Regier *et al.* 1978) is to ensure that those services and agencies are appropriately coordinated. Without effective coordination there will probably be wasteful overlaps and, more commonly, yawning gaps in the spectrum of support. Even in the best health systems there are people who 'fall through the net'.

Consequently, 'mental health services', as *narrowly* defined and as conventionally viewed, actually sit in the middle of a complex, dynamic multi-service, multi-budget world. When we use a term such as 'mental health system' we therefore need to remember that many resources – indeed, an increasing proportion of resources – are not actually in the health care system as conventionally defined but are provided by social welfare, housing, employment, criminal justice, education and other systems. Countries will differ in their service and agency definitions, responsibilities and arrangements, and consequently in their inter-agency boundaries. One of the biggest challenges in trying to establish effective and cost-effective mental health promotion, community-based care and rehabilitation is managing these organizational and inter-professional interfaces and the various incentives and disincentives that characterize them.

A mixed economy

Multiple provider sectors

Some of the services used by people with mental health problems are provided by or located within the state (public) sector, some by private (commercial) or non-governmental (civil society) entities, and some by families or through informal community arrangements. This multiplicity of sectors and services – what we can call the *mixed economy of provision* – is characteristic of all mental health systems in Europe. Even formal mental health promotion strategies, which tend to be dominated by the state (locally, regionally or nationally), as are other public health initiatives, still need inputs from employers and local communities (the 'social capital' effect). Treatment and rehabilitation services may be dominated by the public sector, both quantitatively and strategically, but non-governmental organizations are often also major providers of day and residential care in some countries. They are certainly key providers of advocacy services through user and family groups. Private businesses may provide residential and some specialist psychiatric care; for example, psychotherapy is widely offered by private practitioners. Patterns of provision vary from country to country. In central and eastern Europe, for instance, the public sector has historically dominated service provision; the absence of civil society structures over the last half century has meant that emerging voluntary sector activities remain weak (see Chapter 17).

Another source of provision, still quite marginal today but growing in importance, has arisen from non-contributory, directly-funded employer programmes. Some companies in Europe are themselves funding, and in some cases also providing, on-site mental health support for their staff and families, recognizing the importance of workforce stability (Gabriel and Liimatainen 2000; Cox *et al.* 2004; Jane-Llopis and Anderson 2005; McDaid *et al.* 2005a).

Underpinning most of these organizational responses, and often substituting for them, are the many and various contributions of family carers and volunteers. Policy frameworks sometimes give the impression that these contributions can be treated as 'free' inputs, but they can clearly impose quite high opportunity costs on families. Evidence shows that they have great value in reducing the demands on formal service providers (see Chapter 16).

Policy-makers need not only to recognize these multifarious contributions, but also to make distinctions between the sectors in which they are located, because providers with different legal forms may behave differently in responding to incentives. For instance, a government-run hospital will have different objectives and constraints from a private hospital run on a profit-seeking basis or a charitable hospital tied to a religious community. This may affect their *modus operandi*, their patterns of resource dependency and chosen styles of governance and management. They are likely to have distinctive motivations, influencing their ability and willingness to respond to changes in market opportunities, pricing regimes and competition (Frank and McGuire 2000). They might therefore also have divergent costs, casemix, quality of care and perhaps even user outcomes (Schlesinger and Dorwart 1984; Knapp *et al.* 1998, 1999). Different provider types may also vary with respect to the routes along which they initiate and cultivate trust and reputation, with implications for the kind of commissioning environment that can be put in place.

There are, then, potentially a number of reasons for anticipating inter-sectoral differences in resource-related behaviour. However, simple or rigid demarcations between sectors are neither possible to establish nor sensible to maintain. In terms of perspective, motivation and behaviour there may be wider differences *within* sectors than between them.

Multiple funding sources

Each element in this mixed economy of provision could have a number of funding sources. In mapping or seeking to understand a mental health system and what it can offer to individuals and families, it is therefore also helpful to distinguish the various routes by which these services are financed or purchased, linked to the forms of revenue collection.

The provision and financing dimensions of a mixed economy are clearly not independent. Their inter-connections can be complex and certainly will vary from country to country. Whereas one health care system may have developed on the basis of tax-based finance or compulsory social insurance, and may deliver its services primarily through the state sector, another might be more reliant on insurance policies chosen by individuals, with services dominated by commercial sector companies and self-employed clinicians. We discuss the main types of mental health service financing in a moment.

The mixed economy matrix

A useful starting point for understanding the resource base of a mental health system and its component services is to chart these mixed economies of provision and financing. Cross-classification of the main funding and provider types generates the matrix representation of Figure 4.2, a simple framework describing just the broad inter-connections that characterize pluralist care systems and their constituent transactions.

What do the cells of the matrix contain? A relatively straightforward task for a given country or region – although not attempted here – would be to locate services (e.g. counselling, inpatient facilities, community nurses, primary

REVENUE COLLECTION (FUNDING)	MODE OR SECTOR OF PROVISION			
	Public/state sector	Voluntary/NGO sector	Private (for-profit) sector	Informal sector
General taxation				
Social insurance				
Voluntary insurance				
Charitable				
Foreign governments				
Out-of-pocket				
No exchange				

Figure 4.2 The mixed economy matrix for mental health

Source: Adapted from Knapp (1984)

care doctors, sheltered work schemes) and their funding arrangements in the appropriate cells of the matrix. More demanding but also more informative would be to record the volumes of provision and their associated expenditure levels. Given the multiplicity of service types often active in supporting people with mental health problems, it would be preferable (but again probably quite a difficult task) if the completed matrix ranged quite widely and was not confined to the (narrow) health care system.

Charting the broad contours of the mixed economy of mental health care would therefore help to identify the range and volume of services offered to and used by people with mental health problems, and the means by which they are funded. Identifying the budget base for a country's mental health system is obviously a necessary starting point for considering any major policy or practice changes. For example, tax revenues that support private providers could be linked through contracts, tax incentives or lump-sum cash subsidies. Each transaction type has accompanying needs for appropriate legislative frameworks to control, audit and monitor the links between funding and provision. Mapping the mixed economy also draws attention to services that need coordination. This could be at a macro level, for example bringing together government or health system decision-makers to ensure that national efforts in pursuit of equity and efficiency are not undermined by contradictory actions by constituent parts of the wider system. Or it could be done at a micro level, through the efforts of case managers or other service 'brokers'. But even without the fine detail, the matrix has the signal virtue of reminding us of the inherent economic complexity of most mental health systems.

Financing mental health

How is mental health care financed? We begin with a brief overview of methods of financing used for health care in general, and then consider whether there are distinctive issues impacting on the funding and delivery of mental health-related services in particular, including those external to the health sector. For a comprehensive guide to the general funding of health care see (Mossialos *et al.* 2002).

Methods of financing health care

Although most countries finance their health care through more than one source, there is usually one dominant approach. European countries rely principally on publicly financed systems, typically through some form of taxation or contribution to social health insurance. Other funding sources, such as voluntary health insurance (often called private health insurance), out-of-pocket payments and international aid, play smaller roles.

Funds for health services may be generated through taxation that is raised at national, regional or local level, either directly (e.g. from income) or indirectly (e.g. from sales). Progressive taxation, such as income tax across most economically developed countries, where those with higher incomes contribute at a higher rate, helps to redistribute resources from the better off in a society to the less well off.

The main alternative to taxation in Europe is social health insurance (SHI), which dominates health care financing in, for example, Austria, Belgium, the Czech Republic, France, Germany, the Netherlands and Romania. Although SHI systems differ there are a number of common features. Contributions are usually linked to salaries, with employers typically also making a contribution. In some countries there may be just one or two sickness funds collecting contributions, while in others the choices may be many and perhaps linked to profession. Transfers from general taxation to sickness funds are made to provide cover for unemployed, retired and other disadvantaged or vulnerable people (Normand and Buse 2002). Premiums are not usually based on risk; but risk-adjustment mechanisms are often used to ensure that no one sickness fund is unduly disadvantaged (or indeed advantaged) from the 'risk mix' of its population.

Enrolment is compulsory in most countries with SHI, although there may be some opportunities to opt out, dependent on income, as in Germany. Thus, the use of additional voluntary health insurance (VHI), offered by for-profit or non-profit companies, and taken up and paid for at the discretion of individuals or their employers, is relatively limited in Europe. VHI usually fulfils one of three principal roles: a substitute for SHI (as in Germany for higher paid workers), a complement to public entitlement (as in France to cover co-payments within the public health system) or a supplement (as in Ireland to reduce the time before receiving treatment and to increase service choice) (Mossialos and Thomson 2002). Unlike social insurance, VHI may be risk-rated, offering lower premiums to low-risk individuals, which could mean that higher risk groups in society (such as those with mental health problems) find it unaffordable, especially as mental health problems are more prevalent among lower income groups (see, for example, Weich and Lewis 1998).

Charges are often levied on a selection of health care services, such as pharmaceuticals, dentistry or primary care consultations. They may be in place to raise revenue, and/or also to discourage excessive or inappropriate utilization. However, user charges can be costly to administer and may deter patients from accessing the care they need. One recent study reported that the introduction of user charges for previously exempt vulnerable groups can lead to a reduction in the use of services (Tamblyn *et al.* 2001). Of course, such a reduction in utilization may be a false economy; in the medium term costs may increase if individuals more frequently present themselves at secondary and emergency care facilities, as Soumerai *et al.* documented in their New Hampshire study (1994).

Other financing arrangements are possible. There may be 'informal' or 'under-the-counter' payments for services that are supposedly fully funded, most commonly seen in central and eastern Europe (Lewis 2002). Funds to invest in health – in central and eastern Europe in particular – might be boosted by bilateral aid programmes, contributions from non-governmental organizations (NGOs) and other international bodies. There are some modest specialist health insurance schemes, for instance hospital cash plans, which pay out predetermined cash benefits when individuals use health care services. Others – quite uncommon – are employer accident insurance schemes, motor vehicle insurance and schemes to protect against loss of earnings.

Trends in mental health financing

So does mental health financing differ from financing for the general health system? And if so, what are its impacts?

Where mental health is financed through the health care sector the methods of financing appear to be consistent with the dominant method of health care financing in each country (Knapp *et al.* 2003; Dixon *et al.* 2006). Tax and social insurance-dominated systems both take account of ability to pay and cover vulnerable and low-income groups. Entitlement to health care services through taxation or social insurance is commonplace in most European countries, and in fact accounts for over 70 per cent of total health spending in most west European states. In contrast, changes to health care financing systems in parts of central and eastern Europe are clearly reducing coverage under either taxation or social insurance, increasing still further the already worryingly high proportion of costs met from out-of-pocket payments and VHI (Dixon *et al.* 2006). For example, only 41 per cent of health care expenditure in Armenia and 38 per cent in Georgia comes from public sources. The consequences for people with mental health problems could be grave if the VHI that might fill some of this public finance gap excludes mental health or sets excessively high premiums.

Even where universal entitlement under tax or SHI predominates, entitlement to mental health services may be limited, and arguably inequitable. In supposedly universal systems there can be significant limitations in covering mental health. For instance, some community care services may be the responsibility of social protection budgets, and – as we will show – there is evidence of an increased shift of services out of the health sector. High co-payment levels for services both within and outside the health sector can inhibit access. We explore the implications below.

VHI and mental health

Despite recent trends in some central and eastern European countries, generally speaking VHI does not yet play a significant role in funding mental health services. Reimbursement through such schemes in most cases is strictly limited, and risk-related premiums are high. Indeed, many enduring mental health problems are explicitly excluded from benefit packages in some countries, due to the chronic nature and high cost of some interventions. In Austria, for instance, although private insurers are prohibited from refusing to insure someone with a chronic illness, they can charge higher premiums or impose cost-sharing for hospital care (see Box 4.1). The limitations of VHI in covering long-term chronic problems have been recognized in the Netherlands where even those individuals who choose to opt out of SHI schemes have had to enrol in an exceptional medical expenses insurance scheme. The scheme has covered some of the costs of treatment beyond the first year for chronic conditions and it is estimated that approximately 85 per cent of the costs of mental health care facilities are paid for from this budget, with a further 11 per cent from taxation (Evers 2004).

Box 4.1 Mental health care financing in Austria

Ingrid Zechmeister

Austria is a federal country with nine provinces and around 8 million inhabitants. The country's federal structure and corporatist traditions have led to a complex pattern of health care financing with mixed public responsibilities, heterogeneous service providers and service components, and diverse funding and reimbursement arrangements. This complexity is even stronger in mental health care as the boundaries between the health and social care sectors are quite vague.

Mental health care includes primary and secondary services, psychotherapy, community services such as psychosocial services, housing and day care, institutional long-term care and employment-related services. Hospital care, GP and specialist psychiatrist care as well as psychotherapy legally belong to the health care sector, whereas social services, including long stay institutions, are part of the social care sector. Most service providers are public or private non-profit providers, but there are some self-employed providers, and to a small extent, private for-profit providers.

Figure 4.3 gives a schematic overview of mental health care financing in Austria, which is primarily based on social health insurance. This system is based on the principle of solidarity, i.e. insurance premiums are independent of individual risk, and access to health care is independent of income. Currently, around 98 per cent of the population is included in this scheme. However, social health insurance funds cover around 50 per cent of total health care expenditure. Taxes account for a further 25 per cent of funding and out-of-pocket payments 24 per cent, including co-payments (e.g. prescription fees), private payments for certain services and private insurance (Badelt and Osterle 2001).

Health care providers are reimbursed in a variety of ways for their services. While a performance-related DRG system is used in the hospital sector, reimbursement of GPs and specialist psychiatrists is based on a combination of flat rates and fee for services, negotiated annually. Finally, psychotherapy services are mostly private, although clients can apply for a partial refund from social health insurance for a limited period.

Financing and reimbursement are organized quite differently in the social care sector. In contrast to health care, financing in social care is primarily based on the principle of subsidiarity, resulting in a mix of private and public funds. For most services, out-of-pocket payments using pensions, long-term care allowances or private equity are the key sources of finance, with the difference financed through taxation. Relatives may also have to make a contribution to the costs of care. Provincial laws mean that there can be great differences between and within provinces (Pfeil 2001). Only a few psychosocial services are entirely publicly financed (e.g., in Lower Austria, mobile and ambulatory psychosocial services and employment-related services such as special assistance, consulting or educational training).

The current financing system causes several difficulties. Firstly, according to the General Social Security Act (*Allgemeines Sozialversicherungsgesetz*), social health insurance schemes cover acute health problems whereas people with long-term (mental) health problems are 'transferred' or allocated to the social care and social assistance sector. This is not only disadvantageous in terms of rehabilitation (due to changes in providers, treatment and often a lack of rehabilitation services) but also because of the different financing patterns.

Secondly, reform documents emphasize the reduction in hospital care in favour of non-institutionalized care in the community. The latter is mostly within the social care sector. Without reform more community mental health care will lead to increased out-of-pocket payments for users and their relatives. Compared to people with somatic illnesses, these contributions are likely to be disproportionately higher for mentally ill people (Zechmeister and Osterle 2004).

Thirdly, some incentives in the current financing system actually create obstacles to reform aims. Extended coverage in the health care sector favours hospital care rather than social care. This runs contrary to shifting the focus to community care and to providing complex person-oriented service arrangements (Zechmeister *et al.* 2002). These conflicting incentives may, and in fact partly do, lead to transinstitutionalization rather than deinstitutionalization.

So far, Austria has not generally brought together the objectives stipulated in its mental health care reform plans and the question of how to finance mental health care. Linking these spheres, however, will be crucial for the future development of mental health care provision and financing. As a first step, it is particularly important to discuss what the different concepts of mental health care (such as individualization, normalization, person-oriented care, needs-based care, customer orientation etc.) exactly require in terms of Austrian financing and reimbursement structures. Current arrangements that are characterized by a fragmentation of responsibilities between public authorities and between service sectors often hinder rather than support new developments in mental health care or innovation in the mix between institutional and community-based services. For an effective allocation of funds it is necessary to overcome the strict division between health and social care. This requires the pooling of funds and a redefinition of public responsibilities.

However, there is evidence of growth of niche areas where private insurance is one way of generating additional funding for mental health. For example, in both the United Kingdom and Germany, VHI provides some coverage for addiction programmes (Dixon 2002). Accident and unemployment insurance schemes funded privately by individuals or employers may provide benefits in

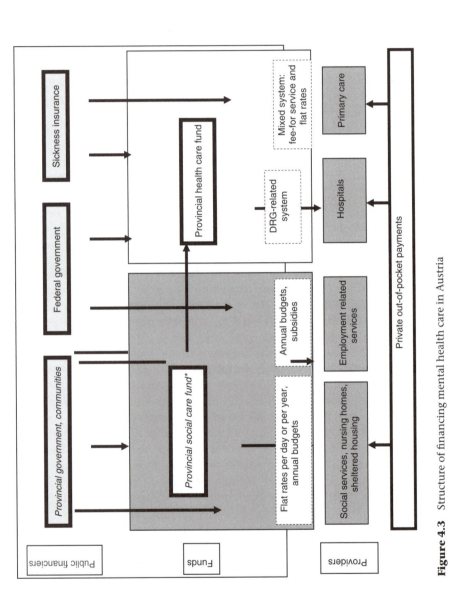

Figure 4.3   Structure of financing mental health care in Austria

Source: Adapted from Zechmeister *et al.* (2002)
* Does not exist in every Austrian province.

kind, cover for critical illness or long-term care, and some of the costs of vocational rehabilitation; for instance, this kind of funding is available in Ireland to get individuals back into work when they are suffering from stress-related health problems. One insurance company in the United Kingdom has reported around 1000 new claims for income protection per year, of which 300 (particularly from teachers) are related to stress or mental illness. This number has been increasing over recent years (Aviva Plc 2005).

In summary, while the role of voluntary health insurance in the mental health area currently remains modest, it cannot be ignored. This is not just because of the growth of specialist coverage in areas such as addiction treatment, work-related stress and rehabilitation – areas where publicly funded coverage may have been modest – it is also because, as publicly financed mental health services are increasingly being delivered by providers from outside the state, opportunities open up for additional private sector financing. The challenge is to protect coverage for mental health problems. Experience from the United States, where the VHI market is most developed, illustrates the difficulty that mental health has in achieving parity with physical health, despite recent significant political pressure. This has allowed a situation to develop where insurance plans provide strictly limited coverage for mental health, with much of the burden falling on (the often under-funded) state mental health systems. Given the significant stigma associated with mental illness and – compared to America – rather weak civil society structures in some parts of central and eastern Europe, there may not be sufficient political and public pressure to safeguard mental health. This is in spite of the welcome Declaration at Helsinki in January 2005 affirming the responsibility of national governments to ensure that there are 'sufficient resources for mental health, considering the burden of disease, and to make investment in mental health an identifiable part of overall health expenditure, in order to achieve parity with investments in other areas of health' (World Health Organization 2005b: 5).

Out-of-pocket payments

User charges are significant in some parts of Europe. In Portugal, for instance, they account for approximately a third of all health costs. Given the strong correlation between mental health problems, unemployment and deprivation, user charges for mental health services could prove to be highly inequitable: those needing services will often be the least able to pay. Even without financial barriers to access, as many as two-thirds of individuals with mental health problems with capacity to benefit do not come into contact with formal services, often because of stigma. The often poor rate of diagnosis of mental health problems in primary care is certainly not going to improve if access is discouraged by user charges. Moreover, people with mental health problems have poorer physical health than the general population, further exacerbating the disincentive effects of out-of-pocket payments.

User payments are not restricted to the health sector; indeed they can be quite high in social care and other sectors, and certainly entitlement to services may be subject to very different rules (see below). The Mental Health Economics

European Network (MHEEN) reported that 8 out of 17 west European countries levied some out-of-pocket charges for specialist mental health services within their publicly funded health systems (Knapp *et al.* 2006b). In Ireland, for instance, while the bottom third of the population are exempt from charges, the remainder of the population will pay a variable fee for primary care consultations and indeed pay a hotel charge towards the costs of inpatient stays. Access to mental health services under private health insurance is limited so there may also be out-of-pocket payments for behavioural and occupational therapy (O'Shea and NiLeime 2004). In Iceland, individuals must make co-payments for most services, although there are reductions for those who are registered as having a disability (Tomasson 2004), while in Belgium there are fixed fees for specialist mental health services, but these are reimbursable under the social health insurance scheme (Dierckx 2004). Out-of-pocket payments have been introduced for psychiatric services in Poland as one consequence of economic transition (Zaluska *et al.* 2005). We return later in the chapter to the issue of low utilization of services when discussing equity.

Donor aid for mental health

Donor aid can be an important source of health system funding in countries undergoing economic transition or recovering from conflict. The proportion of donor aid allocated to mental health is not known for most countries, but there is little evidence to indicate that mental health has been much of a priority, despite its major contribution to the overall disease burden.

Even where funding has been made available for mental health, there can be problems in the way that these funds are used. In Bosnia and Herzegovina, all the major international aid organizations, as well as over 50 NGOs, were working directly or indirectly on mental health issues. While there were a number of positive aspects to this aid, such as placing mental health on the health reform agenda and providing technical support and training to local professionals, some negative consequences have also been highlighted (Funk 2005). Because most funding for reform came from abroad, the proposed changes were resisted either actively or passively by local agencies. In any case, some of the projects were inappropriate for local population needs. This lack of consideration of local circumstances, together with fragmentation and lack of coordination between donors, often meant that the sustainability of mental health reforms was not considered. No realistic national plan for mental health reform was developed. Ideally governments would take an interest in the funding priorities of external donors, and work in partnership to ensure that funds are allocated in ways that are consistent with the immediate and longer-term aims of national mental health policy.

Movement out of the health sector

We have already noted how many services used by people with mental health problems are both funded and delivered *outside* the health sector. As the emphasis on community care has gathered pace, there has also usually been an accompanying shift of services and responsibilities from health care to social care bodies. This has potentially marked implications for both entitlement and access. In contrast to the universality and solidarity found in health care systems, access to social care may be restricted, subject to means testing, perhaps subject also to a disability threshold, and sometimes requiring significant co-payments. In Austria, as summarized in Box 4.1, social health insurance excludes most mental health disorders on the grounds that they are chronic rather than curable, and as much as a third of social care expenditure for mental health is realized through private out-of-pocket payments (Zechmeister *et al.* 2002).

Similarly, in Germany only the medical aspects of psychosocial care are covered under health insurance. Long-term care needs for people with chronic mental health problems are classed as social rehabilitation or social reintegration and are the responsibility instead of social welfare agencies, which are tax-financed and operate means-testing to decide what payments must be made by service users or their families. The Exceptional Medical Expenses Act in the Netherlands (now being phased out) required patients to make a contribution to inpatient care, psychotherapy and sheltered accommodation once they move beyond one year of treatment. In 2003 individuals in long-stay facilities could incur charges of up to €1600 per month, while outpatient psychotherapy involved a co-payment of around €10 per session (Evers 2004). In Russia, individuals living in social care homes (*internats*) lose most (if not all) of any disability pension to which they are entitled (McDaid *et al.* 2006).

Access to supported housing – widely recognized as a key component of any attempt to provide more community-oriented care – and to long-term care may be subject to assessment of financial means. Service users may even be expected to contribute most of their income, as well as use up any capital, savings and other assets before – as a last resort – they become eligible for public assistance. Within the 15 countries of the pre-expansion European Union (EU), only Sweden appeared to fund all social care services *fully* through taxation subject to assessment of need but regardless of income.

Mental health budgets

Regardless of the mechanism used to collect funding in the mixed economy, the scope for resource provision is clearly constrained by the underlying budget allocations to mental health care. Of course, given the inherent multiplicity of services and agencies, decision-makers would need to understand constraints in a number of budgets (health care, social care, housing, etc.) if they are to view the full picture. They should also explore the scope for addressing a budget constraint or funding shortfall in one service or sector by more generous funding in another.

Headline figures

The percentage of gross domestic product (GDP) spent on health care is widely deployed as a marker of a country's commitment to the promotion of health and health-related quality of life. That percentage varies widely across Europe, although it is hard to make valid inter-country comparisons because of differences in the definition of health systems and their expenditures. Notwithstanding these difficulties, it is clear that west European countries have tended to devote higher proportions of national product to health care than most countries in eastern Europe. According to data collected by the World Health Organization (WHO), the range among the countries of the WHO European region is from less than 1 per cent of GDP in Azerbaijan and Tajikistan to 11.2 per cent in Switzerland and 10.9 per cent in Germany (World Health Organization 2005a).

There is apparently greater variation across Europe in the percentage of the health budget spent on *mental* health care, but also much greater uncertainty about whether the boundaries are drawn consistently around 'mental health' from one country to another to place much credence on such figures. Social care, supported housing and secure provision could all variously be included or excluded from calculated mental health proportions. One recent study conservatively estimated that the percentage of the health care budget devoted to mental health in the Czech Republic was 3.5 per cent (Dlouhy 2004), while the proportion in England has hovered between 11 per cent and 13 per cent for the last ten or more years. But, while it is undoubtedly the case that the health system in England has given greater priority to mental health than is the case in the Czech Republic, the *precise* difference is difficult to calculate and probably not accurately reflected in these statistics. From the work of the Mental Health Economics European Network, the percentage of the health budget devoted to mental health in 17 western countries appeared to vary between 4 per cent in Portugal to 13 per cent in England and Luxembourg (Knapp *et al.* 2006b). Data from the WHO *Atlas* suggests, however, that eastern European countries spent higher/lower proportions of their health budgets on mental health. The range, as revealed by those WHO data, is from 1.6 per cent in Azerbaijan and 2.3 per cent in Portugal to 13.4 per cent in Luxembourg and 11 per cent in Sweden (World Health Organization 2005a), but it is understandably difficult to know how much confidence we can have in these differences given that standard definitions were not employed across countries.

Breadth of impact

The EPSILON multi-country study of people with schizophrenia demonstrated how service systems and availability varied greatly between study sites using the European Service Mapping Schedule (ESMS) (Becker *et al.* 2002), and that use of, for example, inpatient care is closely related to supply. A higher proportion of inpatient care was used in the research site in Denmark compared to England and Italy, Spain and the Netherlands, but more beds were available for use. In contrast, the research site in Spain had many fewer inpatient beds and the overall budgetary contribution of inpatient care was therefore lower (Knapp *et al.* 2002). Similarly the ERGOS multi-country study of services used by people with schizophrenia, employing a different data collection approach, also found distinct differences in patterns of treatments across centres, with for instance, family therapy rarely used in French, Portuguese or Dutch centres but frequently provided in the Italian and Spanish sites. Differences were found within as well as across countries and among sites with similar levels of resources. In this study home visits were commonly suggested in the Irish and Portuguese sites but there were differences in use across the French centres in the study (Kovess *et al.* 2005).

What these and many other studies demonstrate is the breadth of economic impact. Evidence from some English studies provides illustrations. Thomas and Morris (2003) calculated the broad costs for depression, finding that the impact on employment (and hence on national productivity), expressed in cost terms, was 23 times larger than the costs falling to the health service. This is an enormous 'hidden' impact. Sizeable 'hidden' costs are not unique to depression. In a study of children with persistent antisocial behaviour in London, only 5 per cent of the total cost was carried by the health service, the remainder falling to schools (special educational needs), social care agencies, community voluntary organizations, families (disrupted parental employment, household damage) and the welfare system (disability and similar transfer payments) (Romeo *et al.* 2006). Another study found that adults, who as children had a conduct disorder, generated costs for a range of agencies that were significantly higher than the costs for a non-morbid control group; most noticeable were the criminal justice system costs, which were 18 times greater (Scott *et al.* 2001). Crime costs are another important consideration when looking at the social impact of addictions. A few years ago, for every GBP£1 of health service expenditure spent on people referred for addiction treatment, it was calculated that another GBP£3 is incurred by the criminal justice system and GBP£10 by the victims of crimes (Healey *et al.* 1998). In old age, mental health problems can often lead to expensive admissions to nursing homes, but a big impact is often felt in the family. Although it is difficult to put a figure on the opportunity costs of informal care, there is no doubt that they are high and often overlooked in policy and practice discussions (McDaid 2001). Overall, therefore, it is clear that the lion's share of the broad social costs of mental illness will often fall outside the health sector.

Silo budgeting

As countries come to rely less on psychiatric inpatient facilities and more on community-based options, the balance of expenditure ought to shift away from health care (as conventionally and narrowly defined) to other areas (especially social welfare and housing). Similarly, as a country's overall commitment to mental health grows – and with it the better recognition of the diversity and multiplicity of individual needs – so again we might expect the balance between health and non-health expenditures to alter. In order to effect change there might therefore be a need to shift funds from one budget to another. But professional rivalry, myopic budget protection, performance assessment regimes or simple stultifying bureaucracy could mean that one agency is unwilling or unable to spend more of their own resources in order for another agency or service to achieve savings or for the broader system overall to achieve effectiveness or cost-effectiveness improvements.

A fair share of the pie?

A pervasive policy challenge across most of Europe and across many decades has been to try to ensure that mental health services and interventions receive a fair share of available health funding. It is obviously difficult and indeed contentious to try to define 'fairness' in this context, but the historically low level of funding for mental health in many European countries is surely both inefficient and inequitable. The assertion of insufficiency follows from the observation of substantial hidden morbidity – often because of stigma and shame – and because of the substantial health and quality of life benefits that wider availability of evidence-based interventions would bring. The argument that present mental health funding levels are inequitable has similar roots: morbidity is not well recognized by many health systems, and it is unevenly distributed across the population. Mental health problems account for nearly 20 per cent of the total disease burden in Europe and are disproportionately experienced by people in lower socioeconomic and other disadvantaged groups. Even in countries such as Norway, with its strong long-term national commitment to mental health system development, there can be threats to sustainability and consistency – in this case because most resource allocation decisions are taken at regional or local level (see Box 4.2).

Box 4.2   Financing mental health services – the case of Norway

Vidar Halsteinli

Norway has a predominantly tax-financed health care system, with only a modest role for out-of-pocket payments. Mental health services are the responsibility of five regional health authorities (RHAs), which provide specialized hospital and community services, and local municipalities which deliver a range of relevant primary health and social care services, including GP care, nursing care and housing. RHAs are funded through grants from central government while municipalities are funded by both central government grants and local taxes. Local decisions and priorities on the way resources are allocated to mental health, other health sector and other public sector interventions may mean that resources intended by central government to be used for mental health can, in fact, be used for other purposes, leading to much debate.

For instance, there has been widespread concern that general government grants to municipalities may mean that a lower share of resources than intended is made available for mental health. One reason for this is that other local areas of concern, such as education, may be supported by strong pressure groups that influence local political decision-making, while mental health service users are less successful in lobbying for improved local services.

One solution has been the introduction of earmarked grants for mental health services, theoretically preventing funds from being used for different purposes. However, this does not entirely solve the problem as mental health services delivered at the municipality level are integrated with other services, making it difficult in practice to ensure that earmarked grants are, in fact, spent on specified mental health plans.

A second challenge in Norway concerns the way in which general hospitals run by RHAs are financed. These are partly financed through a cost-per-case reimbursement basis from central government for somatic health conditions using a system of DRGs. These conditions accounted for 60 per cent of average costs in 2003. A block grant is used to fund other specialist services including mental health. The per case reimbursement system, however, provides strong incentives to increase activity (which has been a major objective so as to reduce waiting lists). The fear among mental health service professionals (and central government staff) is that these incentives have led to a reallocation of budgets and resources away from mental health services to somatic care. The impact of the DRG system has not been empirically documented (Halsteinli *et al.* 2001) but despite the existence a national plan calling for a major increase in the level of resources for mental health services, the annual growth rate has been higher for somatic care since the late 1990s (Bjoerngaard 2002).

Again, as a second-best solution RHAs also receive earmarked grants to increase both the level and quality of mental health services. Unlike the situation in the municipalities, central government has less of a problem in controlling the use of these earmarked grants as they have for specialized, and to a large extent, separate services. Major changes to the way RHAs fund services have been discussed at the national level. One suggestion has been to use the same funding mechanism for both somatic and psychiatric care (Ministry of Health 2003). This would initiate a process that will make activity-based reimbursement of psychiatric services possible in future.

The dominance of institutions

The large, now generally maligned, psychiatric asylums have dominated the European landscape for many decades, both literally and metaphorically. They have certainly dominated mental health finances. Consequently, a major budgetary challenge in many countries has been how to fund the move away from continued heavy reliance on institutional care, whether in psychiatric hospitals or indeed in the very institutional forms of social care found in some parts of central and eastern Europe. It is still the case in some countries today that the lion's share of expenditure on mental health is taken up by institutional care: for instance, around 70 per cent of the mental health budget in Lithuania is used to maintain social care homes and psychiatric inpatient facilities (Bankauskaite and Middtun 2005).

Unfortunately, many countries in central and eastern Europe still link funding for services directly to bed occupancy rates, allowing little flexibility and certainly little incentive to develop community-based alternatives. Worse still are perverse incentives such as that created by the Russian policy of financing psychiatric hospitals with more than 1000 occupied beds more generously than smaller hospitals (McDaid *et al.* 2006).

Deinstitutionalization has been national policy in many countries for some years, as well as an international emphasis through efforts and guidance of bodies such as the European Commission and the World Health Organization (see Chapter 18). Community-based arrangements tend to be preferred to hospital-dominated approaches on the grounds of human rights, relative effectiveness, social inclusion and the expressed preferences of service users. Whether it is more cost-effective is less clear. In principle, as beds, wards and eventually whole hospitals close, so resources should be released to help the development of community-based services. But implementing an appropriate resource-release process is fraught with difficulty. Investments in psychiatric or social care institutions are often effectively 'sunk costs' in the sense that they have little value in any alternative use. Even if the closure of an institution might eventually release resources that could support other mental health service developments, the management of facility closure takes time and will need extra short-term resources. There could be both *hump costs* – initial investment in the new facilities to get them underway and in training staff in new ways of working – and *double running costs* – to resource both the old and the new services in parallel for a few years until one has been closed down and the other has been built up. (Quite probably, average costs will look high in one or both settings because of the diseconomies of operating below optimal scale.) Smaller in size but similar in their incidence and effects are the sunk costs and 'lumpiness' of *human* capital. An institution may be the major employer in an isolated community, in which case its closure will have huge repercussions for the local economy. More generally, there is the question of the extent to which employees can be retrained to work within a more community-oriented system and, if not, what support should be provided during their own 'economic transition'.

The *rate* of funding transfer is another challenge. In some instances hospitals have been closed by moving the most able residents out first: these are the people whose skills, abilities and behavioural characteristics are best suited for a new and more independent life in the community. But these people cost much less than the average hospital inpatient – they have fewer needs and need less staff support – in which case transferring an average amount from the hospital budget to community services risks stripping the hospital of resources (Knapp 1990). In complete contrast, the economic climate in some countries has created an incentive to discharge the *most* costly individuals first, without transferring any or sufficient funds to community-based care. More able residents – who also tend to be less costly because they need less staff supervision – may be kept in institutions in order to provide a supply of unpaid or very low-paid workers.

Deinstitutionalization raises another potential resource difficulty. There is a danger that funds released by hospital closures are not transferred to community-based mental health services: 'leakage' of funds from psychiatric hospital budgets into other parts of the health care system and to non-psychiatric specialties seems common. For instance, Hungary has seen a 50 per cent decline in the number of beds in mental hospitals with apparently little development of community services (Harangozò and Kristòf 2000). Ring-fencing funds for mental health has some disadvantages, as we discuss later, but during the deinstitutionalization process this may be essential for the success of an embryonic community-dominated care system, particularly in the face of local resistance to the 'release' of what may be seen as 'dangerous' individuals (see Chapter 3).

Resource targeting

Because there are not enough resources to meet population needs, choices must be made about how to use available resources – whether, for example, to provide a hospital-based or a community-based service, whether to use one particular drug rather than another, or whether to offer treatment to people with mild depression or to focus available services on people with schizophrenia or Alzheimer's disease. Local decision-makers need information to help them make these choices. In a world that is increasingly embracing evidence-based approaches to policy and practice, a number of resource-related criteria are likely to be invoked to structure or guide decisions. Such criteria might include maximizing the therapeutic impact from a set of resources, getting more people with mental health problems back to work, broadening access to effective care, improving fairness in relation to payment for treatment or its utilization, and improving targeting of services on needs. We can group these resource-related criteria under two heads: efficiency and equity.

Efficiency

In its simplest incarnation, efficiency means achieving the maximum effects in terms of services delivered or outcomes achieved (such as symptom alleviation or quality of life improvement) from a given volume of resource inputs (or a given budget). This concept of productive or technical efficiency links us back to the *production of welfare framework* set out earlier in the chapter. It is also helpful to distinguish *target efficiency* (Bebbington and Davies 1983): the degree to which available services are delivered to people who need them, and the ability of the system to ensure that people in need get the available services. A third and more macro concept is *allocative efficiency*: the extent to which an economy delivers the goods and services that people want.

Many factors might prevent a mental health system from being fully efficient. It may be that too many resources are used up in the administration of the system itself: that is, the so-called *transaction costs* are too high. For example, it may be argued that there are too many bureaucrats deciding how to allocate resources, or too many people monitoring the quality of services, or too many managers overseeing the professional staff who actually deliver care and treatment. Another source of inefficiency may be that resources are used in inappropriate combinations: a highly qualified psychiatrist is likely to be more effective, for example, if he or she has access to a suitable range of psychological and pharmacological therapies and is based in a multidisciplinary team. Poor target efficiency is inevitable if efforts are not made to identify and prioritize needs and to encourage people to come forward for treatment. Another reason for inefficiency could simply be that little is known about the relationship between resources expended and outcomes achieved. This is where cost-effectiveness analyses can contribute.

Cost-effectiveness evidence

Although our primary concern when looking at a new policy or intervention should be to ask whether it is effective in terms of symptom alleviation and quality of life enhancement, we clearly also need to know what it would cost to implement. If two options are equally effective, which of them uses the fewer resources? Or if they cost the same amount, which is the more effective? Or if one of them is simultaneously more effective and more costly, does society consider that it is worth paying the additional amount in order to achieve those better outcomes?

These are the questions which cost-effectiveness analysis was designed to address. Such analyses look at both outcomes and costs for two or more promotion strategies, treatments, service arrangements or policies. In the terms of the production of welfare framework, they compare the two ends of the chain in Figure 4.1 that links what gets spent to what gets achieved.

Given what we have discussed already in this chapter, it is obviously important that any evaluation in the mental health field should be measuring both costs and outcomes quite broadly:

- Have all the relevant costs been taken into account? As we have seen, there are many and various inputs to a mental health system – from health, social care, housing, social security and other agencies – plus economic impacts in terms of lost productivity, premature mortality and family 'burden'. It might be necessary to measure all of these, depending on the policy or practice question that needs to be addressed.
- Are all the dimensions of effectiveness taken into account? Good mental health care is not just about tackling clinical symptoms, but also about improving an individual's ability to function in ways that are valued by them (such as getting back to work) and of course about promoting quality of life.

What do we know?

Had there been a version of this book published 30 years ago, it would have taken very little time or space to summarize what was known about the cost-effectiveness of mental health treatments, interventions or policies because at that time there was virtually no evidence at all. Nowadays, robust evidence is accumulating at an encouraging rate, although not evenly across countries or diagnostic areas.

Most studies have been undertaken in North America, some parts of western

Europe or Australia. This geographical unevenness is relevant because the results of economic evaluations may not transfer readily from one country to another because of differences in health systems, financing arrangements, incentive structures and relative price levels. There might also be differences in the choice of comparator: a service model might look an attractive option compared to standard arrangements in one country but not in comparison to the norm elsewhere. It is infeasible and indeed unnecessary to carry out an evaluation every time a policy decision needs to be taken, but evidence-based decisions should generally be better than evidence-free decisions. This could mean using the results from a study carried out in another country, or updating a previous study, or carrying out a modest adaptation to adjust for context.

There is also an imbalance in the topic coverage of the economic evidence base: with more on pharmaceutical treatments than on psychotherapies, little on service organization and almost nothing on mental health promotion (Knapp *et al.* 2004). For example, one recent review of interventions to tackle depression identified 58 studies, half of which were evaluations of drug therapies, with only two on promotion or screening (Barrett *et al.* 2005). Many of these studies – certainly most of the better studies – had been completed quite recently. Enhanced primary care management of depression pushes up health care costs but leads to larger savings in productivity losses by reducing absenteeism (Rost *et al.* 2004). Some recent studies have begun to look at combination treatments, multi-professional interventions and collaborative care models, many of which look relatively cost-effective (Simon *et al.* 2001; Neumeyer-Gromen *et al.* 2004; Pirraglia *et al.* 2004). There are also attempts to pool evidence from across different treatment options by looking more broadly at cost-effective intervention strategies and their impact on morbidity (Andrews *et al.* 2004; Chisholm *et al.* 2004, 2005).

As we noted earlier, the volume of cost-effectiveness evidence has grown noticeably in the past couple of decades. We are not going to attempt to review or summarize that evidence, but some general comments are pertinent. There have tended to be more cost-effectiveness studies in diagnostic areas where new classes of medication have been launched. A lot of depression studies followed the licensing of the early Selective Serotonin Reuptake Inhibitors (SSRIs) and later antidepressants with other mechanisms of action. Similarly, the arrival of the atypical antipsychotics and the cholinesterase inhibitors stimulated a lot of economic research on, respectively, the treatment of schizophrenia (Basu 2004) and Alzheimer's disease (Jonsson 2004). In each of these diagnostic areas today's evidence base is dominated by drug trials, most of them industry-sponsored. Not all of the research is of an adequate standard, and arguments abound as to the validity of industry-sponsored trials. The National Institute for Health and Clinical Excellence for England and Wales (NICE) somewhat controversially considered the new drug treatments for Alzheimer's disease to be effective but not cost-effective (Loveman *et al.* 2004). Diagnostic areas with relatively less recent psychopharmacological developments appear to have attracted fewer cost-effectiveness analyses. For instance, there have been very few evaluations of interventions for child and adolescent mental health problems (Romeo *et al.* 2005), bi-polar disorder (Knapp *et al.* 2004), most anxiety disorders (Andlin-Sobocki and Wittchen 2005) or personality disorders.

Service evaluations tend to cut across the various diagnostic groups. Economic evidence has usefully contributed to the debate on community versus institutional care. While again evidence is limited to a few countries, it suggests that community-based services do not necessarily reduce overall service-related costs, but could redistribute them between budgets and agencies, however, – importantly – quality of care, quality of life and patient satisfaction with services are usually improved. There is also evidence that quality of care is closely related to expenditure on services. One long-term study looked at the costs of moving from hospital to community-based care in London, finding that the community programme was more cost-effective in the short to medium term (Knapp *et al.* 1995), while an even longer study found continuing economic and quality of life advantages over a 12-year period (Beecham *et al.* 2004). Research in Germany found that the one-year costs for those living in the community with schizophrenia were more than 40 per cent lower than for those in long-term care, but emphasized that this was dependent on the characteristics of the study population (Salize and Rossler 1996).

A number of specific community care interventions have been evaluated, examining different ways in which services can be organized to support people. For example, reviews of economic evidence on assertive community treatment (or assertive outreach) teams or approaches suggest that these do not have a systematic impact on the overall costs of care, but are associated with improved service user quality of life and satisfaction outcomes, implying that they can be cost-effective. Evidence on the cost-effectiveness of home treatment more broadly appears still to be inconclusive (Burns *et al.* 2001). Acute day hospitals that provide intensive psychiatric care without the high overheads and restrictions on liberty may be a cost-effective alternative to inpatient care when demand for inpatient beds is high (Marshall *et al.* 2001).

As we emphasized earlier, the economic consequences of poor mental health are wide-ranging and often the costs associated with work-related difficulties considerably outweigh the costs of delivering health services. Naturally, therefore, policy-makers are keen to find ways to increase economic activity (employment) rates and to decrease absenteeism and so-called 'presenteeism' (reduced productivity when actually at work because of the impact of mental health symptoms). Some North American studies have suggested that programmes providing treatment for depression and support to return to work are fully offset by savings made in the reduction of lost workdays (Rizzo *et al.* 1996; Dewa *et al.* 2003; Rost *et al.* 2004). Economic benefits may be realized by investing in effective workplace mental health promotion strategies. One employee assistance programme run by the McDonnell-Douglas company in the US reduced work loss days by 25 per cent and turnover by 8 per cent of people with mental health problems (Alexander 1990).

Equity

How are the benefits and burdens of a health care system distributed across the population? Society may be willing to sacrifice some efficiency gains in order to allocate more resources to vulnerable or disadvantaged populations. This is the familiar efficiency-equity trade-off. However, equity can be defined in many, sometimes contradictory, ways, including in relation to how services are funded, how they are accessed and what outcomes they achieve (Oliver 2001). For example, one important issue is whether individual contributions to a health insurance system (or through taxes) are linked to ability to pay, indeed whether there may be a redistributive effect, so that those with higher incomes contribute at a proportionately higher rate. We have touched on this question already and discuss it no further here. Similarly, we shall say no more about equity in final health outcomes, primarily because there is so little evidence and because health care is just one of a number of things that exert an impact: outcomes are influenced by many factors over and above mental health services and therapies, including income and its distribution, education, nutrition, housing and lifestyle. Consequently, equity in access – such as equal access to mental health for equal need – is perhaps a more appropriate focus when looking at mental health services alone. One argument is that access or utilization should not be influenced by 'extraneous' factors, such as ability to pay for the service, or geographical location.

It is clear that rates of service utilization by people with mental health problems remain low. For instance, in the Netherlands more than 40 per cent of people with bi-polar disorder are estimated not to come into contact with mental health services (ten Have *et al.* 2002). The ESEMED study, covering six European countries (Belgium, France, Germany, Italy, the Netherlands and Spain), concluded that there was insufficient use of both general and specialist mental health services relative to the prevalence of mental health problems in the population, with only one in four people in need coming into contact with services, although contact rates were higher for some problems such as mood disorders. The lowest rates of service use were found in Italy and Belgium (Alonso *et al.* 2004b). This study also formed part of the WHO Mental Health Survey Consortium which found that up to 85 per cent of people with serious mental disorders across all regions of the globe did not receive treatment in the previous 12 months (World Mental Health Survey Consortium 2004).

Why do individuals with mental health needs not utilize services? An important reason is because of the stigma widely associated with mental illness, which will sometimes – for example, in periods of crisis – be compounded by an impaired ability to make informed choices on whether or not to seek and receive treatment. Utilization of mental health services can also be complicated by involuntary detention and treatment in some settings, which may or may not be justified in terms of protecting the individual against self-harm and/or society against potential risk. Many factors contribute to inequality and numerous solutions have been propounded (McDaid *et al.* 2005b). For example, various safeguards may be required for the protection of human rights, influencing the consumption of services (see Chapter 13), and actions needed to improve public awareness and reduce stigma and discrimination.

Therefore, if one of the goals in a country is to ensure that there is an equal opportunity for all to access services on the basis of need, the methods used to distribute resources will be critical. The MHEEN group looked at resource allocation methods for mental health funding in 17 west European countries (Knapp *et al.* 2006b). With a few notable exceptions, where local budgets are provided, these were determined by reference to historical precedent or political judgement rather than on the basis of an objective measure of population health needs. The methods used are unlikely to target resources on areas where they have the greatest chance of being effective and may also allow inequities to persist, for instance if resources continue to be concentrated in major cities, neglecting rural areas within a country. Stigma could mean that mental health does not receive a fair share of the budget, and there may also be prejudice against funding non-institutional programmes.

Methods of resource allocation can be even more complex in countries dominated by social health insurance systems. Some funding, for example for public health and health promotion services, will be provided through taxation, but the majority of funding may be in the form of direct reimbursements from sickness funds to service providers. The MHEEN group reported an increasing use of diagnosis-related group (DRG) tariffs to reimburse service providers for mental health-related services in both social insurance and tax-dominated countries of western Europe. The use of such DRGs in some countries has led to underfunding for mental health, as reimbursement rates have not always fully taken into account all of the costs associated with chronic mental health problems.

Resource challenges

Reflecting on the frameworks, structures and evidence described in this chapter it is clear that there are a number of resource challenges facing mental health systems in Europe, as indeed there are globally (Knapp *et al.* 2006a).

Resource barriers

One of the most common of the challenges to be addressed across Europe is *resource insufficiency*: not enough financial resources are made available for mental health. This is clearly a major issue for countries where the percentage of GDP devoted to health care is low, or where the percentage going to mental health is limited. If few funds are allocated to mental health there is clearly limited scope for building an effective, accessible system of services. But regardless of a country's GDP, attitudes can put up a powerful barrier to the allocation of resources to mental health. A population survey in Germany found that the public were far less willing to safeguard spending on mental health compared with other health conditions (Matschinger and Angemeyer 2004). Only 10 per cent and 7 per cent of respondents placed schizophrenia and depression, respectively, within their top three areas where budgets would be protected, compared with 89 per cent prioritizing cancer, 51 per cent HIV/AIDS and 49 per cent cardiovascular disease. The low priority accorded mental health was attributed in part to ignorance that conditions could be treated, a belief that they were self-inflicted and an underestimation of individual susceptibility to mental illness. The public may also have prioritized immediate life-threatening conditions over other health concerns.

Current shortages of skilled staff in many countries, and the future likelihood of further short- or long-term difficulties in recruiting appropriate personnel, represent the reality of such resource insufficiency as experienced by people with mental health problems. Such shortages must surely energize both new training initiatives and the search for alternatives to face-to-face treatment modalities. Is it possible to develop effective self-administered, manualized or computer-based psychotherapies that can reduce the demands on clinical psychologists, psychiatric nurses and psychiatrists and can be delivered cost-effectively? Will there be developments in pharmacological treatments that will alleviate symptoms, reduce rates of relapse and improve quality of life, without unacceptable side-effects? And will they be affordable across the world? Will there be genetic or other breakthroughs that could revolutionize preventive strategies as well as symptom alleviation?

An issue less often focused on when thinking of the mental health system is workforce capacity within the primary care sector. National mental health plans and strategies increasingly recognize the importance of primary care, but is capacity sufficient? In addition to looking at the function and need for specialist personnel working in the primary care setting, another staffing issue involves knowledge and skills. To what extent do primary care staff have sufficient training to recognize mental health problems and to interact effectively with other agencies? Chapter 9 discusses a number of primary care training strategies. There are, of course, training needs for individuals working in other front-line areas such as social care, schools and prisons.

Available services are often poorly distributed, being available in the wrong place and at the wrong time relative to population needs and preferences. They may be concentrated in large cities or available only to certain groups of the population (usually those with higher incomes), or – as we noted earlier – tied up in large, old asylums. This *resource distribution challenge* is not at all easy to resolve, as it is often related to the very fundamental precepts of a health system or society. The difficulties encountered in trying to redistribute resources away from the large hospitals illustrate the embeddedness of many resources. Of course, it is inevitable and proper that countries will exhibit marked differences in their patterns of service provision. Many examples could be given:

- Italy famously passed legislation to close its psychiatric hospitals, and the Italian health system today relies much less on inpatient care than, say, Germany's or Belgium's.
- The Netherlands and Finland have invested heavily in psychiatric social work whereas Denmark has given proportionately much greater emphasis to clinical psychology.
- Patterns of medication use reflect different licensing and reimbursement arrangements (see Chapter 7) as well as local cultures of prescribing, professional education, marketing and research. For example, France has a threefold greater rate of psychotropic utilization than the Netherlands (Alonso *et al.* 2004a).
- The family is generally seen to be a more important source of support to people with mental health problems in Mediterranean societies than in northern Europe (see Chapter 16).
- The position and role of primary care is also rather different from one health

system to another, with clear implications for the ways that common mental disorders get recognized and treated (see Chapter 9).

The distributional barrier is therefore going to vary from country to country in its nature and impact.

What none of the data already presented describe is the distribution of services *within* a country. For example, Bulgaria's national mental health programme, launched in 2001, stated very clearly that a problem with its then existing mental health care system was a very uneven distribution of hospital beds. As in some other countries, there were also problems of inpatient psychiatric beds being used as a substitute for nursing home beds. This may be due to lack of nursing home resources, or poor care management of the individual patient. As part of its mental health programme:

> psychiatric beds [should] come closer to the patient's place of residence, each catchment area of 150,000 people will have inpatient, outpatient and rehabilitative services, and the average number of beds per catchment will be between 50 and 75. A reduction in hospital beds is to take place in parallel with the introduction of specific units, offering psychiatric rehabilitation in the community.
>
> (Government of Bulgaria 2000; Tomov *et al.* 2004)

In Spain, there are enormous differences between the autonomous regions (Haro *et al.* 1998). In England, local variations in both health and social care spending on mental health services appear to be associated only in part with variations in need and input prices (Bindman *et al.* 2000; Moscone and Knapp 2005).

The need to consider patterns of resource provision within countries may thus be more important to the development of mental health policy across Europe than simple national comparisons, helping to identify appropriate differences in service mix between localities. A recent comparison between nine Italian and four Spanish areas, geographically dispersed across the two countries, demonstrated that there was great variation in the use of beds – for example, urban Turin had a utilization rate of hospital beds 7.6 times higher than rural Andalucia. Overall, the use of community beds was much higher in Italy: all sites had higher utilization rates than those in Spain. Wide variation was also found in use of a range of community services (Salvador-Carulla *et al.* 2005).

This variability is linked to the more general difficulty of *resource inappropriateness*: available services do not match what is needed or preferred. A clear example to which we inevitably return is the dominant position in many systems of large psychiatric asylums. While undoubtedly seen at the time they were originally opened as the appropriate service response to mental health needs, and while these large and often remote facilities might still provide 'asylum' in the proper sense of the word for people experiencing considerable distress, many do so under conditions of very poor quality of care (see Chapter 10). In cost terms, these hospitals also account for high proportions of available mental health budgets while supporting small proportions of the total population in need. One of the quandaries, as we noted earlier, is that closing a large psychiatric inpatient facility can lead to the leakage of resources out of the mental health system into other parts of the health system or elsewhere. Inadequate as they may be, and often scandalously poor in terms of quality, one argument sometimes voiced in favour of retaining the large, specialist institutions is that they do at least provide a recognizable and ring-fenced mental health resource. Whether this is really a defensible argument is debatable: protecting a decrepit, dehumanizing facility just because it has the label 'mental health' may be a hard case to sustain.

Care or support arrangements may also be too rigidly organized, leaving the system unable to respond to differences or changes in individual needs or preferences, or to community circumstances. Such *resource inflexibility* is common when there is scant information on population or individual needs, or when service users and their families have few opportunities to participate in decision-making about their treatment, or (again) when bureaucratic procedures dominate. Inflexibility is also seen in systems characterized by (perverse) incentives to keep inpatient beds full: the introduction of a new therapy or service model that reduces the need for hospital admission might not lead to savings in the hospital budget if there are financial or other advantages in keeping the beds filled. Services may potentially be available to meet the multiple needs of individual people or families, but they may be poorly coordinated. Such a situation can be compounded by 'silo budgeting', as we noted above.

One final challenge or barrier is the *resource timing* problem: most desired improvements to mental health practice take a long time to work their way through to improved health outcomes or cost-effectiveness gains. Moreover, evidence for improved practice may have been gathered under experimental circumstances and the savings suggested by the research may not actually get realized in a non-experimental setting. For instance, even when funds are made available for mental health there may be a short-term or transitional problem of a lack of suitable professionals, treatment facilities or other resources. If a country has only one psychiatrist per 100,000 population (as is the case in Albania), or if there are no or very few psychologists or other staff trained in some of the psychosocial interventions for which there is good evidence of effectiveness and cost-effectiveness, then even a dramatic increase in mental health funding may still not lead to improved access to suitable services. This supply inelasticity barrier may be only a question of time delays, but could nevertheless prove quite problematic.

Overcoming the barriers

Overcoming these resource barriers is one of the major challenges facing every mental health system in Europe. In most countries far too few resources are allocated to the prevention, identification and treatment of mental health problems. Indeed, there cannot be a single country in Europe that can justify its current investment in mental health care on the grounds of need, efficiency, equity or human rights. Such funding insufficiency is often combined with the other resource problems of poor distribution, inflexibility in allocation or use and lack of affordability. Left unchecked, these resource barriers could both worsen problems of inequity in access to services and also increase allocative and productive inefficiencies, because they make it harder for services to respond to the needs and preferences of service users. Possible steps to address these challenges will not be applicable or appropriate in every country. Each needs to be considered for its local relevance and to assess its potential for improving the level, distribution, appropriateness, flexibility, coordination and ready availability of resources in meeting mental health needs.

Fundamental to any action is the need to improve awareness of mental health issues and to address stigma and discrimination. Some members of the general public may believe that mental illness is self-inflicted and less deserving of attention. They may believe that problems are difficult to treat. They may be ignorant of the high prevalence of illness. They may be unsympathetic towards people whose 'ill health' they attribute to weakness or hypochondria. Improving mental health awareness or literacy may lead to a greater willingness to support mental health initiatives and develop national mental health policies and action plans (Jorm 2000). This is an ambitious aim, of course, for while there are examples of policies and practices that are successful in reducing stigma (Sartorius 2002), many attitudes about mental illness have deep cultural and religious roots. National anti-stigma programmes have nevertheless been introduced and are being evaluated in several European countries, such as in Scotland.

Increasing the resources available for mental health care would not remove all of the barriers, but it would represent an important start. Some governments certainly need to consider giving greater priority to meeting mental health needs. The contribution of mental health problems to overall disease or disability burden, combined with the availability of effective and cost-effective interventions to prevent, treat and/or rehabilitate individuals, would appear to justify a significant increase in funding for mental health in many countries. This makes sense from both social justice and efficiency perspectives.

Another argument for increased investment is to support implementation of a mental health reform process. As is abundantly clear from other chapters in this book, there have been dramatic changes to many systems of mental health care over recent decades, with most western and some other European countries moving from an era dominated by the old asylums to one that is much more proactively focused on community-based support arrangements. Such shifts require *additional* resources, at least in the short term. There is obviously a need to invest in new physical capital and human capital resources in the community prior to the closure of a hospital, to ensure the smooth and effective movement from one system to another. Secondly, community and hospital systems will need to run in parallel for some time, resulting in double running costs. Consequently, mental health reformers will almost certainly need to invest in order to save. Many countries will definitely need injections of additional resources in order to promote quality of life. Reforms that are introduced in a cost-neutral way – or, worse that are intent on saving money – could result in many people being denied care, or offered substandard support. This case needs to be forcefully made.

Evidence on cost-effectiveness can support the case for investment in mental health across many sectors of society; benefits from greater investment could include reduced reliance on social welfare payments, increased productivity, reduced contact with the criminal justice system and improved family and community cohesion. However, this should not be interpreted as meaning that cost savings must be found before there can be investment in mental health. Many cost-effective interventions are also cost *increasing*, so reformers should not need to be defensive about requiring increased levels of expenditure for better outcomes (Knapp 2005).

As we saw in the section on resource targeting, some areas of mental health practice are relatively well provided with evidence; for example, many of the most frequently used treatments for schizophrenia and depression have been the subject of cost-effectiveness evaluations. On the other hand, there have been relatively few economic evaluations of mental health promotion strategies. Given the general finding that economic evidence, unlike most of the evidence coming from clinical studies, does not generalize well from one health system or country to another, there needs to be encouragement for research endeavours that can generate solid platforms of *local* cost-effectiveness and related evidence on the range of therapeutic and service options available within a mental health care system. Given the cost and time needed to generate new evidence, serious consideration needs to be given to how these results might be adapted from another setting or country. This is one of a number of tasks now being explored by the European Commission-supported Mental Health Economics European Network.

The WHO's ongoing CHOICE (Choosing Interventions that are Cost Effective) programme has put together a database on cost-effectiveness evidence for many mental health interventions in Europe. This information, while not at a country-specific level, is provided for three European sub-regions in a transparent manner so that data can potentially be adapted to take account of local priorities, costs and resource availability (Chisholm *et al.* 2004, 2005). This database confirms that cost-effective treatments are available for all of Europe, even where resources for health are very limited.

Assuming that policy-makers can be convinced of the merits of greater investment in mental health, how might this be achieved? Options include expansion of the overall health budget, prioritization of mental health and/or the protection of mental health funds via ring-fenced budgets. There are, of course, disadvantages as well as advantages in the latter, for ring-fenced budgets can stop resources flowing *in* as well as *out*, and can encourage isolationism and reinforce *negative* images of the 'special' nature of mental illness. Another option in some countries, where there is sufficient data on resource utilization and costs, may be to introduce diagnosis-related group (DRG) unit costs. In principle, well constructed DRGs can be an effective way of ensuring that sufficient resources are transferred to secondary and specialist mental health related services. There is, of course, a danger, as highlighted by recent experiences in Austria (see Box 4.1), that the complexity of mental health might mean that DRG costs are underestimated (Zechmeister *et al.* 2002). This is a general problem with chronic conditions.

Resource inequity is another major challenge. Information gathering and lobbying on local prevalence data, cost-of-illness studies, disability burden figures, quality of life descriptions, cost-effectiveness evidence and anti-discrimination efforts could all assist. Fairer allocation of resources is likely to be achieved through the reduction of income-related inequity, finding ways of better serving rural areas and encouraging patient decision-making (McDaid *et al.* 2005b). None of these is remotely easy, but might be supported through an equity audit (Who gets what? At what personal cost?) and surveys of service users' needs, satisfaction levels and preferences, as well as explicit national or regional allocation formulae for the appropriate and transparent allocation of funding and capital investment. Mapping the mixed economy of mental health – both provision and the arrangements for financing – has potentially many uses, as discussed earlier. Mappings are obviously not solutions in themselves, but they provide a platform for discussions about how to improve the availability, distribution and deployment of resources.

Where information is available on the level of psychiatric need within countries, this can be used to allocate resources more equitably from central to local level, as in England (see Box 4.3). Local purchasers or service providers would then receive a share of the national health budget, based not only on the age and gender composition of their local populations but also on the basis of mental health need. With regular surveys, particular areas of concern might be addressed and budgets adjusted to reflect the changes. Nowhere might such an approach be more appropriate than in some of the countries that still are heavily reliant on institution-based services, with funding tied up in beds. Funding tied to individuals rather than institutions would help to break down one of the barriers to deinstitutionalization.

Box 4.3 Funding mental health care in England

The annual budgets of local purchasers (primary care trusts) for health care are determined on the basis of weighted populations, assignment of recurrent resources, together with some special allocations and redistributions. Weightings are based on age profiles and measures of health care need, including a specially developed mental health need index. This index combines a number of indicators of population need used to allocate funding to local government together with evidence on patterns of mental health care need from the Health Survey of England. Mental health as a proportion of total local purchaser allocations in 2003/4 varied from 22.5 per cent to 8.1 per cent, around an average of 11.6 per cent (Glover 2004). Some of this variation is due to the additional finance provided for remaining long-stay institutions.

Local purchasers are free to spend more or less on mental health than determined by the mental health needs allocation, but in providing services, local planners must ensure that services are available that meet the needs of the National Service Framework for Mental Health (Department of Health 1999), ensuring that resources are targeted in evidence-based ways to mental health. Small amounts of additional money for mental health can be earmarked through special allocations: in recent years these have included funds for mentally disordered offenders and to help implement mental health aspects of the NHS Plan.

Available resources could be deployed more efficiently in every health system. Although somewhat clichéd, much can be improved by ensuring that money follows the patients or service users. Supportive actions might include proper needs assessments, creating opportunities for patients to be involved in decision-making, shifting responsibility for arranging and purchasing services to localities while ensuring that national policies and treatment fidelity are followed, and that good standards are achieved.

Improved coordination might be obtained by reducing budgetary conflicts between ministries, seeking compensation between budgets for greater overall efficiency and again encouraging patient decision-making. This would certainly be aided through cross-ministry discussions and perhaps even the transfer of funds into joint budgets and the introduction of case management or similar case-finding, brokerage and micro coordinated efforts. These arrangements have their own (transaction) costs, of course, and a careful spending balance must be struck between resources that deliver mental health care and resources that simply coordinate. However, such initiatives are only going to be remotely possible in countries that already have some degree of coordination and strategic policy steer. In fragmented multi-provider health care systems with little centralized control the challenge is likely to be huge, although may be more feasible in regions with devolved powers.

Another way of helping to ensure that funds are allocated to meet needs, particularly within the community, is by encouraging 'direct payments' or 'individual budgets' (consumer-directed care). Individuals are given cash with which to purchase some or all of their services. This not only empowers individuals, but promotes independence and inclusion, and offers greater opportunities for rehabilitation, education, leisure and employment. This system has only been introduced in a few countries, for example in England, Scotland and the Netherlands. While not fully evaluated, if experience is similar to that when such payments have been used for people with physical or sensory disabilities it may avoid some of the problems of funding and coordinating services across different provider sectors.

Looking forward

The last decade has seen a significant increase in the attention given to mental health by many supra-national bodies, including WHO, the European Commission and many European governments, most notably with the recent commitment by all European governments to providing a 'fair and adequate' level of resources for mental health (World Health Organization 2005b). There is now substantial evidence that greater resource investment in many areas of mental health is not only justified on the grounds of tackling inequalities, the high degree of social exclusion and adverse consequences, but also that it represents a more efficient use of health (and other) resources. Efficiency gains can be both immediate and long-term. There remain gaps in knowledge, however, and international initiatives aimed at improving awareness, and looking at the transferability of the results of cost-effectiveness and related studies, such as the work of the WHO CHOICE programme globally and the MHEEN network in Europe, can help build capacity and fill some of these gaps. These initiatives may serve to strengthen the case further for investment.

Of course, on their own, these positive developments will not lead to a level of funding of mental health consistent with its individual and societal impact. Effective communication and ongoing engagement are needed with stakeholders in all sectors, including policy-makers, service users and families, employers, trade unions and schools. Any discussion of funding must therefore also consider other sectors, where in comparison with European health care systems, there may be even greater barriers to access, with higher levels of co-payments and use of income-related means-testing. NGOs and international donors will also need to continue to play important roles both in funding and delivering services. The long-term sustainability of effective initiatives needs to be an important goal.

It is crucial to recognize that it is not just a question of the level of funding for mental health, but also of the way in which these funds are used. Moving towards greater reliance on community care requires resources to be shifted away from institutional care. But as we have seen, there can be many barriers to achieving this. Financial incentives can be a powerful tool to improve the flow of funds to and within a mental health system, broadly defined, and to create incentives and disincentives to better action and performance. Making decision-makers aware of the cost implications of their decisions can be quite illuminating; making them financially responsible in a direct way can be particularly influential in changing behaviour. These incentives can also be used to empower service users through consumer-directed payment schemes to make their own decisions on service needs.

References

Alexander, A.C.G. (1990) *McDonnell Douglas Corporation Employee Assistance Program Financial Offset Study 1985–1989*. Westport, CT: Alexander Consulting Group.

Alonso, J., Angermeyer, M.C., Bernert, S. *et al.* (2004a) Psychotropic drug utilization in Europe: results from the European Study of the Epidemiology of Mental Disorders (ESEMeD) project, *Acta Psychiatrica Scandinavica Supplementum*, 420: 55–64.

Alonso, J., Angermeyer, M.C., Bernert, S. *et al.* (2004b) Use of mental health services in Europe: results from the European Study of the Epidemiology of Mental Disorders (ESEMeD) project, *Acta Psychiatrica Scandinavica Supplementum*, 420: 47–54.

Andlin-Sobocki, P. and Wittchen, H.U. (2005) Cost of anxiety disorders in Europe, *European Journal of Neurology*, 12(supplement): 39–44.

Andrews, G., Sanderson, K., Corry, J. and Lapsley, H. (2004) Utilising survey data to inform public policy: comparison of the cost-effectiveness of treatment of ten mental disorders, *British Journal of Psychiatry*, 184: 526–33.

Aviva Plc (2005) http://www.aviva.com.

Badelt, C. and Osterle, A. (2001) *Grundzüge der Sozialpolitik*. Vienna: Manz.

Bankauskaite, V. and Middtun, N.G. (2005) Mental health care reform in Lithuania: development and challenges, *Eurohealth*, 11(1): 19–23.

Barrett, B., Byford, S. and Knapp, M. (2005) Evidence of cost-effective treatments for depression: a systematic review. *Journal of Affective Disorders*, 84(1): 1–13.

Basu, A. (2004) Cost-effectiveness analysis of pharmacological treatments in schizophrenia: critical review of results and methodological issues, *Schizophrenia Research*, 71(2–3): 445–62.

Bebbington, A.C. and Davies, B. (1983) Equity and efficiency in the allocation of the personal social services, *Journal of Social Policy*, 12(3): 309–30.

Becker, T., Hulsmann, S., Knudsen, H. *et al.* (2002) Provision of services for people with schizophrenia in five European regions, *Social Psychiatry and Psychiatric Epidemiology*, 37(10): 465–74.

Beecham, J., Hallam, A., Knapp, M., Carpenter, J.S.W., Cambridge, P., Forester-Jones, R., Tate, A., Woolf, D.A. and Coulen-Schrijner, P. (2004) Twelve years on: service use and costs for people with mental health problems who left psychiatric hospital, *Journal of Mental Health*, 13(4): 363–77.

Bindman, J., Glover, G., Goldberg, D. and Chisholm, D. (2000) Expenditure on mental health care by English health authorities: a potential cause of inequality, *British Journal of Psychiatry*, 177: 267–74.

Bjoerngaard, J. (2002) *SAMDATA Psykisk helsevern Tabeller 2001*. Unimed Report 1/02. Trondheim: SINTEF.

Burns, T., Knapp, M., Catty, J., Healey, A., Henderson, J., Watt, H. and Wright, C. (2001) Home treatment for mental health problems: a systematic review, *Health Technology Assessment*, 5(15): 1–146.

Chisholm, D., Sanderson, K., Ayuso-Mateos, J.L. and Saxena, S. (2004) Reducing the global burden of depression: population-level analysis of intervention cost-effectiveness in 14 world regions, *British Journal of Psychiatry*, 184: 393–403.

Chisholm, D., van Ommeren, M., Ayuso-Mateos, J.L. and Saxena, J. (2005) Cost-effectiveness of clinical interventions for reducing the global burden of bipolar disorder, *British Journal of Psychiatry*, 187: 559–67.

Cox, T., Leka, S., Ivanov, I. and Kortums, E. (2004) Work, employment and mental health in Europe, *Work and Stress*, 18(2): 179–85.

Dewa, C., Hoch, J., Lin, E., Paterson, M. and Goering, P. (2003) Pattern of antidepressant use and duration of depression-related absence from work, *British Journal of Psychiatry*, 183: 507–13.

Dierckx, H. (2004) *Financing Mental Health Systems – Belgium*. Report prepared for the Mental Health Economics European Network. London: LSE.

Dixon, A. (2002) Dilemmas in mental health, *Eurohealth*, 8(1): 25–8.

Dixon, A., McDaid, D., Knapp, M. and Curran, C. (2006) Financing mental health services in low and middle income countries: equity and efficiency concerns, *Health Policy and Planning*, 21(3): 171–82.

Dlouhy, M. (2004) Mental health care system and mental health expenditures in the Czech republic, *Journal of Mental Health Policy and Economics*, 7(4): 159–65.

Evers, S. (2004) *Financing Mental Health Systems – The Netherlands*. Report prepared for the Mental Health Economics European Network. www.mhe-sme.org/en/projects_mheii.htm.

Frank, R.G. and McGuire, T. (2000) Economics and mental health, in A.J. Culyer and J.P. Newhouse (eds) *Handbook of Health Economics*. Amsterdam: Elsevier.

Funk, M. (2005) Promoting social inclusion in an enlarged Europe – international cooperation and involving stakeholders in the mental health reform process, in *Global Health Challenges: European Approaches and Responsibilities*. Gastein: European Health Forum Gastein.

Gabriel, P. and Liimatainen, M.-R. (2000) *Mental Health in the Workplace*. Geneva: International Labour Organization.

Glover, G. (2004) *Mental Health Care Funding in England*. Durham: Centre of Public Mental Health, Durham University.

Government of Bulgaria (2000) *National Mental Health Programme of the Citizens of the Republic of Bulgaria 2001–2005.* Sofia: Government of Bulgaria.

Halsteinli, V., Torvik, H. and Hagen, T. (2001) *Vekst og virkemidler.* Tondheim: SINTEF.

Harangozò, J. and Kristòf, R. (2000) Where is Hungarian mental health reform? *Mental Health Reforms,* 2: 14–18.

Haro, J.M., Salvador-Carulla, L., Cabases, J., Madoz, V. and Vazquez-Barquero, J.L. (1998) Utilisation of mental health services and costs of patients with schizophrenia in three areas of Spain, *British Journal of Psychiatry,* 173: 334–40.

Healey, A., Knapp, M., Astin, J., Gossop, M., Marsden, J., Stewart, D., Lehmann, P. and Godfrey, C. (1998) Economic burden of drug dependency: social costs incurred by drug users at intake to the National Treatment Outcome Research Study, *British Journal of Psychiatry,* 173: 160–5.

Jane-Llopis, E. and Anderson, P. (2005) *Mental Health Promotion and Mental Disorder Prevention: A Policy for Europe.* Nijmegen: Radboud University Nijmegen.

Jonsson, L. (2004) Economic evidence in dementia: a review, *European Journal of Health Economics,* 5(Suppl 1): S30–5.

Jorm, A. (2000) Mental health literacy: public knowledge and beliefs about mental disorders, *British Journal of Psychiatry,* 177: 396–401.

Knapp, M. (1984) *The Economics of Social Care.* London: Macmillan.

Knapp, M. (1990) Economic barriers to innovation in mental health care, in I. Marks and R. Scott (eds) *Mental Health Care Delivery: Innovations, Impediments and Implementation.* Cambridge: Cambridge University Press.

Knapp, M. (1995) The economic perspective: framework and principles, in M. Knapp (ed.) *The Economic Evaluation of Mental Health Care.* Aldershot: Arena.

Knapp, M. (2005) Money talks: nine things to remember about mental health financing, *Journal of Mental Health,* 14(2): 89–93.

Knapp, M., Beecham, J. and Koutsogeorgopoulou, V. (1995) Service use and costs of home-based versus hospital-based care for people with serious mental illness, *British Journal of Psychiatry,* 166(1): 120–2.

Knapp, M., Chisholm, D., Astin, J., Lelliott, P. and Audini, B. (1998) Public, private and voluntary residential mental health care: is there a cost difference? *Journal of Health Services Research and Policy,* 3(3): 141–8.

Knapp, M., Hallam, A., Beecham, J. and Baines, B. (1999) Private, voluntary or public? Comparative cost-effectiveness in community mental health care, *Policy and Politics,* 27: 25–41.

Knapp, M., Chisholm, D., Leese, M., Amaddeo, F. *et al.* (2002) Comparing patterns and costs of schizophrenia care in five European countries: the EPSILON study. European psychiatric services: inputs linked to outcome domains and needs, *Acta Psychiatrica Scandinavica,* 105(1): 42–54.

Knapp, M., Novick, D., Genkeer, L., Curran, C. and McDaid, D. (2003) Financing health care in Europe: context for the Schizophrenia Outpatient Health Outcomes Study, *Acta Psychiatrica Scandinavia Supplementum,* 416: 30–40.

Knapp, M., Barrett, B., Romeo, R., McCrone, P., Byford, S., Beecham, J., Patel, A. and Simon, J. (2004) *An International Review of Cost-Effectiveness Studies for Mental Disorders.* Washington, DC: Fogarty International Centre of the National Institutes of Health.

Knapp, M., Funk, M., Curran, C., Prince, M., Grigg, M. and McDaid, D. (2006a) Economic barriers to better mental health practice and policy, *Health Policy and Planning,* 21(3): 157–70.

Knapp, M., McDaid, D. and Ammadeo, F. (2006b) Financing arrangements for mental health in Western Europe, *Journal of Mental Health,* forthcoming.

Kovess, V., Caldas de Almeida Jose, M., Carta, M. *et al.* (2005) Professional team's choices of intervention towards problems and needs of patients suffering from schizophrenia across six European countries, *European Psychiatry*, 20(8): 521–8.

Lewis, M. (2002) Informal health payments in central and eastern Europe and the former Soviet Union: issues, trends and implications, in E. Mossialos, A. Dixon, J. Figueras and J. Kutzin (eds) *Funding Health Care: Options for Europe*. Buckingham: Open University Press.

Loveman, E., Green, C., Kirby, J., Takeda, A. *et al.* (2004) *The clinical and cost-effectiveness of donepezil, rivastigmine, galantamine and memantine for Alzheimer's disease. Technology Assessment Report*. London: National Institute for Health and Clinical Excellence.

Marshall, M., Crowther, R., Almaraz-Serrano, A., Creed, F. *et al.* (2001) Systematic reviews of the effectiveness of day care for people with severe mental disorders: (1) acute day hospital versus admission; (2) vocational rehabilitation; (3) day hospital versus outpatient care, *Health Technology Assessment*, 5(21): 1–75.

Matschinger, H. and Angemeyer, M. (2004) The public's preference concerning the allocation of financial resources to health care: results from a representative population survey in Germany, *European Psychiatry*, 19(8): 478–82.

McDaid, D. (2001) Estimating the costs of informal care for people with Alzheimer's disease: methodological and practical challenges, *International Journal of Geriatric Psychiatry*, 16(4): 400–5.

McDaid, D., Curran, C. and Knapp, M. (2005a) Promoting mental well-being in the workplace: a European policy perspective, *International Review of Psychiatry*, 17(5): 365–73.

McDaid, D., Oliver, A., Knapp, M. and Funk, M. (2005b) *Minding Mental Health: Towards an Equitable Approach*. London: London School of Economics and Political Science.

McDaid, D., Samyshkin, Y., Jenkins, R., Potasheva, A.P. *et al.* (2006) Health system factors impacting on delivery of mental health services in Russia: multi-methods study, *Health Policy*, forthcoming.

Ministry of Health (2003) *St meld 5 (2003–2004): Inntektssystem for spesialisthelsetjenesten*. White paper. Oslo: Ministry of Health.

Moscone, F. and Knapp, M. (2005) Exploring the spatial pattern of mental health expenditure, *Journal of Mental Health Policy and Economics*, 8(4): 205–17.

Mossialos, E. and Thomson, S.M.S. (2002) Voluntary health insurance in the European Union, in E. Mossialos, A. Dixon, J. Figueras and J. Kutzin (eds) *Funding Health Care: Options for Europe*. Buckingham: Open University Press.

Mossialos, E., Dixon, A., Figueras, J. and Kutzin, J. (2002) *Funding Health Care: Options for Europe*. Buckingham: Open University Press.

Neumeyer-Gromen, A., Lampert, T., Stark, K. and Kallischnigg, G. (2004) Disease management programs for depression: a systematic review and meta-analysis of randomized controlled trials, *Medical Care*, 42(12): 1211–21.

Normand, C. and Buse, R. (2002) Social health insurance, in E. Mossialos, A. Dixon, J. Figueras and J. Kutzin (eds) *Funding Health Care: Options for Europe*. Buckingham: Open University Press.

Oliver, A. J. (2001) *Why Care about Health Inequality?* London: Office of Health Economics.

O'Shea, E. and NiLeime, A. (2004) *Financing Mental Health Systems – Ireland*. Report prepared for the Mental Health Economics European Network, http://www.mhe-sme.org/en/projects_mheii.htm.

Pfeil, W. (2001) *Vergleich der Sozialhilfesysteme der österreichischen Bundesländer*. Vienna: BMSG.

Pirraglia, P.A., Rosen, A.B., Hermann, R.C., Olchanski, N.V. and Neumann, P. (2004) Cost-utility analysis studies of depression management: a systematic review, *American Journal of Psychiatry*, 161(12): 2155–62.

Regier, D.A., Goldberg, I.D. and Taube, C.A. (1978) The de facto US mental health services system: a public health perspective, *Archives of General Psychiatry*, 35(6): 685–93.

Rizzo, J., Abbott, T.A. and Pashko, S. (1996) Labour productivity effects of prescribed medicines for chronically ill workers, *Health Economics*, 5(3): 249–65.

Romeo, R., Byford, S. and Knapp, M. (2005) Economic evaluations of child and adolescent mental health interventions: a systematic review, *Journal of Child Psychology and Psychiatry*, 46(9): 919–30.

Romeo, R., Knapp, M. and Scott, S. (2006) Economic cost of severe antisocial behaviour in children – and who pays it? *British Journal of Psychiatry*, 188: 547–53.

Rost, K., Smith, J. and Dickinson, M. (2004) The effect of improving primary care depression management on employee absenteeism and productivity: a randomised trial, *Medical Care*, 42(12): 1202–10.

Salize, H.J. and Rossler, W. (1996) The cost of comprehensive care of people with schizophrenia living in the community: a cost evaluation from a German catchment area, *British Journal of Psychiatry*, 169(1): 42–8.

Salvador-Carulla, L., Tibaldi, G., Johnson, S., Scala, E. *et al.* (2005) Patterns of mental health service utilisation in Italy and Spain. An investigation using the European Service Mapping Schedule, *Social Psychiatry and Psychiatric Epidemiology*, 40(2): 149–59.

Sartorius, N. (2002) Iatrogenic stigma of mental illness, *British Medical Journal*, 324: 1470–1.

Schlesinger, M. and Dorwart, R. (1984) Ownership and mental-health services: a reappraisal of the shift toward privately owned facilities, *New England Journal of Medicine*, 311(15): 959–65.

Scott, S., Knapp, M., Henderson, J. and Maughan, B. (2001) Financial cost of social exclusion: follow up study of antisocial children into adulthood, *British Medical Journal*, 323(7306): 191.

Simon, G., Katon, W., von Korff, M. *et al.* (2001) Cost-effectiveness of a collaborative care program for primary care patients with persistent depression, *American Journal of Psychiatry*, 158: 1638–44.

Soumerai, S.B., McLaughlin, T.J., Ross-Degnan, D., Casteris, C.S. and Bollini, P. (1994) Effects of a limit on Medicaid drug-reimbursement benefits on the use of psychotropic agents and acute mental health services by patients with schizophrenia, *New England Journal of Medicine*, 331(10): 650–5.

Tamblyn, R., Laprise, R., Hanley, A. *et al.* (2001) Adverse events associated with prescription drug cost-sharing among poor and elderly persons, *Journal of the American Medical Association*, 285(4): 421–9.

ten Have, M., Vollebergh, W., Bijl, R. and Nolen, W.A. (2002) Bipolar disorder in the general population in the Netherlands (prevalence, consequences and care utilisation): results from The Netherlands Mental Health Survey and Incidence Study (NEMESIS), *Journal of Affective Disorders*, 68(2–3): 203–13.

Thomas, C. and Morris, S. (2003) Cost of depression among adults in England in 2000, *British Journal of Psychiatry*, 183: 514–19.

Tomasson, K. (2004) *Financing Mental Health Systems – Iceland*. Report prepared for the Mental Health Economics European Network, http://www.mhe-sme.org/en/projects_mheii.htm.

Tomov, T., Mladenova, M., Lazarova, I., Sotirov, V. and Okoliyski, M. (2004) Bulgaria mental health country profile, *International Review of Psychiatry*, 16(1–2): 93–106.

Weich, S. and Lewis, G. (1998) Material standard of living, social class and the prevalence of common mental disorders in Great Britain, *Journal of Epidemiology and Community Health*, 52(1): 8–14.

World Health Organization (2000) *The World Health Report 2000. Health Systems: Improving Performance*. Geneva: World Health Organization.

World Health Organization (2005a) *Atlas. Mental Health Resources Around the World*. Geneva: World Health Organization.

World Health Organization (2005b) *Mental Health Declaration for Europe. Facing the Challenges, Building Solutions.* Copenhagen: World Health Organization.

World Mental Health Survey Consortium (2004) Prevalence, severity and unmet need for treatment of mental disorders in the World Health Organization World Mental Health Surveys, *Journal of the American Medical Association*, 291(21): 2581–90.

Zaluska, M., Suchecka, D., Traczewska, J. and Paszko, J. (2005) Implementation of social services for the chronically mentally ill in a Polish health district: consequences for service use and costs, *Journal of Mental Health Policy and Economics*, 8(1): 37–44.

Zechmeister, I. and Osterle, A. (2004) Dann war auf einmal kein Geld mehr da. Zur Rolle der Finanzierung in der österreichischen Psychiatriereform, *Psychiatrische Praxis*, 31(4): 184–91.

Zechmeister, I., Osterle, A., Denk, P. and Katschnig, H. (2002) Incentives in financing mental health care in Austria, *Journal of Mental Health Economics and Policy*, 5(3): 121–9.

chapter five

The evidence base in mental health policy and practice

Rachel Jenkins, David McDaid, Traolach Brugha, Paul Cutler and Robert Hayward

As we saw in Chapter 1, the burden of ill health attributed to mental illness in Europe is high (Wittchen and Jacobi 2005). There is also a growing appreciation of the particular importance of mental disorders as a result of their relationship with poverty and physical disease. Undoubtedly, mental health has risen up the policy agenda, as can be most clearly seen through the recent World Health Organization (WHO) European Region Declaration and Action Plan for mental health, as well as the publication of the recent European Commission Green Paper (Commission of the European Communities 2005; World Health Organization 2005a). Yet despite this significant burden, the availability of evidence on effective interventions and greater recognition of the importance of good mental health (see Chapter 4), it continues to attract a low share of health budgets in many European countries.

Specific mental health policies setting out strategic goals and the means to achieve them are essential; yet in several European countries such policies are absent or are very old (World Health Organization 2005b). Of course, even if policies are in place they need to be informed by evidence, not only on the size and nature of mental health problems in a country, but also on what is known to be effective in meeting this challenge. This is, of course, not just a mental health issue; across all sectors of public policy there is an increasing recognition of the need to take account of evidence in the decision-making process (Oliver and McDaid 2002).

While evidence-based, or perhaps better described as evidence-informed, policy-making can take many forms in the health sector, there is a tendency to equate it with the concept of evidence-based medicine (EBM), an approach which seeks to rigorously assess effectiveness through experimental controlled trials. However, evidence itself can come from many other sources ranging from experimental trials to surveys and focus groups. It might also come to light as a result of public inquiries and/or media pressure. Each has its own strengths and weaknesses. How can these different approaches be used to facilitate evidence-informed mental health policy?

This chapter will look at how to encourage a more evidence-informed approach to mental health policy. It will begin by considering how approaches adopted in the development of evidence-based medicine may be applied and will draw on experience in developing evidence-based policy across all areas of public policy. It is important to not just focus on the evidence observed in experimental trials; the chapter also looks at how other sources of evidence can inform the policy-making process.

Too often however, evidence has had little impact on policy-making. It can be lost within the myriad of different political and public demands, anecdotes, myths and lobbying that policy-makers have to contend with. In addition to having some capacity for generating evidence, it is important to develop capacity within the policy-making community to make sense of different sources of evidence. Enhancing what is known as 'receptor capacity' can help in filtering the many sources of 'good' and 'bad' information, highlighting the strengths and limitations of different approaches. The chapter ends by looking at ways of involving all stakeholders in the policy-making process, with particular attention given to central and eastern Europe. It looks at how to improve the process of dissemination and diffusion of ideas and thus bridge the gap between research and mental health policy.

The growth of EBM

The EBM movement came to real prominence in the early 1970s, although the term itself would not be coined until some years later in Canada (Evidence Based Medicine Working Group 1992). This followed public concern about the safety of some medications – most notably in Europe with the high number of birth defects in the children of women who had been taking the drug thalidomide in the 1960s. New regulations were introduced requiring that all new medications be the subject of large-scale trials prior to licensing for widespread use. Archie Cochrane, one of the chief architects of the evidence-based health care movement, argued for such regulation to go beyond simply ensuring that interventions were safe. He wanted interventions to be shown to be both effective and efficient, with a much greater focus placed on encouraging the incorporation of empirical evidence on the effect of interventions into the decision-making process (Cochrane 1973).

Thus, EBM emphasized the need to generate knowledge through systematic empirical research. Its mainstay was the randomized controlled trial (RCT) where individuals are randomly placed into an intervention or control group. The idea of such trials was not new – their use had been increasing since the well publicized work on the treatment of tuberculosis undertaken in the immediate postwar period by Bradford-Hill and colleagues (British Medical Research Council 1948). Such carefully controlled experiments, it was argued, minimized the level of internal bias in an evaluation and therefore provided a reliable estimate of the incremental consequences of introducing an intervention in a particular setting.

While initially concentrating on pharmaceuticals, over time, the use of EBM has expanded to evaluate other interventions such as surgical procedures and medical devices. For instance, there are now thousands of experimental studies that have looked at the efficacy of drug therapies for mental disorders,[1] and to a lesser extent, trials for other interventions such as psychotherapy or different approaches to organizing and delivering community-based care. The methodologies of trials have also developed so that there are now initial studies purely on the efficacy of interventions undertaken in ideal clinical settings, followed by naturalistic, larger-scale trials undertaken in everyday conditions intended to increase the generalizability of study findings.

A 'hierarchy of evidence' has developed around EBM, and while there are some variations, the list below presents a typical hierarchy. Under this hierarchy the most powerful sources of evidence are the use of meta-analytical techniques to pool evidence from a number of RCTs, followed by the results of single RCTs. This would be followed by a range of non-randomized, but controlled trials, with single case studies at the bottom of the hierarchy. With minor variations and refinements, most hierarchies follow this basic structure. Examples include the hierarchy outlined in a recent publication from the former Health Development Agency in England (Weightman *et al.* 2005), as well as that of the Cochrane Collaboration.

1 Systematic reviews and meta-analyses.
2 Randomized controlled trials.
3 Non-randomized controlled trials.
4 Cohort studies/time series designs.
5 Case-control studies.
6 Cross-sectional surveys.
7 Case series.
8 Single case reports.

Qualitative approaches to evaluation

Few EBM hierarchies make any mention of qualitative approaches to evaluation, or if they do these are placed at the very bottom. While evidence from the quantitative research methods such as the RCT is very powerful, it is not without its limitations. This has been well documented elsewhere (see Tansella *et al.* 2006) and a detailed analysis of their strengths and weaknesses is not our focus here. However, one key issue, notwithstanding the increased use of naturalistic trials, is that their results cannot be easily generalized. Medications may, for instance, be administered in many different ways in different cultures and in different health system settings. This may have an impact on potential effectiveness. Another limitation may be the exclusion of specific population groups, such as older people or children, or those with co-morbid health conditions, from participation in RCTs.

Regardless of their advantages and disadvantages, some complex non-pharmaceutical, mental health related interventions are difficult to evaluate using RCTs. Looking at community-wide interventions, for instance on stigma campaigns, it may be difficult for a control group not to be 'contaminated' by information they might receive from the individuals enrolled in the intervention group. Different approaches to evaluation are required which, from the perspective of the hierarchy of evidence-based medicine, may be viewed as inferior.

Yet some contend that at least as much value ought to be placed on quantitative observational studies (Black 1996) or on non-controlled qualitative analyses (Newburn 2001). Not only can such approaches be used to explore hypotheses to help in the framing of future quantitative studies, but supporters of qualitative techniques also argue that these methods better reflect the real-world environment within which decision-makers operate, and offer a better understanding of the underlying social mechanisms that cause interventions to succeed or fail (Sanderson 2000).

But what do we mean by qualitative research? This is a broad term that covers a wide range of methods which 'involve the systematic collection, organization, and interpretation of textual material derived from talk or observation. It is used in the exploration of meanings of social phenomena as experienced by individuals themselves, in their natural context' (Malterud 2001: 483). Unlike quantitative studies the aim is not to generate statistically significant results, but to explore themes, patterns and associations within a richer and more diverse data set. As such, qualitative research is useful for addressing a different set of evaluation questions: not 'how many xs?', but 'what is x, how does x vary in different situations and why?' Examples of the approach can include focus groups, the observation of organizational settings and team behaviour, and in-depth interviews.

Such research can help inform the debate on the generalization of findings from studies. It may be used in the assessment of complex outcomes that are difficult to quantify (e.g. changes in organizational culture or sense of community), but which impact on the success of an intervention. They can also be used to identify differences in the importance of outcomes between different stakeholders (Pope *et al.* 2002). One recent systematic review looking at the effectiveness of electroconvulsive therapy (ECT) indicated that service user-led research reported significantly less benefit than clinician-led studies. This, it was argued, may be due to clinical studies obtaining information from those undergoing ECT too soon after treatment and using simplistic questionnaires that did not pick up complex patient views. The study highlighted the need for more qualitative research to identify outcomes of value to those that undergo treatment (Rose *et al.* 2003).

Qualitative approaches should not be viewed as an alternative to quantitative approaches; in fact, they can be seen as complementary. The hierarchy of evidence seen in EBM, which places least value on qualitative research methods (if they are mentioned at all), can be replaced by a matrix which emphasizes the need to match the research design to the research question, as illustrated in Table 5.1 (Muir-Gray 1996; Petticrew and Roberts 2003). While it is clear that the systematic pooling of the findings of many studies generally provides the most robust source of evidence, and that trials best answer questions of efficacy, effectiveness and cost-effectiveness, the matrix indicates that for questions of appropriateness, satisfaction, service delivery processes and acceptability, qualitative research methods provide appropriate research designs.

Is the EBM movement applicable to evidence-informed mental health policy?

In short, the answer is yes, but not in isolation. To link EBM to evidence-informed policy-making it is essential to take into account a myriad of factors including local context, needs, existing structures and human resources, as well as flexibility for system change. The use of evidence from quantitative research methods, such as the RCT on its own, is unlikely to be sufficient to answer many of the questions that policy-makers have to contend with. Policy-makers need more information than the evidence from an RCT on whether symptoms get better with drug A or drug B, and perhaps at what cost. For instance, they need to know the context in which a study was undertaken, the potential for replicability in their own setting, and the perspectives of service users and health care professionals on the merits of these drugs. Complementary qualitative research methods can help to broaden this information to better inform policy-makers on the context in which individual interventions have been shown to work. However, this is only one additional element of the information required for evidence-informed policy-making.

The key questions and contextual issues for policy-making are much broader than simply what works best, and also, must operate at the *macro level* as well as the *individual level*. For instance, while access to new medications and the balance between community and institutional-based care may be the predominant preoccupation in some of the relatively rich countries of western Europe, in other parts of the continent access even to basic older medicines may still be restricted. Moreover, there may be little desire or flexibility within the mental health system to invest in community-based services.

Key policy issues in some countries thus may revolve around ensuring that the medicines used are adequate in terms of their availability and that staff have basic training and continuing professional education on their use, management of side-effects and recognition of early symptoms of relapse. They may also need information on the necessary resources for, and the most effective ways of, delivering new services such as community-based care, rehabilitation, supported employment and risk management. These are but a few of the issues that need to be considered in formulating national mental health policies (Jenkins *et al.* 2002; World Health Organization 2004).

Another key constraint in both the formulation and implementation of policy is the availability of resources. Highly cost-effective interventions that may be included within a mental health policy may be cost-increasing. This can have significant consequences for the health budget; if investing in new cost-effective approaches requires a greater share of the existing health budget, then the number of people that may be treated or the nation's ability to maintain other services or ensure that adequate training is provided may be reduced. Policy solutions need to be tailored to match available resources within countries (see Chapter 4).

Evidence-informed policy thus will not be achieved simply by referring to the disparate elements of effectiveness and cost-effectiveness studies. A number of years ago, a senior figure in the EBM movement stated that since the only RCT on mental health in primary care we had (at that time) was on the benefit of using health visitors to screen for depression in postnatal mothers, our entire policy for primary mental health care should therefore focus on this activity. Such a piecemeal and unstrategic approach is not desirable. Policy, by definition, has to take a broad systemic overview. It has to ensure that connections are made, akin to putting all the elements of a jigsaw puzzle into place, so that the system will work as an integrated and coherent whole, and the policy can be implemented.

What types of information and evidence do policy-makers need?

Policy-makers need to have both qualitative and quantitative information on mental health policy options in a form which is accessible, organized, accurate, triangulated, usable and owned by key stakeholders (Jick 1979; Smith 1989; Kelle 2001). They require information on systemic as well as programmatic issues (Hafner and Heiden 1991) and must analyse the political, economic and institutional contexts carefully if they are to assess the need and potential for reform (Cassells 1995).

Such assessments must cover multiple sectors, not only health but also social welfare, housing, employment, education and criminal justice to name but a few. They must also look at the role, and take account of the views, of different stakeholders including service users, families, professionals within and outside the health system, employers, non-governmental organizations (NGOs) and the general public. The links between these different sectors and stakeholders must be identified; analysis needs to look not just at the potential content of policy, but also at the practicalities of implementation.

In developing mental health policy, experience in the development of generic models for the design and reform of health systems (e.g. Hurst 1991; Roemer 1991; Frenk 1994; Cassells 1995; Murray and Frenk 2000), can be drawn on. It is only recently that there has been interest in looking at mental health-specific systems and the ways in which mental health systems interact with both general health systems as well as broader social policy spheres within countries (Jenkins *et al.* 2002; Goering *et al.* 2003; Gulbinat *et al.* 2004; World Health Organization 2004).

Integrating knowledge

Information on the broad picture of system development, available infrastructure, human capacity, demographic profile and epidemiological trends within a country are required. Such broad information can help to inform decisions, such as how much money should be spent overall and how it should be divided up between promotion, prevention, treatment and rehabilitation services. It can also help to decide the balance that should be sought between public and private health care, generalist and specialist health, mental health and social care. Finally, it can help determine the importance of public policy on mental health. 'Narrow' information on the effectiveness of interventions and specific treatment options emerging from qualitative and quantitative research must complement such information.

Therefore, a key challenge is to integrate what can be very disparate bits of evidence, knowledge, experience and values into a reasonably cohesive whole to respond to the needs of policy-makers. Until recently, few studies were available upon which to base 'broad information' decision-making. Useful information to help build capacity in policy-making across countries is still urgently needed. One helpful approach may be through policy synthesis (see below).

When it comes to 'narrow studies', however, we are on firmer ground as methods exist which allow us to more easily synthesize results. As Table 5.1 illustrates, we can see how powerful such a review can be. The systematic review is a rigorous attempt to identify all relevant studies in both the published and unpublished (grey) literature. Systematic reviews may, but not necessarily, focus on RCTs. Meta-analysis takes things one step further by using statistical techniques to combine the outcomes of a number of RCTs identified through systematic review to come to a more definitive conclusion as to whether an intervention is effective.

There are still limitations with systematic reviews, as with other methods of evaluation. Their quality is entirely dependent on the quality and quantity of the existing investigations upon which they are based (Herbert and Bø 2005). High quality investigations aimed at issues relevant to the proposed policy are not always available, especially in the middle- and low-income countries of central and eastern Europe. There are also issues over the extent to which results can be generalized from high-income countries such as the United Kingdom to other parts of Europe where the context, infrastructure and level of resources may be very different. Another limitation is the difficulty in conducting systematic reviews across the broader health care sector and the interplay of health care, welfare, criminal justice, education and environmental policies. Only a very restricted set of policy questions has been addressed using this approach, although some groups, including the Campbell Collaboration are beginning to do more work in this area (see below).

One potentially powerful way of dealing with some of these cross-sectoral interventions, and indeed some of the 'broader issues', may be through the use of a new approach known as 'policy synthesis'. This goes beyond the boundaries of the traditional systematic review. While still in its infancy, such syntheses have been commissioned by the NHS Service Delivery and Organization Unit in England and also by the Canadian Health Services Research Foundation. They consist of systematic reviews that incorporate information not only from RCTs but also from other sources of evidence, including qualitative research. They also use deliberative approaches such as focus groups, public consultations and citizens juries to capture some of the societal values that will influence whether or not an intervention may be introduced successfully (Lavis *et al.* 2005; Mays *et al.* 2005; Pawson *et al.* 2005; Sheldon 2005). However, until now, these approaches do not appear to have been applied to mental health policy-related questions.

Table 5.1 A matrix of evidence

Research question	Qualitative research	Survey	Case-control studies	Cohort studies	RCTs	Quasi-experimental studies	Non-experimental evaluation	Systematic review
Effectiveness: does this work better than doing that?	++			+	++	+		+++
Process of service delivery: how does it work?	++	+					+	+++
Salience: does it matter?	++	++						+++
Safety: do benefits outweigh risk of harm?	+		+	+	++	+	+	+++
Acceptability: will there be a demand for this service?	++	+			+	+	+	+++
Cost effectiveness: is this a good use of scarce resources?					++			+++
Appropriateness: is this an appropriate intervention to deliver?	++	++						++
Satisfaction with service: are users, providers and other stakeholders satisfied with the service?	++	++	+	+				+

Key: +++ Most robust evidence ++ Reasonable evidence + Can provide some weak evidence

Source: Adapted from Petticrew and Roberts (2003). This matrix was itself adapted from an original by Muir-Gray (1996).

A blueprint for improving the construction of evidence-informed policy

We have looked at EBM and its link with policy-making, setting out some of the informational needs of policy-makers. In this section we set out some of the key elements of a blueprint to help facilitate and improve both the construction and implementation of evidence-informed policy (see Box 5.1).

Box 5.1   Elements of a blueprint for improving the construction of evidence-informed policy

1 Enhance understanding of the kinds of information which are helpful for policy development.
2 Ensure that situation appraisals are undertaken to obtain contextual information that will assist policy being tailored to the local situation. Develop frameworks and methods of synthesis.
3 Enhance accessibility to information.
4 Plan future research and development to support evidence-based mental health policy.
5 Invest in the development of knowledge transfer mechanisms between policy-makers and other stakeholders.

Enhance understanding of how different types of information can be used in policy development

A key first step in the development of policy for mental health is to understand how different types of information can be used in policy development. Policy ultimately is dependent first on identifying the needs of the population, then understanding what current structures and services are available, and finally determining how to augment or change the current service mix. *Epidemiological research* and information obtained from *routine data collection and local surveys* can help inform both our understanding of population needs and the current structure and utilization of services. For policies and their implementation strategies to be credible, they need to be highly tailored to the local situation for which they are intended. *Rapid situation assessment and appraisal* can be used to enhance our understanding of the local context.

Once needs have been identified and local services and structures mapped, policy needs to consider the *evidence base on interventions and strategies to improve mental health*. It is at this stage that information from both qualitative and quantitative studies of specific interventions should be collected. If previous national or local policies and strategies have been evaluated, this information can also be used to inform the policy debate.

Identifying needs using epidemiological research

One powerful way of identifying mental health needs is through the use of epidemiological research (Jenkins 2001). Methods, namely epidemiological interviewing techniques (Wing *et al.* 1990; Lewis *et al.* 1992; Jenkins and Meltzer 2003) can be used to appraise mental health, mental disorders and the accompanying disability in individuals and populations. There are also methods to assess the service needs of sick populations (e.g. Marshall *et al.* 1995; Phelan *et al.* 1995; Avon Measure Working Group 1996). Although epidemiology is crucial for policy-makers (Jenkins 2001), few countries perform national epidemiological studies on the general household population because of the perception that such studies are relatively expensive and time-consuming. This need not be the case; the current world mental health survey has been working with 14 countries worldwide to run national surveys (World Mental Health Survey Consortium 2004). Relatively small-scale, but nonetheless useful, community-based and primary care studies on mental disorders have already been undertaken in many low-income countries (Institute of Medicine 2001).

Identifying needs and mapping service availability

Data from household and service-user surveys (at various levels in the service), routine data on patients, service inputs and processes can also play a vital role. Again, there are limitations in existing health information systems which often focus largely on routine data collection of hospital admissions, consultations and discharges. They may gather little information on specialist outpatient clinics, less still on consultations in primary care or the community, and nothing at all on population rates of illness. They sometimes include mortality data, but they hardly ever include health or social outcomes – although efforts to introduce routine mental health outcome measurements have grown (Jenkins 1990; Wing *et al.* 1998). There have been developments, for instance in England, with the introduction of the mental health minimum data set, which aimed to bring together data covering many aspects of individual patients' personal characteristics, problems and care (Glover and Sinclair-Smith 2000).

Timing and access to this information is also important. In some countries these data are often collected and published much too late to be useful in health planning and decision-making (Smith 1989). They may not be sufficiently synthesized with qualitative information so as to be easily interpreted by decision-makers. Moreover, information and evidence may not always be accessible outside the narrow confines of the specific governmental department in which it was produced (e.g. the prison service).

Obtaining different perspectives on what constitutes evidence of effectiveness

While discussion occurs over what type of evidence should be used to inform policy-making and practice, much less is said about who decides what evidence should be used or which sources of evidence should be given priority. Evidence generated by service users traditionally has had little impact in the development of policy. In England, at least, there is evidence that this is beginning to change where academic-based groups such as the Service Users Research Enterprise at the Institute of Psychiatry, King's College London, exist (Rose *et al.* 2006) (see also Chapter 14). Rose *et al.* have proposed that a multiple perspectives paradigm be used to integrate various sources of evidence generated by different methods of scientific enquiry, including that produced by service users. They also argue that service users should have a greater role in setting research questions, identifying interventions (and by implication, policy strategies) and also ensuring that research designs take account of service-user perspectives.

Undertake situation appraisal and assessment

The process of reform and the difficulty of implementing policy and institutional change have been relatively neglected (Walt and Gilson 1994) compared with the content of reform – both require a detailed prior-situation assessment. Therefore, such a detailed situation assessment should be considered to be a key prerequisite for evidence-informed policy (World Health Organization 2004).

The notion of a mental health situation assessment is similar to the public health concept of situation analysis where population needs and demands, existing services and current resources are assessed in order to effect change and improvement. Such situation assessments provide a background for setting priorities for policy development and a common reference point for the rest of the policy development process (Green 1999). It is particularly useful in countries where routine information collection has not been the norm. There is, therefore, a need for a comprehensive strategy for synthesizing existing evidence on context, needs, inputs, processes and outcomes from multiple sources, disciplines and perspectives.

One such strategy has been developed and piloted in 15 countries worldwide, including three within Europe. The Mental Health Country Profile (MHCP) is one of the tools developed by the International Mental Health Policy and Services Project to assist policy-makers in developing evidence-based mental health policies (Gulbinat *et al.* 2004; Jenkins *et al.* 2004). This project aimed to increase the accessibility, availability and use of information to policy-makers in order to help guide evidence-based mental health policy development around the world.

The mental health situational analysis contained in the MHCP provides information about countries' social and physical context, including their population needs and demands, their available resources and service provision models, and health and social outcomes. The Profile aims to aid mental health policy development in five ways. First, it provides policy-makers with a tool that *gathers and describes local information* that is appropriate for assessing the overall mental health situation in a *standardized* way that, nonetheless, *captures the local sociocultural context*. Second, it is a tool that can be used to review existing mental health policy. Third, it serves as an *enabling tool* that will alert and inform policy-makers, professionals and other key stakeholders on important issues that need to be considered in mental health policy development. Fourth, it provides detailed country-specific information in a *systematic format*, which will facilitate global sharing of experiences of mental health reform and strategies between policy-makers and other stakeholders. Fifth, it is designed to be a *capacity-building tool*, used not by external consultants, but by local stakeholders to enhance their capacity for situation appraisal and hence mental health policy development and implementation. It does not seek to rank countries, nor to produce artificial typologies, but rather to explore in an objective manner the complexity of the relationships within and between countries in relation to context, need, inputs, processes and outcome of the complex social, health and welfare systems as they impact on mental health.

Enhance accessibility of information

It is important to make as much use of the existing evidence base on effective (and cost-effective) interventions as possible. While evaluation undertaken in a specific country may be limited, policy decisions may be informed by the examination of international experience. This must be done carefully; findings in one context may not be generalizable to different settings where structures, resources and culture may be very different. There are also separate issues around the capacity to understand and interpret information even when it is available.

There are a variety of international sources of information that may be of use in the policy development process. These include the work of the Cochrane Collaboration (www.cochrane.org) which publishes systematic reviews of evidence on the effectiveness of health interventions as well as the work of various health technology assessment agencies and research councils including the National Institute for Health and Clinical Excellence in England (NICE – www.nice.org.uk), the Netherlands' Organization for Health Research and Development (www.zonmw.nl) and the National Board for Health and Welfare in Finland (www.stakes.fi).

These sources of evidence are very helpful in increasing access to the evidence base although, as yet, they contain much less information on the broader questions beyond specific medicines, psychological interventions and specific service structures such as 24-hour nursing care and vocational training/ rehabilitation. There is, for instance, less (albeit growing) research related to mental health promotion (a database is being developed at www.imhpa.net), multi-sectoral interventions to tackle stigma and the effective coordination of community-based care by different agencies.

A sister organization to Cochrane, the Campbell Collaboration (www.campbellcollaboration.org), reviews and synthesizes evidence on social and behavioural interventions and public policy, including education, criminal justice and social welfare, among other areas. Its primary concern is evidence on overall intervention or policy effectiveness and how effectiveness is influenced by variations in process and implementation, intervention components and recipients, as well as other factors. Systematic reviews relevant to mental health are underway. Other useful sources of information include the WHO's Health Evidence Network (http://www.euro.who.int/hen) which has produced a number of syntheses on the effectiveness of interventions for mental health (see Gilbody 2004; Guo and Harstall 2004; Thornicroft and Tansella 2004).

As discussed in Chapter 4, information on the cost-effectiveness of interventions can help to make the best use of limited resources and help build the case for investment in mental health. There are a number of different sources of information on the cost-effectiveness of different interventions. Perhaps the most useful of these is the continuously updated WHO Choice (Choosing Interventions that are Cost Effective) database (www.who.int/choice/en/). The database contains information on the most cost-effective approaches to tackle alcohol-related disorders (Chisholm *et al.* 2004a) and depression (Chisholm *et al.* 2004b) across three different regions of Europe (and other regions of the world), each distinguished by their level of available resources. Another useful source of information is the NHS Economic Evaluation Database hosted by the Centre for Reviews and Dissemination at the University of York (www.york.ac.uk/inst/crd/crddatabases.htm). This contains information on several thousand economic evaluations of relevance to the United Kingdom's NHS, including many on mental health-related issues.

Planning future research and development to support evidence-informed mental health policy

It is important to consider how to prioritize and fill in gaps in existing knowledge. National policy is about setting a broad vision and broad brush strategy so it may have to address issues that are as yet unresearched or inadequately researched. How should policy-makers proceed when an evaluative study has not been done, and indeed, may not be able to be done; or has been done in another context which may not be applicable? How can the evidence base be strengthened to begin to plug this gap?

There are many examples of policies being tried out in one or several places in a somewhat ad hoc way, with inferences being drawn from an apparent impact on the ground. Some well-intentioned social policy interventions intuitively thought to be effective have been found to have unfortunate or indeed very harmful consequences when assessed empirically (Petrosino *et al.* 2000). Turning to mental health, within the United Kingdom and Ireland alone, historically, policy initiatives were sometimes tried out within one administrative area before widespread implementation. For example, the first high security psychiatric hospital, Dundrum, was established in Ireland in the nineteenth century in the form of a 'criminal lunatic asylum' (Walsh and Daly 2004). This led to the later establishment of similar hospitals in Scotland and England, all of which are still in operation. However, by present research standards this would be regarded as far from optimal, as the results of a single case study could be open to interpretations that are far from empirically sound. The introduction of 24-hour nursed beds, in contrast, was based on evidence drawn from comparative case evaluations in Worcester and Manchester (Woolf and Goldberg 1988; NHS Executive 1996).

Learning from evaluation of the Care Programme Approach

Past experience can also help us to think carefully about the design of future studies so that they can address questions that policy-makers want to answer. It also emphasizes the importance of careful interpretation of study findings and using caution when drawing conclusions. Again, looking at the United Kingdom, the Care Programme Approach (CPA) is an example of a policy that was introduced in response to public (and hence political) pressure following a clinical incident. It was also introduced in the light of other countries' innovative developments around case management, but was not a direct transportation of other country models; rather this was an approach unique to the United Kingdom. The programme was not based on a prior CPA study, nor was it the same model as that used in case management trials which were subsequently conducted by a number of research teams in the United Kingdom. The key components of the CPA were: the existence of a key worker rather than a case manager; assessment; a care plan; and regular review as necessary.

Case management trials conducted, and subsequently reviewed in a Cochrane review (Marshall *et al.* 1998), were, in fact, about a case management model in which a specific case manager (not a key worker) was assigned to a client. Furthermore, the United Kingdom trials of case management were conducted after the introduction of CPA, and so the control populations were, at least theoretically, (also) in receipt of CPA. The outcome variables chosen for evaluation in the Cochrane review included hospital readmissions and it was assumed that this was an undesirable outcome. Yet, it was just as likely that increased attention to clients led to less neglect; thus for many, if the need for a hospital admission arose, this may have been an appropriate event.

So for all these reasons, the United Kingdom case management trials were not in any sense an evaluation of CPA as used in the United Kingdom, but that was exactly what the Cochrane review claimed them to be. This is a good example of how even rigorous reviews may be flawed by subjective bias. In retrospect, it is a helpful exercise to consider whether trials should have been conducted on the separate and joint components of the CPA, or whether it was reasonable for policy-makers to assume that the key components were sufficiently well understood to be of clinical value.

Making use of multi-level approaches to evaluation

One way in which the strength of the evidence base for policy-making may be improved is to make greater use of evaluation designs such as cluster randomized trials. It is vital to understand the need for multi-level approaches to the design and interpretation of such evaluations of policy changes. In most, if not all, examples one is interested in at least two levels: the effect on individuals (or on households and families) and the effect on a higher-level unit which might be schools, communities, institutions such as prisons and so on. Policy may be implemented at the higher-level unit while the aim may well be to achieve a benefit at the individual level. Clustering is the phenomenon whereby the effect on individuals tends to be similar among individuals who are embedded within a higher-level unit. Thus, outcomes for children will be affected in part by the characteristics of their school, and outcomes for patients by the characteristics of the specialist or primary care clinical service they attend. We are not aware of formal guidance on the use of such methodologies in relation to implementing governmental or administrative policies. However, an excellent guide to multi-level methodologies used in the evaluation of health care systems has been published by Health Technology Assessment (Ukoumunne *et al.* 1999). This guide covers formal randomized experimental evaluations as well as the design and interpretation of naturally-occurring phenomena.

Invest in the development of knowledge transfer mechanisms between policy-makers and other stakeholders

We began this chapter by noting that too often evidence has little impact on policy-making, or such evidence is lost within the myriad of different political and public demands, anecdotes, myths and lobbying that policy-makers have to contend with. Three specific types of questions are likely to arise from policy-makers (Lomas 2005). In addition to the question familiar to those looking at issues in EBM as to whether something works (with greater emphasis on setting and context), policy-makers are also likely to simply want to know whether an issue is something significant that merits attention. If it is significant, what is causing this, how extensive is it, who is it affecting and what are some possible options for addressing it? A third question relates to the consequences of under-taking a specific action. This is, again, a context question to help inform the stakeholder – issues may include identifying those interest groups who support or oppose the action and why, as well as looking at who will be affected, with what consequences and what possible side-effects. It may also consider what other actions should be taken alongside the planned action or reform.

Formulating and implementing mental health policy is thus heavily dependent on political support and building partnerships and coalitions between different stakeholder groups. One key issue is how to improve the linkages and opportunities for exchange of information between those individuals generating evidence and those who wish to make use of evidence. This objective should consider how to ensure that evidence from all perspectives, including those of service users and families, has an opportunity to inform the policy-making process. Structures and mechanisms for user involvement have been particularly weak across most of Europe. In some of the countries of central and eastern Europe, the challenge is even greater still as there has been little culture of community involvement in policy-making with no history of users and families forming themselves into non-governmental bodies to put forward a case for greater attention to mental health. Later in this section we will look at an example of an approach to foster such local participation in the policy-making process.

The context in which evidence is used is crucial; there may be a limited *institutional* and *individual* capacity to interpret and make use of evidence alongside other information sources (Lomas 2000; Oliver and McDaid 2002; Lavis *et al.* 2003). How can we further develop the capacity within the policy-making community (and indeed among other stakeholders) to interpret the different sources of evidence, each using their own methodologies with all their attendant strengths and weakness? How can we ensure that people have a better under-standing of the fact that a lack of evidence on the effectiveness of an interven-tion does not equate with evidence of a lack of effect? Perhaps most critically, how can policy-makers and their advisers more easily identify badly-conducted, poor-quality studies that otherwise erroneously may have an impact on policy and practice and deny scarce resources to other more effective activities? Approaches to improving capacity within the policy community in order to interpret and make use of information will be discussed further below.

Meeting the challenge of knowledge transfer

It is important to recognize that knowledge transfer is complex: decision-making is never a simple linear process where information from knowledge producers and others informs the policy-making process. Rather, there are many competing factors and influences that must be taken into account; for instance, political considerations, industry, service and family group advocacy, as well as ethical and equity concerns. Public inquiries, which sometimes take place over many years, may also be a driver of policy. A series of public inquiries into mental health in New Zealand have been closely linked to the development of mental health policy in that country (Brunton 2005). Policy-making might also be influenced (for better or worse) by the personal experience of policy-makers of mental health problems in their own families, as well as by scandals or events reported in the media. For instance, it was one television documentary about conditions at an asylum on the island of Leros in Greece in the early 1980s rather than any scientific evidence that provided the impetus for mental health system reform (Strutti and Rauber 1994).

With the relatively rare example of the Leros situation and other scandals and sensational events, in most instances it can take much time for evidence to inform the policy-making process – decisions are unlikely to be made in response to one piece of information (a knowledge-driven approach). The many models of research utilization (Hanney *et al.* 2003) also include various political and problem-solving models all the way through to suggesting that informa-tion may have a pervasive 'enlightening' impact over time, helping to build awareness and to promote the future acceptability of pieces of knowledge (Weiss 1979).

It should also be remembered that measuring the impact of evidence in the policy-making process can itself be an extremely complex and difficult task, requiring a high degree of access to the decision-making process in order to truly identify connections between evidence and policy. It is especially difficult when, as a result of new evidence, the status quo is maintained, so on the surface, at least, nothing appears to have changed. Furthermore, even when an apparent link can be observed between the publication of a specific report and changes in policy and practice, such information in fact may simply be used as a justification for a preordained action or something that policy-makers already believe in (Weiss 1999).

Nevertheless, if we are to improve the facilitation of knowledge transfer in the policy-making process it is helpful to understand some of the practical barriers that have to be overcome. These can include the absence of personal contact between those generating evidence and the policy-making community. It may also be the case that evidence does not provide answers to the key policy questions of interest to decision-makers. Reports may be incomprehensible and a lack of transparency in how results are reported may make comparisons between studies with conflicting results difficult.

The environment in which policy development, legislation and implementation operates also needs to be fully understood. This policy environment includes the structures in ministries of health, the dynamics and tensions between ministers, civil servants, professional advisers within government, professional advisers outside government, the influence of users and carers, the influence of the media and of the general public, and the influence of related professionals (e.g. lawyers specializing in mental health legislation). There can be a gulf of understanding between these different groups, who effectively speak different languages, have different conceptual frameworks for their understanding of mental health issues, and have differing degrees of access to the available information. Frequent staff moves and organizational changes compound the difficulty of developing a shared understanding and shared goals and strategies. Frequent personnel moves, especially of ministers, means that there is an inevitable discrepancy between the timescales allowed for policy development and the timescales for research evaluation, so that policy development nearly always runs faster than research timetables.

Building links between stakeholders

Good personal links between researchers and policy-makers allow for an iterative process of dialogue and an exchange of views to take place. Bringing both groups together at an early stage, along with other key stakeholders, in order to identify research questions, which are both of policy relevance and feasible from the point of view of research, has been shown to be effective. Partnerships set up between groups for the purpose of developing and implementing policy can be more effective both in producing research and in its effective dissemination (Walter *et al.* 2003, 2005). A supportive environment can also help in the uptake of research. Such a partnership model has been created with some success in linking a university-based research unit with the mental health policy branch of the Ontario provincial government (Goering *et al.* 2003).

Promoting user involvement in the policy-making process: the example of the Pathways to Policy project

There is increasing recognition that users, families and other grass-roots stakeholders, including informal and formal carers, professionals and managers, historically have been excluded from the existing policy process. Advocacy within the policy-making community by these groups can help promote improved quality and better appropriateness of services; therefore, mechanisms to promote the opportunity for advocacy need to be fostered (Funk *et al.* 2005). Examples of how to tackle this objective include the establishment of local and national policy forums which can now be found in several countries in western

Europe, and increasingly, in some countries of eastern Europe. By involving users and local stakeholders in social change, mental health policy and practice can have greater ownership and investment from all sectors of society, especially those who have been excluded (Barham 1992). Local expertise and real-world knowledge can be harnessed.

While civil society structures are relatively well established in western Europe, their recent development in central and eastern Europe, coupled with greater local democracy and local institutional frameworks for expressing the plurality of views in mental health, provided a new impetus for more transparency in the creation and evaluation of policy options. There has been an opportunity for the promotion of mental health issues to be seen as fundamental to citizenship and human rights; it is no longer seen as a separate issue but an integral part of the wider human-development agenda (Cutler and Hayward 2005, 2006).

The Pathways to Policy project established in partnership with local mental health NGOs in five countries (Estonia, Bosnia and Herzegovina, Romania, Armenia and Kyrgyzstan), focused on the development of new skills and knowledge to build capacity to participate in local service situation appraisal, advocacy, dialogue with professionals on assessments and treatment plans, and the development of strategic multi-sectoral relationships in order to achieve change. The overall aims were to increase active participation in the local policy process and raise public awareness about mental health.

The project evolved as a result of the changing interests and vision of local groups in central and eastern Europe demanding to have a voice at a wider community level (Barham and Hayward 1995). Strategic changes in the region and the development of civil society provided a backdrop to this precedent. A theme emerged of increased confidence and awareness among local grass-roots stakeholders that they had both the right and ability to engage in mental health policy. There was also a recognition that users, families and other local community actors had been excluded from existing policy processes (Cutler and Hayward 2003). The project demonstrated the benefits that can be acquired by local stakeholders as part of the process of participating in the policy-making process. This 'policy-as-process model' highlighted the importance of how policy was made, and focused on the success of the project in building local policy capacity and mechanisms for dialogue rather than on the outcomes of any particular policy. Four fundamental measures of progress in capacity-building were observed.[2]

The first was the development of new skills and knowledge to build local policy capacities. Users of mental health services, their families and carers, their NGOs and other local mental health stakeholders in each of the five Pathways to Policy countries were able to develop new skills and knowledge about advocacy and policy. These skills were used to undertake local action to improve the quality of life of individuals and groups of people with mental health problems. Links with policy-makers meant that this learning experience worked both ways; for example, at a Tallinn policy workshop a member of the mental health section of the Estonian Ministry of Social Affairs was asked to work in a small group with several users. She later commented that she learned more about the reality of local mental health housing projects from that discussion than from a formal evaluation of the service and had become convinced of the value of service-user assessment of services.

The second measure of progress was the development of new strategic relationships for change. Users of mental health services and a wide range of other local stakeholders formed new, stronger and sustainable relationships with each other. This enabled them to learn from each other, form partnerships and alliances, and ultimately have a greater influence on local mental health policies and practices. The Tallinn forum collaborated on a state-led review of mental health policy, contributing to a national mental health policy framework document. As a result of the project, service users also acquired a greater voice in mental health policy at a local level through active and visible participation on the local policy forums and local action plans. The fourth fundamental achievement was the raising of public awareness of mental health issues through both the local policy forums and the positive contribution and expertise of (ex) users of mental health services in working with the media and the public. Some additional, specific examples of other actions which helped develop capacity and facilitated in creating a greater role for service users in the policy-making process are shown in Box 5.2.

Early on in this chapter we emphasized the value of using different research methods to obtain evidence not only on what works, but also on the context, culture and structures within a system. We have also highlighted that the perspectives of service users and families can differ markedly from those of other groups, and it is important that these perspectives are part of the multiple source of information that is used to promote evidence-informed policy. The Pathways

Box 5.2   Examples of capacity developments fostered by the Pathways to Policy project

- Greater knowledge on the state of local services.
- Development of a small network of lawyers providing advocacy for service users.
- Media contact with user groups led to isolated service users coming into contact with policy forums and mental health organizations.
- Service users trained GPs and the police to raise awareness of the needs of people with mental health problems.
- Input into national mental health policy framework documents.
- Service users played a prominent role in leading public consultations, meaning that issues of great importance, such as barriers to employment, were highlighted.
- Increased assertiveness and confidence of users involved in local policy forums.
- Opportunities for dialogue between service users and the judiciary over involuntary admissions procedures.

to Policy project, through its various policy workshops, open forums and public consultations helped to identify not only a number of very specific localized issues, but also a number of broad concerns that applied across all the countries covered, including difficulties in accessing information at a local level on a variety of issues, such as human rights, alternative treatments, medication side-effects and policy alternatives.

Overall, the project demonstrated that it is possible to create linkages for exchange and dialogue between the users of mental health services, carers and families, and other stakeholders including policy-makers in countries where conditions for the development of evidence-informed mental health policy are still limited. New and sustainable relationships were forged, resulting in innovative learning, partnerships and alliances that have been both influential and beneficial to local mental health policy and practices, and have helped to challenge the pervading views on mental health policy and practice.

Building receptor capacity to promote evidence-informed policy-making

One of the challenges that policy-makers have to face is sifting through information arising from numerous studies, each of differing quality and using different research methods. What relevance will a study on community care provision in the United Kingdom have for decision-makers in Poland? If cognitive behavioural therapy works in Madrid, will it work in Oslo or Sofia? If a national programme for suicide prevention works in Scotland, will it work in Bavaria? How can the 'receptor capacity' of the policy-making community – that is, its ability to interpret and assess the relevance of different sources of evidence, as well as engage with those different groups that produce evidence – be strengthened?

Often, reports are long and highly technical, making it unlikely that they will be read by policy-makers. Indeed, those who produce evidence have been described as living in a completely separate community from policy-makers. These two communities can have great difficulty in communicating; they may also harbour a sense of mutual mistrust (Innvaer et al. 2002). There is a clear need for short, concise documents highlighting the key potential outcomes and consequences of any one intervention or strategy.

This is not to say that detailed information on evidence should not be provided; rather, this should be targeted not at time-constrained policy-makers but at their key civil servants and policy advisers. The recommendations of these advisers can play a key role in determining the direction of policy. One further way of improving the 'receptor capacity' of both communities to each others' ideas may be through the use of so-called 'knowledge brokers', individuals with some training in the technical aspects of health service research, but who are also comfortable in a policy-making environment. Typically, these individuals are employed as advisers within ministries of health but may have good links to the research and other stakeholder communities. They can help filter the many different types of information that constantly bombard the political and policy-making process. This type of role may be particularly appropriate if there is a high turnover of civil servants, as occurs in some political systems. Such knowledge brokers have been employed with some success in Canada to link researchers with mental health policy-makers (Goering *et al.* 2003).

Regardless of whether knowledge brokers are employed, it is impossible to make more than the most cursory of assessments of evidence from both quantitative and qualitative research, if it is not presented in a transparent and clear manner. This should include: clearly presenting the research questions a study sought to address; the methodologies used; how study populations and study samples were determined; what exclusion criteria were applied; and whether evaluators and researchers were independent of study funders. Well-developed international guidelines are available for both qualitative and quantitative research methods. A well-known guideline for RCTs is the CONSORT (Consolidated Standards of Reporting Trials) statement which is intended to help authors improve reporting by using a 22-point checklist (Moher 1998). The QUORUM group, using a similar approach, have produced a checklist for the reporting of meta-analyses of RCTs (Moher *et al.* 1999) and there is guidance from the Cochrane Collaboration on methods for reporting the results of systematic reviews. Similarly, the methods and background to survey instruments can be presented while guidelines are also available for qualitative studies which can help indicate, for instance, what the composition of focus groups should be and how the responses to questions are recorded and/or interpreted (Pope *et al.* 2002).

Conclusions

The notion of EBM is frequently understood as a rather narrow concept. It has mostly been applied to medicines, somewhat to psychological interventions, rather less so for complex interventions, and only rarely for whole service structures. EBM, complemented by other sources of information that address issues such as satisfaction and appropriateness of services, is an essential tool in the process of formulating mental health policy. It is, however, but one of a number of inputs into this process.

Evidence-informed policy is not simply a summation of disparate pieces of EBM, but rather an approach with its own unique requirements, processes and constraints. Therefore, it is clear that conceptual tools are needed to help planners and policy-makers design and reform strategies, and to predict and subsequently trace the effects of policy, institutional and health system change (Cassells 1995). It is important that conceptual tools respond to the charge that, historically, attention has been paid to the content of health sector reform, to the extent that the players and processes involved and the context within which the policy is developed have been ignored (Walt and Gilson 1994; Koivusalo and Ollila 1998). It is also critical that sufficient time, resources and attention are invested in creating the conditions for policy dialogue between all stakeholders including service users. In some European countries, where resources and interest in mental health policy are limited, bottom-up advocacy and capacity-building can have an important role in helping to place mental health on the policy agenda, and perhaps also encourage the development of policy at both local and national levels.

Finally, it is important to stress that evidence-informed policy can only occur if those who ultimately take decisions have the skills, or access to support, to interpret and weigh up many different sources of (often conflicting) evidence and information. Knowledge broking represents one potential means of achieving this and will itself require careful evaluation.

Notes

1   For instance one Finnish database has recorded more than 15,000 trials. See http:// psitri.stakes.fi.
2   For fuller accounts see Cutler and Hayward (2005, 2006).

References

Avon Measure Working Group (1996) *The Avon Mental Health Measure. A User Approach to Assessing Need*. London: MIND.

Barham, P. (1992) *Closing the Asylum*. Harmondsworth: Penguin.

Barham, P. and Hayward, R. (1995) *Relocating Madness*. London: FAB.

Black, N. (1996) Why we need observational studies to evaluate the effectiveness of health care, *British Medical Journal*, 312: 1215–18.

British Medical Research Council (1948) Streptomycin treatment of pulmonary tuberculosis, *British Medical Journal*, 2: 768–82.

Brunton, W. (2005) The place of public inquiries in shaping New Zealand's national mental health policy, 1858–1996, *Australia and New Zealand Health Policy*, 2: 24.

Cassells, A. (1995) *Health Sector Reform: Key Issues in Less Developed Countries*. Geneva: World Health Organization, WHO/SH5/NHP/95.4.

Chisholm, D., Rehm, J., van Ommeren, M. and Monteiro, M. (2004a) Reducing the global burden of hazardous alcohol use: a comparative cost-effectiveness analysis, *Journal of Studies on Alcohol*, 65(6): 782–93.

Chisholm, D., Sanderson, K., Ayuso-Mateos, J.L. and Saxena, S. (2004b) Reducing the global burden of depression: population-level analysis of intervention cost-effectiveness in 14 world regions, *British Journal of Psychiatry*, 184: 393–403.

Cochrane, A.L. (1973) *Effectiveness and Efficiency: Random Reflections on Health Services*. London: Nuffield Provincial Hospitals Trust.

Commission of the European Communities (2005) *Improving the Mental Health of the Population: Towards a Strategy on Mental Health for the European Union*. Green Paper. Brussels: Health and Consumer Protection Directorate, European Commission.

Cutler, P. and Hayward, R. (2003) Grass-roots initiatives in mental health policy in Eastern Europe, *Eurohealth*, 8(5): 39–42.

Cutler, P. and Hayward, R. (2005) *Exploring the Usefulness of the Policy-as-process Model to Mental Health NGOs Working in Eastern Europe and Central Asia*. Centre for Reflection on Mental Health Policy Research Paper. Canterbury: Interaction Press.

Cutler, P. and Hayward, R. (2006) Stakeholder involvement: a challenge for intergovernmental organizations, *Journal of Public Mental Health*, 5(1): 14–17.

Evidence Based Medicine Working Group (1992) Evidence-based medicine: a new approach to teaching the practice of medicine, *Journal of the American Medical Association*, 268(17): 2420–5.

Frenk, J. (1994) Dimensions of health system reform, *Health Policy*, 27(1): 119–34.

Funk, M., Minoletti, A., Drew, N., Taylor, J. and Saraceno, B. (2005) Advocacy for mental health: roles for consumer and family organizations and governments, *Health Promotion International*, 21(1): 70–5.

Gilbody, S. (2004) What is the Evidence on Effectiveness of Capacity-building of Primary Health Care Professionals in the Detection, Management and Outcome of Depression? Copenhagen: World Health Organization.

Glover, G. and Sinclair-Smith, H. (2000) Computerized information systems in English mental health care providers in 1998, *Social Psychiatry and Psychiatric Epidemiology*, 35(11): 518–22.

Goering, P., Butterill, D., Jacobson, N. and Sturtevant, D. (2003) Linkage and exchange at the organizational level: a model of collaboration between research and policy, *Journal of Health Services Research and Policy*, 8(Suppl 2): 14–19.

Green, A. (1999) *An Introduction to Health Planning in Developing Countries*. Oxford: Oxford University Press.

Gulbinat, W., Manderscheid, R., Baingana, F., Jenkins, R. *et al.* (2004) The International Consortium on Mental Health Policy and Services: objectives, design and project implementation, *International Review of Psychiatry*, 16(1–2): 5–17.

Guo, B. and Harstall, C. (2004) *For which Strategies of Suicide Prevention is there Evidence of Effectiveness?* Copenhagen: World Health Organization.

Hafner, H. and Heiden, W. (1991) Methodology of evaluative studies in the mental health field, in H. Freeman and J. Henderson (eds) *Evaluation of Comprehensive Care of the Mentally Ill*. London: Gaskell.

Hanney, S.R., Gonzalez-Block, M.A., Buxton, M.J. and Kogan, M. (2003) The utilization of health research in policy making: concepts, examples and methods of assessment, *Health Research and Policy Systems*, 1(2): 1–28.

Herbert, R.D. and Bø, K. (2005) Analysis of quality of interventions in systematic reviews, *British Medical Journal*, 331: 507–9.

Hurst, J. (1991) Reforming health care in seven European nations, *Health Affairs*, 10(3): 7–21.

Innvaer, S., Vist, G., Trommald, M. and Oxman, A. (2002) Health policy makers' perceptions of their use of evidence: a systematic review, *Journal of Health Services Research and Policy*, 7(4): 239–44.

Institute of Medicine (2001) *Neurological, Psychiatric and Development Disorders: Meeting the Challenge of the Developing World*. Washington, DC: National Academy Press.

Jenkins, R. (1990) Towards a system of outcome indicators for mental health care, *British Journal of Psychiatry*, 157: 500–14.

Jenkins, R. (2001) Making psychiatric epidemiology useful: the contribution of epidemiology to government policy, *Acta Psychiatrica Scandinavica*, 103(1): 2–14.

Jenkins, R. and Meltzer, H. (eds) (2003) A decade of national surveys of psychiatric epidemiology in Great Britain: 1990–2000, *International Review of Psychiatry*, 15(1–2): 5–200.

Jenkins, R., McCulloch, A., Friedli, L. and Parker, C. (2002) *Developing a National Mental Health Policy*. Hove: Psychology Press.

Jenkins, R., Gulbinat, W., Manderscheid, R., Baingana, F. *et al.* (2004) The mental health country profile: background, design and use of a systematic method of appraisal, *International Review of Psychiatry*, 16(1–2): 31–47.

Jick, T.D. (1979) Mixing qualitative and quantitative methods: triangulation in action, *Administrative Science Quarterly*, 24(4): 602–11.

Kelle, U. (2001) Sociological explanations between micro and macro and the integration of qualitative and quantitative methods, *Forum Qualitative Sozial Forschung/Forum Quantitative Social Research*, 2(1), available at http://qualitative-research.net/fqs-eng.htm.

Koivusalo, M. and Ollila, E. (1998) *Making a Healthy World: Agencies, Actors and Policies in International Health*. London: Zed Books.

Lavis, J., Robertson, D., Woodside, J.M., McLeod, C.B. and Abelson, J. (2003) How can research organization more effectively transfer research knowledge to decision makers? *Milbank Quarterly*, 81(2): 221–48.

Lavis, J., Davies, H., Oxman, A., Denis, J.L., Golden-Biddle, K. and Ferlie, E. (2005) Towards systematic reviews that inform health care management and policy-making, *Journal of Health Services Research and Policy*, 10(Suppl 1): 35–48.

Lewis, G., Pelosi, A., Araya, R. and Dunn, G. (1992) Measuring psychiatric disorder in the community: a standardized assessment for use by lay interviewers, *Psychological Medicine*, 22(2): 465–86.

Lomas, J. (2000) Using linkage and exchange to move research into policy at a Canadian Foundation, *Health Affairs*, 19(3): 236–40.

Lomas, J. (2005) Using research to inform healthcare managers and policy makers' questions: from summative to interpretive synthesis, *Healthcare Policy*, 1(1): 55–71.

Malterud, K. (2001) Qualitative research: standards, challenges, and guidelines, *Lancet*, 358: 483–8.

Marshall, M., Gray, A., Lockwood, A. and Green, R. (1998) Case management for people with severe mental disorders, *The Cochrane Database of Systematic Reviews*, 2: Art. No.: CD000050. DOI: 10.1002/14651858.CD000050.

Marshall, M., Hogg, L.I. and Lockwood, A. (1995) The Cardinal Needs Schedule – a modified version of the MRC Needs for Care Assessment Schedule, *Psychological Medicine*, 25(3): 605–17.

Mays, N., Pope, C. and Popay, J. (2005) Systematically reviewing qualitative and quantitative evidence to inform management and policy-making in the health field, *Journal of Health Services Research and Policy*, 10(Suppl 1): 6–20.

Moher, D. (1998) CONSORT: an evolving tool to help improve the quality of reports of randomized controlled trials: consolidated standards of reporting trials, *Journal of the American Medical Association*, 279(18): 1489–91.

Moher, D., Cook, D.J., Eastwood, S., Olkin, I., Rennie, D. and Stroup, D.F. (1999) Improving the quality of reports of meta-analyses of randomized controlled trials: the QUOROM statement: quality of reporting of meta-analyses, *Lancet*, 354(9193): 1896–900.

Muir-Gray, J.M. (1996) *Evidence-based Healthcare*. London: Churchill Livingstone.

Murray, C. and Frenk, J. (2000) A framework for assessing the performance of health systems, *Bulletin of the World Health Organization*, 78(6): 717–39.

Newburn, T. (2001) What do we mean by evaluation? *Children and Society*, 15(1): 5–13.

NHS Executive (1996) *24 Hour Nursed Care for People with Severe and Enduring Mental Illness*. Leeds: NHS Executive.

Oliver, A. and McDaid, D. (2002) Evidence-based health care: benefits and barriers, *Social Policy and Society*, 1(3): 183–90.

Pawson, R., Greenhalgh, T., Harvey, G. and Walshe, K. (2005) Realist review – a new method of systematic review designed for complex policy interventions, *Journal of Health Services Research and Policy*, 10(Suppl 1): 21–34.

Petrosino, A., Turpin-Petrosino, C. and Finckenauer, J. (2000) Well meaning programs can have harmful effects! Lessons from experiments of programs such as Scared Straight, *Crime & Delinquency*, 46(3): 354–79.

Petticrew, M. and Roberts, H. (2003) Evidence, hierarchies, and typologies: horses for courses, *Journal of Epidemiology and Community Health*, 57(7): 527–9.

Phelan, M., Slade, M., Thornicroft, G., Dunn, G., Holloway, F., Wykes, T., Strathdee, G., Loftus, L., McCrone, P. and Hayward, P. (1995) The Camberwell Assessment of Need: the validity and reliability of an instrument to assess the needs of people with severe mental illness, *British Journal of Psychiatry*, 167: 585–9.

Pope, C., van Royen, P. and Baker, R. (2002) Qualitative methods in research on healthcare quality, *Quality and Safety in Health Care*, 11(2): 148–52.

Roemer, M. (1991) *National Health Systems of the World*. Oxford: Oxford University Press.

Rose, D., Wykes, T., Leese, M., Bindman, J. and Fleischman, P. (2003) Patients' perspectives on electroconvulsive therapy: systematic review, *British Medical Journal*, 326: 1363–8.

Rose, D., Thornicroft, G. and Slade, M. (2006) Who decides what evidence is? Developing a multiple perspectives paradigm in mental health, *Acta Psychiatrica Scandinavica Supplementum*, 429: 109–14.

Sanderson, I. (2000) Evaluation in complex policy systems, *Evaluation*, 6(4): 433–54.

Sheldon, T.A. (2005) Making evidence synthesis more useful for management and policy-making, *Journal of Health Services Research and Policy*, 10(Suppl 1): 1–5.

Smith, G. (1989) Development of rapid epidemiologic assessment methods to evaluate health status and delivery of health services, *International Journal of Epidemiology*, 18: S2–15.

Strutti, C. and Rauber, S. (1994) Leros and the Greek mental health system, *International Journal of Social Psychiatry*, 40(4): 306–12.

Tansella, M., Thornicroft, G., Barbui, C., Cipriani, A. and Saraceno, B. (2006) Seven criteria for improving effectiveness trials in psychiatry, *Psychological Medicine*, 36(5): 711–20.

Thornicroft, G. and Tansella, M. (2004) Components of a modern mental health service: a pragmatic balance of community and hospital care. Overview of systematic evidence. *British Journal of Psychiatry*, 185: 283–90.

Ukoumunne, O., Gulliford, M., Chinn, S., Sterne, J. and Burney, P. (1999) Methods for evaluating area-wide and organization-based interventions in health and health care: a systematic review, *Health Technology Assessment*, 3(5): 1–92.

Walsh, D. and Daly, A. (2004) *Mental Illness in Ireland 1750–2002: Reflections on the Rise and Fall of Institutional Care*. Dublin: Health Research Board.

Walt, G. and Gilson, L. (1994) Reforming the health sector in developing countries: the central role of policy analysis, *Health Policy and Planning*, 9(4): 353–70.

Walter, I., Davies, H. and Nutley, S. (2003) Increasing research impact through partnerships: evidence from outside health care, *Journal of Health Services Research and Policy*, 8(Suppl 2): 58–61.

Walter, I., Nutley, S. and Davies, H. (2005) What works to promote evidence-based practice? A cross-sector review, *Evidence and Policy*, 1(3): 335–63.

Weightman, A., Ellis, S., Cullum, A., Sander, L. and Turley, R. (2005) *Grading Evidence and Recommendations for Public Health Interventions: Developing and Piloting a Framework*. London: Health Development Agency.

Weiss, C. (1979) The many meanings of research utilization, *Public Administration Review*, 39(5): 426–31.

Weiss, C. (1999) The interface between evaluation and public policy, *Evaluation*, 5(4): 468–86.

Wing, J.K., Babor, T., Brugha, T., Burke, J., Cooper, J., Goel, R., Jablensky, A., Regier, D. and Sartorius, N. (1990) SCAN schedules for clinical assessment in neuropsychiatry, *Archives of General Psychiatry*, 47(6): 586–93.

Wing, J.K., Beevor, A., Curtis, R., Park, S., Haddon, S. and Burns, A. (1998) Health of the Nation Outcome Scales (HoNOS), research and development, *British Journal of Psychiatry*, 172: 11–18.

Wittchen, H.-U. and Jacobi, F. (2005) Size and burden of mental disorders in Europe – a critical review and appraisal of 27 studies, *European Neuropsychopharmacology*, 15(4): 357–76.

Woolf, K. and Goldberg, D. (1988) Further observations on the practice of community care in Salford. Differences between community psychiatric nurses and mental health social workers, *British Journal of Psychiatry*, 153: 30–7.

World Health Organization (2004) *Mental Health Policy, Plans and Programmes* (updated version). Geneva: World Health Organization.

World Health Organization (2005a) *Mental Health Declaration for Europe: Facing the Challenges, Building Solutions*. Copenhagen: World Health Organization.

World Health Organization (2005b) *Atlas. Mental Health Resources Around the World*. Geneva: World Health Organization.

World Mental Health Survey Consortium (2004) Prevalence, severity and unmet need for treatment of mental disorders in the World Health Organization World Mental Health Surveys, *Journal of the American Medical Association*, 291(21): 2581–90.

chapter six

Developments in the treatment of mental disorders

Ville Lehtinen, Heinz Katschnig, Viviane Kovess-Masféty and David Goldberg

Introduction

This chapter begins with an introduction defining and briefly describing mental disorders, and outlines the most important intervention categories for their treatment. This is followed by a presentation of some epidemiological data on the need (and especially unmet need) for psychiatric treatment. The development of each treatment category is then described in more detail – covering the categories of pharmacological and other somatic treatments, psychotherapies and psychosocial interventions – with a special focus on the impact that some of these developments have had on health and mental health policies. The importance of integrating the different modes of treatment is underlined throughout the chapter. Finally, we consider possible future developments in treatment.

Definitions of mental health conditions

The understanding and classification of mental illness has changed over time. Traditionally, the main categories have been: psychoses, neuroses, personality disorders, alcoholism and other substance use disorders, and organic mental disorders. Intellectual disability (mental retardation) and even epilepsy have sometimes been regarded as mental disorder categories, particularly in the past and occasionally are still referred to as such in some World Health Organization (WHO) documents. This practice is no longer appropriate as it helps to maintain old prejudices both toward epilepsy and mental health problems. The most recent classifications of diseases, the *International Classification of Diseases – 10* (*ICD-10*) (World Health Organization 1992) and the *Diagnostic and Statistical Manual-IV* (DSM-IV) (American Psychiatric Association 1994), use broadly the same categories as above, although the term 'neurosis', for example, is no longer in widespread use.

The *ICD-10* defines mental disorders as: 'the existence of a clinically recognizable set of symptoms or behaviour, associated in most cases with distress and with interference with personal functions'. The *DSM-IV* classification gives a fuller definition:

a clinically significant behavioural or psychological syndrome or pattern that occurs in an individual and that is associated with present distress (e.g. a painful symptom) or disability (i.e. impairment in one or more important areas of functioning) or with a significantly increased risk of suffering death, pain, disability, or an important loss of freedom. In addition, this syndrome or pattern must not be merely an expectable and culturally sanctioned response to a particular event, for example, the death of a loved one. Whatever its original cause, it must currently be considered a manifestation of a behavioural or biological dysfunction in the individual. Neither deviant behaviour (e.g., political, religious, or sexual) nor conflicts that are primarily between the individual and society are mental disorders unless the deviance or conflict is a symptom of a dysfunction in the individual, as described above.

For most mental health problems aetiology is not fully known. It is clear that for the so-called 'functional' (non-organic) conditions, like schizophrenia or depression, the causes are multiple and heterogeneous. However, from epidemiological and other research we know that many factors contribute to the occurrence of mental illness. These determinants or risk factors can be grouped into the following categories:

- biological factors (like heredity, pre-, peri- and post-natal hazards, physical diseases);
- psychological factors (like early separation, traumatic experiences, low sense of coherence);
- social factors (like lack of social support, low social status, unemployment, societal disintegration).

The stress-vulnerability model, which was originally developed by Zubin and Spring (1977) for schizophrenia, seems to be the most appropriate for explaining most mental disorders. Some of the determinants increase vulnerability, while others function as precipitating or maintaining factors. Increased vulnerability can be caused by hereditary factors, by biological factors affecting brain development during pregnancy, by factors associated with delivery (for example diseases or injuries), but evidently also by psychosocial factors like insecure attachment and maternal separation. In later childhood, physical abuse, sexual abuse and neglect are major causes of mental health problems. Precipitating factors usually include adverse life events or developmental challenges (for example, entering school or leaving the parental home).

The treatment of mental health problems

The treatment of mental illness can be categorized in a similar way to determinants:

- biological treatments: the most important are psychotropic drugs but other treatments can be mentioned, such as electro-convulsive therapy (ECT) and bright light treatment;
- psychological treatments or psychotherapies;
- psychosocial interventions like case management, daily life activities, family interventions, network therapy and counselling.

Although there were some treatment developments in the first half of the twentieth century, there have been enormous developments in the past 50 years (see also Chapter 2). These developments have had an enormous impact on people with mental health problems and their families, as well as on mental health professionals, the care system and the general public. Below, we describe the most important developments in the different treatment categories during the last few decades, and their impacts (both positive and negative).

According to epidemiological surveys in many countries, mental disorders are quite common among the general population (Goldberg and Huxley 1980, 1992; Bland et al. 1994; Kessler et al. 1994; Meltzer et al. 1995; Almeida-Filho et al. 1997; Bijl et al. 1998; Andrews et al. 2001; Jacobi et al. 2004; Kessler et al. 2005; Pirkola et al. 2005). Summarizing these studies, one can conclude that, generally, the prevalence of all mental disorders during the previous month varies between 10 and 15 per cent of the general population, the 6–12-month prevalence rate is 15 to 25 per cent, and the lifetime prevalence rate has reached up to 50 per cent. Studies conducted with children have also shown high prevalence rates: from 10 to 20 per cent among school-aged children (e.g. Fombonne 1994; Puura et al. 1998). Depression and anxiety disorders are the most prevalent mental health problems, followed by substance use disorders among adults. Among children the most common are attention deficit and conduct disorders.

However, the occurrence of mental illness does not always mean the need for treatment, which must be assessed separately (Lehtinen 1985; Bebbington 1990). Assessing the need for treatment is not necessarily an easy task. This is especially true when it comes to the mode of treatment to be offered, despite the publication of several treatment guidelines in the last 20 years (e.g. American Psychiatric Association 2002; National Collaborating Centre for Mental Health 2005). There still exist different schools in psychiatry, for example, with regard to whether psychotherapy or drug treatment should be the treatment of choice. Assessing the need for treatment is therefore easier than deciding what kind of treatment is needed. In epidemiological surveys one also encounters situations where the people in question are either not aware of their mental health problem – and thus are not ready to seek any help – or are aware of somatic symptoms for which no physical cause can be found, and seek help for these rather than the accompanying mental condition. Should such people be counted among those who need treatment?

These problems have certainly contributed to the fact that studies which have explicitly assessed the need for mental health treatment are far rarer than surveys on the occurrence of mental disorders. Table 6.1 gives an overview of some of these studies. As can be seen, according to these studies, about 10 per cent of the population have some self-perceived need for treatment, but many more people who are unaware of their mental health problems can benefit from treatment by their general practitioner (GP) or other staff in primary care.

Epidemiological studies have also shown that the need for treatment of mental health conditions is often unmet (Goldberg and Huxley 1980, 1992; Howard *et al.* 1996; Flisher *et al.* 1997; Kessler *et al.* 2001; McConnell *et al.* 2002; Bebbington *et al.* 2003; World Mental Health Survey Consortium 2004). In the case of depression or anxiety disorder, usually only 20 to 30 per cent receive some treatment, but in psychoses this figure may rise to 80 per cent. The lack of treatment is partly due to insufficient availability of services, partly to unrecognized need, and partly to fear of stigma or other negative societal attitudes.

There are some studies that buck this trend, where higher rates of utilization for common mental health disorders have been observed. The Netherlands Mental Health Survey and Incidence Study (NEMISIS) reported, overall, that in any one 12-month period a third of those with any mental health problem would use either primary care or specialist mental health services. Rates for some sub-groups of the population were much higher than those observed in

Table 6.1 Need for treatment due to mental disorders in some selected population studies

Authors, year	Country	Sample size	Age ranges	Self-perceived need for treatment (%)	Clinical assessment of need for treatment (%)
Weyerer and Dilling (1984)	Germany	1,536	0	8.7	–
Shapiro *et al.* (1984)	USA	3,481	18	13.6	–
Regier *et al.* (1988)	USA	18,571	18	11.2	–
Lehtinen *et al.* (1990)	Finland	7,217	30	8.6	17.2
Lehtinen *et al.* (1993)	Finland	743	31–80	9.6	20.6
McConnell *et al.* (2002)	Northern Ireland	1,242	18–64	–	14.4
Narrow *et al.* (2002)	USA	28,959	18	–	18.5

many other studies. Over 60 per cent of people with mood disorders received some help, and for anxiety disorders this figure was over 40 per cent. One reason put forward to explain such utilization rates was the low financial threshold to access services (Bijl and Ravelli 2000). In Finland, the Mini-Finland Health Survey revealed that almost everyone who received a psychiatric diagnosis had at some time in their life been in contact with a mental health service (Lehtinen *et al.* 1990). These studies illustrate that caution must be exercised when drawing conclusions in cross-country comparisons; some may use very divergent methodologies and focus on different population groups, while health system structures may also have an impact on results.

Pharmacological and other somatic treatments

Somatic treatments for mental disorders can be divided into pharmacological treatment, convulsive therapies, psychosurgery and other treatments such as bright light therapy. Undoubtedly, the most important of these are the psychopharmacological or drug treatments.

Psychotropic drugs

The era of modern psychopharmacology is now about 50 years old (see Chapters 2 and 7). Before 1950 clinical psychiatry had available only a few and very non-specific substances, like opium, chloral, barbiturates and paraldehyde. The 1950s were clearly a turning point. The first neuroleptic drug, chlorpromazine, was synthesized in 1950, the first 'minor tranquillizers' like chlordiazepoxide were launched some years later, and the first antidepressant drugs – imipramine and phenelzine – were in use before the end of that decade. Today, there are more or less specific drugs available for almost every mental disorder, and new psychotropic drugs come onto the market every year. For many psychiatrists psychotropic drugs form the main basis for all treatment of mental illness, and one cannot imagine a modern mental health service system that could manage without them (Bazire 1997; Sussman 2005). Pharmacological treatment has also had the greatest impact on the mental health care system. In the following, the most important psychotropic drugs are described very briefly, although we cannot offer a fully comprehensive account of what is a complex and challenging context.

Antipsychotic drugs or neuroleptics are mainly for the treatment of schizophrenia and other psychoses, conditions in which these are seen as the drugs of choice, although their effect is relatively unspecific and mainly symptomatic (American Psychiatric Association 1997). These drugs decrease hallucinations and delusions, and partly also decrease distorted thinking as well as anxiety and restlessness in patients. Additionally, most of these drugs have a specific mitigating effect which justifies the name 'neuroleptic'. One big problem, especially with the 'old' neuroleptics, is the many side-effects that these drugs cause, especially on the muscular system (tremors and stiffness). Most are disturbing to the patient, some can be life-threatening (malignant neuroleptic syndrome), and some of the long-term effects can be permanent (tardive dyskinesia). Therefore, the classic neuroleptics have been largely replaced by so-called atypical or 'second generation' drugs that have fewer side-effects and perhaps also a better effect on so-called 'negative symptoms' and 'depressive symptoms' (Thomas and Lewis 1998). One of these, clozapine, is often effective when other neuroleptics have failed but it also has a number of side-effects.

Antidepressants are the other important group of psychotropic drugs. They stimulate the psychomotor activity of a depressed person, raise the mood and improve negative thinking. The mode of action of different types of antidepressants is different but their main effect is to increase the amount of serotonin and/or noradrenaline in specific parts of the brain. During the 1990s a group of 'new' antidepressants were launched, with fewer and less severe side-effects but seemingly with no better therapeutic effect (Perry 1996). The increase in the use of these drugs has been enormous in many countries during the last ten or more years (see below). Recently, concerns have been raised about adverse events associated with some of the newer antidepressants (Healy 1998; and see Chapter 7), although generally they are seen to be safer than the older, 'tricyclic' medications they have largely replaced. Another group of drugs useful in the treatment of recurrent depressions are the mood stabilizers (for example, lithium).

Other psychotropic drugs include the anxiolytics or minor tranquillizers, and the hypnotics. One problem connected with these drugs is that they can produce what is called 'low-dose dependence' which makes it difficult for patients to stop their medication. Sometimes they introduce tolerance, meaning that drug doses need to be increased in order to have the required effect. Because of this, there is a risk of misuse or overuse, especially when these drugs are used on a regular or long-term basis.

Other somatic treatments

Convulsive treatments have been used in psychiatry since the 1930s. The use of these treatments has gradually decreased, partly due to ethical problems and partly because more effective and less controversial treatments have been developed. Among these, ECT is the only one still in use to treat severe depressive symptoms. ECT has been shown to be the most effective treatment in severe recurrent depression, especially if associated with a somatic syndrome, severe suicidal ideation or psychotic features (Olfson *et al.* 1998). A relatively new mode of somatic treatments is bright light therapy in the treatment of a specific disorder – seasonal affective disorder or SAD (Lam 1994). Regular daily exposure to bright light seems to both prevent and alleviate these symptoms. Transcranial magnetic stimulation (TMS) and vagus stimulation (VS) also show some promise in treating depression.

Policy impacts and consequences

The launch of modern psychotropic drugs brought about dramatic changes for the whole mental health care system during the post-war period. They have undoubtedly facilitated the reduction in the number of psychiatric hospital beds, often contributing to the closure of mental hospitals. They have also facilitated the building of alternative, community-based treatment systems, and the adaptation of other forms of interventions, like psychotherapies and psychosocial rehabilitation. These developments have improved the situation and quality of life of many people with mental health problems. Adequate drug treatment, often combined with other modes of treatment and rehabilitation, allows patients who were previously bound to mental hospitals as long-term patients to live more or less independently in the community. Of course, drug developments alone cannot explain all of these positive changes, but it seems justified to state that without pharmacological treatments they would not have been possible. Certainly, other factors have been influential, such as the development of other treatment modes, better understanding of, and knowledge about, mental disorders, and broader societal changes, such as more positive attitudes toward people with mental disorders and toward mental health issues in general (see Chapters 3 and 14).

However, the situation is not always as positive as described above. These developments have also produced new problems. The closure of hospitals and the failure to introduce adequate community care systems has marginalized a substantial number of mental health service users in some countries (see Chapter 10). Homelessness of people with mental health problems has become an increasing problem (Gill et al. 2003), especially in many of our large cities. All this seems to exacerbate other problems like alcoholism and drug abuse, criminality and the risk of violence. Mentally ill patients have an increased risk of committing violent acts, but they often also become victims of violence by others. An increasing number of mentally ill people are in prison which, of course, is not the right place for ensuring their proper care (Lader et al. 2003) (see Chapter 3 for a discussion of social exclusion).

Other consequences have accrued from these developments. For families the burden of care in looking after long-term, mentally ill relatives has increased, although for many families the possibility to live again with a close family member is felt to outweigh the greater care responsibilities (see Chapter 16). For society the closure of many mental hospitals has brought savings, but on the other hand, building up the alternative community care system also needs resources. The problem in many European countries has been that the money saved from hospital closures has not been transferred to the development of community care, leading to an increased reliance on families and the transfer of financial responsibility to social care systems (often with fewer entitlements), plus the risk of marginalization.

Use of antidepressants has increased dramatically during the last 20 years. For example, in Finland the use of these drugs increased fivefold during the 1990s (Lehtinen et al. 1993; see also Chapter 7). There are certainly several reasons for this development: the better recognition of depression both by the general public and by primary care physicians, the new antidepressants available with milder and fewer side-effects, and better acceptance by patients – and certainly, also, the rather aggressive marketing efforts by the drug industry. One positive consequence has been that, today, people with depression are less likely to go untreated. According to epidemiological surveys from the 1990s, a third or less of people with a depressive disorder have had any treatment (Lin and Parikh 1999; McConnell *et al.* 2002; Ialongo *et al.* 2004). Among the negative consequences of the growth in antidepressant use are the increased prescribing of these new drugs for people without any real indications – as some kind of 'happiness pill' – and perhaps too, the neglect of other modes of treatment of depression, especially psychotherapy.

Psychotherapies

Psychotherapies are widely used and favoured by the public, but there are many providers with quite diverse training – if indeed they have any at all – who claim to be psychotherapists. In most countries, little has been done to regulate and evaluate providers, which makes psychotherapy very much a public concern. Yet public demand is very high: in general population surveys, most people declared that, in the case of psychological or behavioural problems, they thought psychotherapy to be the appropriate treatment (Angermeyer and Matschinger 1996; Jorm *et al.* 1997; Saragoussi *et al.* 2005). Many fewer people thought that psychotropic drugs would work, and they expressed a fear of addiction to medication (Angermeyer *et al.* 1993; Saragoussi *et al.* 2006).

In many countries there have been attempts to clarify the situation in order to protect the public, especially from sects which claim to provide psychological help. Paying for psychotherapies (either total or partial payment) through the health care system is also an issue that has prompted some European countries to establish guidelines for clinical indications, as well as for the qualifications of providers (see Chapter 4).

The many faces of psychotherapy

To define psychotherapy is not an easy task. In general, it can be defined as a psychological procedure, the aim of which is to achieve favourable psychological changes in an individual or in a group of people by specific psychosocial interaction that must be scientifically validated and acquired by a specific training. This definition considers four different aspects of psychotherapy: the target, the goal, the method and the training:

- the target is people with a mental health problem;
- the goal is to alleviate or cure the disorder;
- the psychological method used is based on the goal-oriented and systematic application of a scientifically validated psychological theory; and
- sufficient training in the specific technique is a prerequisite to utilization of that technique.

In its modern, scientific meaning psychotherapy has been used for more than 100 years in the treatment of mental health problems. One of its most prominent pioneers was, without doubt, Sigmund Freud, the founder of psychoanalysis in the early twentieth century. Since Freud's day, hundreds of psychotherapy techniques, based on a variety of theories, have been developed. In most of the reviews and meta-analyses of psychotherapies, such as that recently conducted for the French National Institute of Research (INSERM 2004), six major theoretical frameworks of psychotherapy are usually identified for operational purposes:

1 Analytic/psychodynamic approach.
2 Behavioural approach.
3 Cognitive-behavioural approach.
4 Humanistic (Rogerian) approach.
5 Systems theory approach (including most of the group and family therapies).
6 Problem/solution-oriented psychotherapies, which are not based on a specific theory, but are standardized and research-based interventions for specific disorders (such as schizophrenia, depression, eating disorders etc.).

In addition to this theoretical categorization, psychotherapies can also be grouped according to their target, intensity or expected duration. Thus, we have individual psychotherapies, family therapies and group therapies, as well as long-term (with a duration of several years) and short (some six to ten visits) therapies. The most intensive psychotherapy (psychoanalysis) can have five visits weekly for years, while some supportive long-term therapies are conducted with very infrequent visits.

In a survey to compare psychotherapies across Europe, conducted by the European Commission, 195 psychotherapists in eight European countries (Belgium, Italy, Poland, United Kingdom, Sweden, Portugal, France and Switzerland), working in mental health outpatient centres, were approached to fill in questionnaires (Power 1997). The results of this offer some interesting insights, even though they may not be truly representative of these countries. According to their own estimation, the respondents identified nine types of psychotherapy: psychoanalysis, behavioural therapy, cognitive-behavioural therapy, family therapy, brief psychodynamic therapy, group therapy, counselling, humanistic therapy (Rogers, bio-energetic), marital/sex therapy, in addition to an open category which included a variety of approaches. In some areas, subcategories have to be specified; for example, the psychoanalytic category can be subdivided into classical psychoanalysis and psychoanalytic psychotherapy. Group therapy can be psychoanalytic, too, but can also be based on some other psychological theory. This illustrates the diversity of techniques even when using a relatively precise definition of psychotherapy, as in this survey ('a therapeutic approach and practice, either individual or group orientated, relating to a specific, standardized technique which makes use of a programmed strategy in terms of section planning and expected outcome definition').

The providers of psychotherapy

Psychotherapy is not considered to be a purely medical treatment. Thus, the provider of psychotherapy need not to be a medical doctor. In practice, psychotherapy is provided by people from a variety of professional backgrounds. The European survey revealed that the diversity of psychotherapies is paralleled by an even larger diversity of providers, in terms of professional background:

33 per cent of the psychotherapists were psychiatrists, 47 per cent psychologists, 4 per cent social workers, 6 per cent nurses and 10 per cent had some other training. Moreover, this therapist mix varied considerably across countries: in France 78 per cent were psychiatrists whereas in Sweden and the United Kingdom there were no psychiatrists. On the other hand, 12 per cent provided 'counselling' in Belgium, Italy, Switzerland and Sweden, whereas this never happened in the other participating countries.

In the European Commission survey most of the psychotherapists were members of a scientific society. A third of them had training in psychoanalysis, a third in behavioural therapy and another third in family or couple therapy, but again, these proportions varied markedly by country: in France 79 per cent had training in psychoanalysis whereas in Italy this proportion was zero. The average length of training was about five years with a supervision of about five to six years. However, it should be noted that in this survey the respondents came from the public sector health system, and the above results may not apply to the private sector where a far larger range of professional backgrounds can be found among persons calling themselves psychotherapists. In most European countries a list of the diverse societies claiming to train psychotherapists has been established in order to protect the public, although they are not necessarily coordinated or unified, and in some countries no such list is available. This means that the label of psychotherapist could be used in some countries by any professional or even by a person without any acceptable training.

In most countries no clear and explicit regulations exist about the professional requirements of people who may claim to call themselves psychotherapists. One problem is also the diverse training of the many providers of help called psychotherapy. Health systems should have some control over the training and qualifications of a psychotherapist. In recent years there have been attempts to clarify the situation e.g. in many countries a psychotherapist is a legalized professional, and only those who have been authorized can use that title.

Evidence of the effectiveness of psychotherapy

There have been tentative efforts to evaluate psychotherapies since the pioneering work of Knight (1952) who retrospectively studied 592 patients treated by psychoanalysis for more than six months. The evaluation focused on symptoms, patients' productivity, adaptation (including sexual pleasure, coping and problem-solving ability) and interpersonal relations. The main finding was that 56 per cent of patients improved or were cured. However, if those who left therapy within the first six months were included in the results, this rate was only 30 per cent. (It should be noted that around 30 per cent of patients in any controlled trial may report some improvement due to the placebo effect – Miller and Rosenstein 2006.)

This historical attempt was followed by many others. In later studies researchers have tried to set standards for evaluation, including control groups, randomization and long-term follow-up. Several studies have demonstrated the efficacy of psychotherapeutic treatment in parallel with pharmacological treatment for a number of mental disorders (Katschnig and Windhaber 1998; Marder *et al.*

2003; Stiles *et al.* 2006), contributing to a growth in credibility and popularity of psychotherapeutic intervention. In recent years, it has been possible to summarize the results of several studies through meta-analyses, providing estimates of efficacy by type of disorders and type of psychotherapy (Bateman and Fonagy 2000; Roth and Fonagy 2004; INSERM 2004).

The following conclusions can be drawn from these reviews:

- psychodynamic psychotherapies have proved to be effective, especially in personality disorders;
- cognitive-behavioural therapies have shown their effectiveness in treating depression, anxiety, schizophrenia, bipolar disorder, alcohol abuse disorders, bulimia and personality disorders;
- family therapies have worked in anorexia, schizophrenia and bi-polar disorder;
- psychoeducational interventions have been effective in bi-polar disorder and schizophrenia.

In most cases psychotherapy was evaluated in conjunction with, or compared to psychotropic drug treatment.

Psychotherapy and policy issues

Psychotherapies are effective in treating a variety of mental health problems, but there are still many controversies concerning their most appropriate place in the treatment of these conditions. One problem is the large number of schools of psychotherapy, with their own traditions and training systems, which do not always understand each other, and may even fight each other. Similar misunderstandings exist between psychotherapists and professionals favouring somatic treatments, especially drugs, although in most cases an appropriate combination of psychotropic drugs and psychotherapy would be the most effective treatment.

It is also clear that the development of different psychotherapeutic techniques has greatly influenced public attitudes towards mental illness, as reflected in the media, and the development of mental health service systems. The psychological theories behind these techniques have helped us to gain a better understanding of mental health problems, and to accept them as part of our normal everyday life, like physical illnesses. Today, psychotherapy is an essential and appropriate part of the range of treatments required for the comprehensive treatment of mental disorders. The provision of psychotherapies should be an integral part of the mental health plan or strategy of every country, region and treatment unit.

The financing of psychotherapy is also an important issue. In many countries, treatment is provided mainly by private psychotherapists, raising questions about the range of indications and conditions that should be partially or totally reimbursed to allow patients to cover their treatment costs. The type of provider is also essential since non-medical providers are less costly and are often more accessible than psychiatrists – provided the former have been trained adequately. One policy recommendation is to set up national guidelines for the types of conditions for which psychotherapies are beneficial, as well as for the type of psychotherapy that should be provided and the training required (Roth and Fonagy 2004). This also calls for large-scale evaluations of different types of psychotherapy with long enough follow-up analyses.

Psychosocial interventions

Over the last 30 years there has been a trend towards differentiating between psychotherapy and various psychosocial interventions, the distinction being that the former deals with the inner world of individual patients or small groups of patients, while the latter deals with the context in which the individual is living. In practice, the distinction may not be that clear (e.g. in the case of family therapy), but it is important to keep these two types of interventions separate, since the skills required are different. While psychotherapy is treatment with psychological methods, irrespective of whether it occurs on a one-to-one basis or in a group setting, psychosocial interventions are not primarily directed at individual people but at the context in which they live, in order to change this context or to make it instrumental to improving symptoms and quality of life. The systematization of psychosocial interventions is still as open as the field of psychotherapy, perhaps even more so, as no formal 'schools' have been established. Most developments have simply occurred through personal practitioner initiatives locally and have spread via publications to other locations. More often than in the case of psychotherapy, psychosocial approaches are problem-oriented and well evaluated, especially in the field of working with the families of people with mental health problems.

Often, psychosocial interventions are not clearly separated conceptually from mental health services and some of the psychosocial measures listed below, in fact, can also be subsumed under mental health services (e.g. structuring daily life by day hospital attendance). Quite a few chapters in the *Textbook of Community Psychiatry* by Thornicroft and Szmukler (2001) demonstrate this overlap. One way of classifying psychosocial interventions is to look at the size of the social network involved. Thus, one could distinguish interventions at the micro-level (i.e. a service user's family and friends), the meso-level (organizations and institutions such as schools) and the macro-level (society as a whole with its norms and values in different cultures and subcultures). The closer we approach the macro-level, the less clear and the less well researched the interventions become.

Specific psychosocial interventions include:

- Case management, i.e. providing a care coordinator to the service user and his or her family in order to help to coordinate all possible helping resources.
- Assertive community treatment (ACT) and assertive outreach programmes for people with severe mental disorders.
- Help to structure daily life, including contact opportunities for individuals who would otherwise remain inactive – day hospitals, day centres, clubs and the like offer these opportunities.
- Support for independent living arrangements wherever possible or provision of sheltered living (residential facilities, group homes etc.).

- Assisting service users to find appropriate jobs in the labour market or in sheltered settings, whereby the principle of 'first place, then train' is increasingly pursued (in contrast to the traditional principle of 'first train, then place'). An interesting development in this area is the creation of patient-run companies and social firms.
- Offering participation in normal societal (especially cultural) activities.
- Providing a satisfactory standard of living, including access to health care and legal help.
- Working with the service user's family. This has become *the* psychosocial intervention at the micro-level. The types of activities are numerous and include family therapy, psychoeducational groups for the individual's relatives, multiple family groups, family self-help groups and family self-help organizations. Many interventions are standardized and documented. The concept of expressed emotion, as elaborated during the 1970s, kicked off this development (Brown *et al.* 1962; Kuipers 1979; Bogren 1997) (see also Chapter 16).

Usually, such interventions are combined with pharmacotherapy, and integrated treatment plans should be worked out, especially for people with persistent mental health problems living in the community (see Herz and Marder 2002). Practically no intervention is possible at a macro-level but it is important to recognize, especially in times of increased migration (for example, in cases of displaced refugees but also due to globalization impacts – see Chapter 15), that – at this level – cross-cultural differences have to be taken into account for each type of psychiatric treatment. At the macro-level we can also locate the type of health care system in a country, and particularly how these health care structures (tax-funded or social health insurance systems) influence the availability and quality of psychiatric care. Health services research and mental health policy could therefore also be classified as psychosocial endeavours at the macro-level.

On the meso-level the restructuring of psychiatric services themselves constitutes an important intervention, but is not dealt with here (see Thornicroft and Tansella 2004 and Chapter 10). As far as other organizations are concerned, such as schools, the military or companies, their structure has to be considered; but intervention in these structures is not the task of psychiatry proper. Since people with mental health problems today largely live outside psychiatric institutions and are integrated into 'normal' organizations and institutions, they need to be taken into account within comprehensive mental health plans and strategies.

The most important developments in psychosocial interventions concern the inclusion of family members in the management and treatment processes, especially for people with chronic conditions, and particularly those with schizophrenia. The role of the professional is somewhat blurred in psychosocial interventions, and the term 'professional' itself may even need reconsideration. Many approaches are more educational than therapeutic and since most service users live outside psychiatric institutions, aspects of daily quality of life have come to the forefront. Concepts such as disability, quality of life, empowerment and self-help play increasingly prominent roles and wherever professionals are involved, their role is to take these concepts into consideration.

NICE guideline on the treatment of depression

The National Institute for Health and Clinical Excellence (NICE) in England and Wales has commissioned a series of guidelines in which the methods of evidence-based medicine are used to formulate policies for health care workers in both generalist and specialist settings. The guideline on depression (National Collaborating Centre for Mental Health 2005) illustrates many of the points discussed in this chapter. Although depressive illnesses of all grades of severity are treated in primary care in the United Kingdom, it is generally the case that less severely depressed people are treated in primary care rather than in specialist care. It is also true to say that as the severity of depression increases, there is a lower prevalence: so, there are far more people with mild depression than moderate depression, and so on. In terms of available human resources, there are not enough trained staff to provide psychotherapy to everyone who might benefit from it. The NICE guideline makes detailed recommendations not only about drug treatments and psychological treatments, but also on the best service arrangements; the three-tier model advocated in this chapter is therefore echoed in the document.

In view of staffing and service constraints, the guideline uses a 'stepped care' approach, in which each step up the hierarchy indicates a need for a more specialized (and usually much more expensive) treatment. Having provided, in the *first step*, detailed guidance on how GPs can improve their detection rates for depression, the guideline moves to the *second step*, which is the best-practice management of mild depression (just diagnosable on *ICD-10* criteria, with four symptoms, in addition to entry symptoms). This is done in primary care, by GPs or practice nurses. There is no difference between active antidepressant drug and placebo in mild depression, so primary care staff are advised to use other treatment interventions, such as self-help, physical exercise, 'watchful waiting' and problem-solving. To the extent that drugs have any role here, it is not as antidepressants but as aids to the restoration of sleep and as daytime sedatives. Computerized cognitive-behaviour therapy has also been shown to be effective in mild depression. However, antidepressants may have a place if mild depression persists after treatment of a more severe episode, or where the individual has a past history of depression.

The *third step* is the management of moderate depression, defined as five or six additional symptoms, and severe depression defined as seven or more additional symptoms. Here, antidepressants have been shown to be effective, and are recommended on the basis of their relatively low toxicity, low cost, generally low discontinuation syndrome and tolerability – as there is no evidence that any one antidepressant is more effective than another. SSRIs (selective serotonin reuptake inhibitors) are recommended in view of these considerations. Examples of recommended antidepressants are citalopram and fluoxetine; or sertraline if heart disease is present. Simple psychological interventions like problem-solving by primary care staff may be effective, but are somewhat more expensive than drugs. Single episodes of moderate and severe depression are best treated in primary care. Patients with chronic depression should be offered a combination of antidepressants and cognitive-behaviour therapy.

The *fourth step* is the treatment of treatment-resistant, recurrent, atypical and psychotic depression. These illnesses should be treated by mental health professionals either in specialist settings or in primary care. Detailed advice is offered for each of these kinds of illness, and antidepressants are again recommended. Expensive psychological interventions such as cognitive-behavioural therapy or interpersonal psychotherapy are recommended, if necessary in combination with an antidepressant. A wide range of specialist mental health staff may participate in treatment plans. The *fifth step* is inpatient care, where patients should be admitted if there is a risk of self-harm or to life. In addition to all interventions described in Step 4, nursing care and ECT are available in this setting.

NICE guidelines are issued for many mental health conditions, and are available in several different formats. The guideline on depression is downloadable at www.nice.org.uk/pdf/word/CG023NICEguideline.doc.

Future perspectives

The twentieth century witnessed an enormous development in the treatment and management of mental health problems. Effective and well-studied treatment methods are now available, especially in pharmacology but increasingly also in the field of psychotherapy and psychosocial interventions. It would seem that the most important innovations were launched between the 1950s and 1970s, and since then nothing really revolutionary has happened in the field of treatment. What we now have, however, is more evidence-based knowledge on the effectiveness of the different methods, although generally we still need to know more on how they work in the real world.

The newer-generation drugs are widely seen to have fewer side-effects and to be better tolerated by patients, but progress with regard to effectiveness has been modest. The modality of these drugs is mainly symptomatic, and a substantial proportion of users (30 to 40 per cent) do not benefit from them. One major reason is that the aetiology of the so-called 'functional mental disorders' is still somewhat unclear and is in any case multi-faceted. Therefore, there is still considerable need for further research in this field.

One important area will certainly be in biological research of mental health problems, and there have been substantial developments in recent years. Spin-off effects from this research, particularly in developing treatments, may also be expected. But many experts have warned that we should not be too optimistic here (Hedgecoe 2004). It seems very unlikely that we could ever find a biological mode of treatment which, on its own, could cure such long-term developmental conditions as schizophrenia. We will always need a combination of many different modes of therapy adapted according to the specific and often changing needs of individual patients and also of those within their close networks, especially family members (Alanen 1997).

Modern brain research has, however, given some new perspectives on the possibility of developing and even discovering new modes of biological treatments. The most promising areas of research have undoubtedly been in molecular biology and gene technology, as well as in the use of new research techniques such as brain imaging. Gene research has developed enormously in recent years, revealing some specific genes susceptible to, for example, schizophrenia and bi-polar disorder (Levinson *et al.* 2003). However, in the case of schizophrenia, it seems most likely that it is not caused by a single gene disturbance but that several genes can increase the risk of developing the condition. It also seems evident that genetic errors are neither necessary nor sufficient causes. The aetiology of schizophrenia must still be regarded as multi-faceted, including psychosocial risk factors. However, based on this new research of the biological causes, it is likely that new and more specific treatment methods may be developed.

Psychological and psychosocial treatments are also expected to develop in the future. New research will reveal new understandings of, for example, the meaning of social interaction in promoting mental health and preventing mental health problems. Already, specific interventions to foster good parenting and early infant-parent interaction have produced evidence in the prevention of mental health problems in growing children (Stewart-Brown *et al.* 2004; Barlow *et al.* 2005; Brown and Sturgeon 2006).

Concluding remarks

There is a good deal of evidence-based knowledge on integrated approaches where pharmacotherapy and some kind of psychotherapy and/or psychosocial intervention are combined. In a number of trials on schizophrenia and on anxiety disorders the superiority of such combined approaches has been demonstrated (Katschnig and Windhaber 1998; Marder *et al.* 2003).

Increasingly, outcome measures encompass not only psychopathological symptoms but also disabilities, quality of life and functioning (Katschnig *et al.* 2005). For schizophrenia, studies have indicated that the new antipsychotic drugs help to motivate users to also take part in psychosocial programmes (Rosenheck *et al.* 1998).

In sum, what was evident in common sense now has been demonstrated by scientific research to be true: that the therapeutic approach centred on the individual, i.e. pharmacotherapy and psychotherapy, should be supplemented by treatment approaches that focus on the life context of people living with mental health conditions. Family interventions, counselling, network interventions, community work, psychosocial rehabilitation and other psychosocial measures must be considered when designing new services. Moreover, what is urgently needed is the evaluation of the 'real world' effectiveness of all treatment methods described in this chapter whenever they are provided in a given health care system. Effective (combined) treatment methods still have to be implemented in many places.

References

Alanen, Y.O. (1997) *Schizophrenia: Its Origins and Need-adapted Treatment*. London: Karnac Books.

Almeida-Filho, N., de Jesus, M. J., Coutinho, E., Franca, J.F., Fernandes, J., Andreoli, S.B. and Busnello, E.D. (1997) Brazilian multicentric study of psychiatric morbidity, *British Journal of Psychiatry*, 171: 524–9.

American Psychiatric Association (1994) *Diagnostic and Statistical Manual of Mental Disorders, DSM-IV*. Washington, DC: American Psychiatric Association.

American Psychiatric Association (1997) Practice guideline for the treatment of patients with schizophrenia, *American Journal of Psychiatry*, Supplement, 4, 154: 1–63.

American Psychiatric Association (2002) *Practice Guidelines for the Treatment of Psychiatric Disorders, Compendium 2002*. Washington, DC: American Psychiatric Association.

Andrews, G., Henderson, S. and Hall, W. (2001) Prevalence, comorbidity, disability and service utilisation: overview of the Australian National Mental Health Survey, *British Journal of Psychiatry*, 178: 145–53.

Angermeyer, M.C. and Matschinger, H. (1996) Public attitude towards psychiatric treatment, *Acta Psychiatrica Scandinavica*, 94(5): 326–36.

Angermeyer, M.C., Daumer, R. and Matschinger, H. (1993) Benefits and risks of psychotropic medication in the eyes of the general public: results of a survey in the Federal Republic of Germany, *Pharmacopsychiatry*, 26(4): 114–20.

Barlow, J., Parsons, J. and Stewart-Brown, S. (2005) Preventing emotional and behavioural problems: the effectiveness of parenting programmes with children less than 3 years of age, *Child: Care, Health and Development*, 31(1): 33–42.

Bateman, A.W. and Fonagy, P. (2000) Effectiveness of psychotherapeutic treatment of personality disorder, *British Journal of Psychiatry*, 177: 138–43.

Bazire, S. (1997) *Psychotropic Drug Directory 1997: The Professionals' Pocket Handbook and Aide Memoire*. Wiltshire: Quay Books.

Bebbington, P.E. (1990) Population surveys of psychiatric disorder and the need for treatment, *Social Psychiatry and Psychiatric Epidemiology*, 25(1): 33–40.

Bebbington, P., Meltzer, H., Brugha, T., Farrell, M., Jenkins, R., Ceresa, C. and Lewis, G. (2003) Unequal access and unmet need: neurotic disorders and the use of primary care services, *International Review of Psychiatry*, 15(1–2): 115–22.

Bijl, R.V. and Ravelli, A. (2000) Psychiatric morbidity, service use, and the need for care in the general population: results of the Netherlands Mental Health Survey and Incidence Study, *American Journal of Public Health*, 90(4): 602–7.

Bijl, R.V., Ravelli, A. and van Zessen, G. (1998) Prevalence of psychiatric disorder in the general population: results of the Netherlands Mental Health Survey and Incidence Study (NEMESIS), *Social Psychiatry and Psychiatric Epidemiology*, 33(12): 587–95.

Bland, R.C., Newman, S.C., Russell, J.M. and Orn, H.T. (eds) (1994) Epidemiology of psychiatric disorders in Edmonton: phenomenology and comorbidity, *Acta Psychiatrica Scandinavica*, Supplement, 376: 1–70.

Bogren, L. (1997) Expressed emotion, family burden and quality of life in parents with schizophrenic children, *Nordic Journal of Psychiatry*, 51(4): 229–33.

Brown, G.W., Monck, E.M., Carstairs, G.M. and Wing, J.K. (1962) Influence of family life on the course of schizophrenic illness, *British Journal of Preventive and Social Medicine*, 16: 55–68.

Brown, H. and Sturgeon, S. (2006) Healthy start of life and reducing early risks, in C. Hosman, E. Jané-Llopis and S. Saxena (eds) *Prevention of Mental Disorders: Effective Strategies and Policy Options*. Oxford: Oxford University Press.

Flisher, A.J., Kramer, R.A., Grosser, R.C., Alegria, M. *et al.* (1997) Correlates of unmet need for mental health services by children and adolescents, *Psychological Medicine*, 27(5): 1145–54.

Fombonne, E. (1994) The Chartres study I: prevalence of psychiatric disorders among French school-aged children, *British Journal of Psychiatry*, 164: 69–79.

Gill, B., Meltzer, H. and Hinds, K. (2003) The prevalence of psychiatric morbidity among homeless adults, *International Review of Psychiatry*, 15(1): 134–40.

Goldberg, D.P. and Huxley, P.J. (1980) *Mental Illness in the Community: The Pathway to Psychiatric Care*. London: Tavistock.

Goldberg, D.P. and Huxley, P.J. (1992) *Common Mental Disorders: A Bio-social Model*. London: Routledge.

Healy, D. (1998) *The Anti-depressant Era*. Cambridge, MA: Harvard University Press.

Hedgecoe, A. (2004) *The Politics of Personalised Medicine: Pharmacogenetics in the Clinic*. Cambridge: Cambridge University Press.

Herz, M.I. and Marder, S.R. (2002) *Schizophrenia: Comprehensive Treatment and Management*. Philadelphia, PA: Williams & Wilkins.

Howard, K.I., Cornille, T.A., Lyons, J.S., Vessey, J.T. *et al.* (1996) Patterns of mental health service utilization, *Archives of General Psychiatry*, 53(8): 696–703.

Ialongo, N., McCreary, B.K., Pearson, J.L., Koenig, A.L. *et al.* (2004) Major depressive disorder in a population of urban, African-American young adults: prevalence, correlates, comorbidity and unmet mental health service need, *Journal of Affective Disorders*, 79(1–3): 127–36.

INSERM (2004) Psychotherapie: trois approches évaluées, in INSERM (ed.) *Expertise Collective*. Paris: INSERM.

Jacobi, F., Wittchen, H.U., Holting, C., Hofler, M. *et al.* (2004) Prevalence, co-morbidity and correlates of mental disorders in the general population: results from the German Health Interview and Examination Survey (GHS), *Psychological Medicine*, 34(4): 597–611.

Jorm, A.F., Korten, A.E., Rodgers, B., Pollitt, P. *et al.* (1997) Belief systems of the general public concerning the appropriate treatments for mental disorders, *Social Psychiatry and Psychiatric Epidemiology*, 32(8): 468–73.

Katschnig, H., Freeman, H. and Sartorius, N. (eds) (2005) *Quality of Life in Mental Disorders*, 2nd edn. Chichester: Wiley.

Katschnig, H. and Windhaber, J. (1998) Die Kombination einer Neuroleptika-Langzeitmedikation mit psychosozialen Massnahmen, in P. Riederer, G. Laux and W. Pöldinger (eds) *Neuro-Psychopharmaka – Ein Therapie-Handbuch. Band 4: Neuroleptika. 2. Auflage*. Vienna: Springer-Verlag.

Kessler, R.C., McGonagle, K.A., Zhao, S., Nelson, C.B. *et al.* (1994) Lifetime and 12-month prevalence of *DSM-III-R* psychiatric disorders in the United States: results from the National Comorbidity Survey, *Archives of General Psychiatry*, 51(1): 8–19.

Kessler, R.C., Berglund, P.A., Bruce, M.L., Koch, J.R. *et al.* (2001) The prevalence and correlates of untreated serious mental illness, *Health Services Research*, 36(6): 987–1007.

Kessler, R.C., Demler, O., Olfson, F. M., Pincus, H.A. *et al.* (2005) Prevalence and treatment of mental disorders, 1990 to 2003, *New England Journal of Medicine*, 352: 2515–23.

Knight, R.P. (1952) An evaluation of psychotherapeutic techniques, *Bulletin of the Menninger Clinic*, 16: 113.

Kuipers, L. (1979) Expressed emotion: a review, *British Journal of Social and Clinical Psychology*, 18(2): 237–43.

Lader, D., Singleton, N. and Meltzer, H. (2003) Psychiatric morbidity among young offenders in England and Wales, *International Review of Psychiatry*, 15(1–2): 144–7.

Lam, R.W. (1994) Seasonal affective disorders, *Current Opinion in Psychiatry*, 7(1): 9–13.

Lehtinen, V. (1985) Assessment as to the need for psychiatric treatment, *Nordic Journal of Psychiatry*, 39: 463–9.

Lehtinen, V., Joukamaa, M., Jyrkinen, E., Raitasalo, R. *et al.* (1990) Need for mental health services of the adult population in Finland: results from the Mini Finland Health Survey, *Acta Psychiatrica Scandinavica*, 81(5): 426–31.

Lehtinen, V., Veijola, J., Lindholm, T., Väisänen, E. *et al.* (1993) *Mielenterveyden pysyvyys ja muutokset suomalaisilla aikuisilla* (with English summary: *Stability and Changes of Mental Health in the Finnish Adult Population*). Turku: Kansaneläkelaitoksen julkaisuja AL: 36.

Levinson, D.F., Levinson, M.D., Segurado, R. and Lewis, C.M. (2003) Genome scan meta-analysis of schizophrenia and bipolar disorder, part I: methods and power analysis, *American Journal of Human Genetics*, 73(1): 17–33.

Lin, E. and Parikh, S.V. (1999) Sociodemographic, clinical, and attitudinal characteristics of the untreated depressed in Ontario, *Journal of Affective Disorders*, 53(2): 153–62.

Marder, S.R., Glynn, S.M., Wirshing, W.C., Wirshing, D.A. *et al.* (2003) Maintenance treatment of schizophrenia with risperidone or haloperidol: 2-year outcomes, *American Journal of Psychiatry*, 160(8): 1405–12.

McConnell, P., Bebbington, P., McClelland, R., Gillespie, K. and Houghton, S. (2002) Prevalence of psychiatric disorder and the need for psychiatric care in Northern Ireland: population study in the District of Derry, *British Journal of Psychiatry*, 181: 214–19.

Meltzer, H., Gill, B., Pettiecrew, M. and Hinds, K. (1995) *The Prevalence of Psychiatric Morbidity Among Adults Living in Private Households. OPCS Surveys of Psychiatric Morbidity in Great Britain. Report 1*. London: HMSO.

Miller, F.G. and Rosenstein, D.L. (2006) The nature and power of the placebo effect, *Journal of Clinical Epidemiology*, 59(4): 331–5.

Narrow, W.E., Rae, D.S., Robins, L.N. and Regier, D.A. (2002) Revised prevalence estimates of mental disorders in the United States: using a clinical significance criterion to reconcile two surveys' estimates, *Archives of General Psychiatry*, 59(2): 115–23.

National Collaborating Centre for Mental Health (2005) *Depression: Management of Depression in Primary and Secondary Care*. London: Gaskell.

Olfson, M., Marcus, S., Sackeim, H.A., Thompson, J. and Pincus, H.A. (1998) Use of ECT for the inpatient treatment of recurrent major depression, *American Journal of Psychiatry*, 155(1): 22–9.

Perry, P.J. (1996) Pharmacotherapy for major depression with melancholic features: relative efficacy of tricyclic versus selective serotonin reuptake inhibitor antidepressants, *Journal of Affective Disorders*, 39(1): 1–6.

Pirkola, S., Isometsä, E., Suvisaari, J., Aro, H. *et al.* (2005) *DSM-IV* mood, anxiety and alcohol use disorders and their comorbidity in the Finnish general population: results from the Health 2000 Study, *Social Psychiatry and Psychiatric Epidemiology*, 40(1): 1–10.

Power, M. (1997) First results on the psychotherapist questionnaire in psychotherapies in Europe on seven countries. European Commission mimeo.

Puura, K., Almqvist, F., Tamminen, T., Piha, J. *et al.* (1998) Psychiatric disturbances among prepubertal children in southern Finland, *Social Psychiatry and Psychiatric Epidemiology*, 33(7): 310–18.

Regier, D.A., Boyd, J.H., Burke, J.D., Rae, D.S. *et al.* (1988) One-month prevalence of mental disorders in the United States. Based on five epidemiologic catchment area sites, *Archives of General Psychiatry*, 45(11): 977–86.

Rosenheck, R., Tekall, J., Peters, J., Cramer J. *et al.* (1998) Does participation in psychosocial treatment augment the benefit of clozapine? *Archives of General Psychiatry*, 55(7): 618–25.

Roth, A. and Fonagy, P. (2004) *What Works for Whom: A Critical Review of Psychotherapy Research*. Guilford: The Guilford Press.

Saragoussi, D., Kovess, V., Suchocka, A., Sevilla-Dedieu, C. *et al.* (2006) Help-seeking intentions among the public for mental health disorders: a French study. In submission.

Shapiro, S., Skinner, E.A., Kessler, L.G., von Korff, M. *et al.* (1984) Utilization of health and mental health services: three epidemiologic catchment area sites, *Archives of General Psychiatry*, 41(10): 971–8.

Stewart-Brown, S., Patterson, J., Mockford, C., Barlow, J. *et al.* (2004) Impact of a general practice based group parenting programme: quantitative and qualitative results from a controlled trial at 12 months, *Archives of Disease in Childhood*, 89(6): 519–25.

Stiles, W.B., Barkham, M., Twigg, E., Mellor-Clark, J. and Cooper, M. (2006) Effectiveness of cognitive-behavioural, person-centred and psychodynamic therapies as practised in UK National Health Service settings, *Psychological Medicine*, 36(4): 555–66.

Sussman, N. (2005) General principles of psychopharmacology, in B.J. Sadock and V.A. Sadock (eds) *Kaplan & Sadock's Comprehensive Textbook of Psychiatry*, 8th edn. Philadelphia, PA: Lippincott Williams & Wilkins.

Thomas, C. and Lewis, S. (1998) Which atypical antipsychotics? *British Journal of Psychiatry*, 172: 106–9.

Thornicroft, G. and Szmukler G. (eds) (2001) *Textbook of Community Psychiatry*. Oxford: Oxford University Press.

Thornicroft, G. and Tansella, G. (2004) The components of a modern mental health service: a pragmatic balance of community and hospital care, *British Journal of Psychiatry*, 185: 283–90.

Weyerer, S. and Dilling, H. (1984) Prävalenz und Behandlung psychischer Erkrankungen in der Allgemeinbevölkerung. Ergebnisse einer Feltstudie in drei Gemeinden Oberbayerns, *Nervenartzt*, 55: 30–42.

World Health Organization (1992) *The ICD-10 Classification of Mental and Behavioural Disorders: Clinical Descriptions and Clinical Guidelines*. Geneva: WHO.

World Mental Health Survey Consortium (2004) Prevalence, severity, and unmet need for treatment of mental disorders in the World Health Organization World Mental Health Surveys, *Journal of the American Medical Association*, 291: 2581–90.

Zubin, J. and Spring, B. (1977) Vulnerability: a new view of schizophrenia, *Journal of Abnormal Psychology*, 86(2): 103–26.

chapter seven

Psychopharmaceuticals in Europe

Nikolas Rose

Introduction

Over the last half of the twentieth century, health care practices in developed, liberal and democratic societies, notably in the United States and Europe, have become increasingly dependent on commercially produced pharmaceuticals.[1] This is especially true in relation to psychiatry and mental health. We could term these 'psychopharmacological' societies. While it is difficult to assess the precise value of the market, estimates based on ex-manufacturers' prices put the European market at US$4741 million in 2000 – up from US$2110 million in 1990 – which compares with a total US market of US$11,619 million – up from US$2502 million in 1990.[2] In many different contexts, in different ways, in relation to a variety of problems, by doctors, psychiatrists, parents and by ourselves, human subjective capacities have come to be routinely reshaped by psychiatric drugs. The aim of this chapter is to describe the kinds of thinking that underpin such developments, and to examine the impact of these ways of thinking on the prescribing of psychiatric drugs in Europe, through an analysis of comparative data on the use of psychiatric drugs in different countries.

The rise of the psychopharmacological paradigm

It is well known that the first widely used psychiatric drug was chlorpromazine (Largactil, Thorazine), developed from antihistamines in the years after the Second World War.[3] Two French psychiatrists, Pierre Deniker and Jean Delay, who administered it to a group of psychotically agitated patients at the Hôpital Sainte-Anne in Paris in 1952, are credited with the discovery of its psychiatric effects. Its use spread through the asylums of Europe and North America, and made Smith, Kline and French, who held the US patent, US$75 million in 1955 alone (Healy 2001: 97). The drug was thought not to be a sedative like barbiturates or chloral, but to act specifically on the symptoms of mental illness. Nonetheless, up to the late 1960s, most psychiatrists thought of it as a general 'tranquillizer', and many thought that its main use was to make patients more open to the kind of therapeutic rapport necessary for psychotherapy. Indeed, many suggested that the effects of the drugs were not to remove the symptoms, such as hallucinations, let alone to produce a cure for schizophrenia, but to reduce the disturbance – thus, the patients might still hear the persecutory voices but would be disinterested in them. But in the 1960s, large-scale double-blind trials were adopted as the most convincing mode of proof in psychopharmacology, and they seemed to demonstrate that neuroleptic drugs specifically targeted the symptoms of schizophrenia. They also seemed to show that the drugs produced a low level of adverse effects – a finding that was later overturned with the gradual acceptance that the drugs were linked to an irreversible dysfunction of movements known as tardive dyskinesia (Gelman 1999). The drugs now appeared to be more than mere 'tranquillizers' – they seemed to target the specific symptoms of psychotic disorder.

Soon after the clinical effects of the drugs were accepted, attempts were made to identify their mode of action. Experiments in rats seemed to show that chlorpromazine and related drugs – often termed 'neuroleptics' – antagonized the action of L-dopa and enhanced the accumulation of the metabolites of dopamine and noradrenaline in the rat brain. On this basis, the researchers began to argue that the neuroleptics in some way prevented, or blocked, dopamine, and to some extent noradrenaline, from being taken up by the receptors after its secretion into the synapse. By 1963, a fully formed 'dopamine hypothesis' was articulated by Carlsson and Lindqvist for the specific mode of action of neuroleptic drugs. By a simple reversal of the causal chain, it also seemed that we had a dopamine hypothesis for schizophrenia itself – if antipsychotic drugs had their effect by blocking the action of dopamine, then schizophrenia must be linked to an excess of, or hypersensitivity to, dopamine. It seemed obvious that there was a reciprocal relation between the mode of action of the drug and the mode of causation of the condition. As more refined psychopharmacological experimental techniques were developed, it became accepted that all the drugs thought to be clinically effective as antipsychotics blockaded one particular type of dopamine receptor – the so-called D_2 receptor – in one particular area of the brain – the mesocortical regions. The problem was that the apparently firm pharmacological evidence linking the clinical efficacy of a particular 'antipsychotic' to its affinity for postsynaptic D_2 receptors was not matched by firm evidence that those diagnosed with schizophrenia had anything abnormal in their dopamine system. Despite the unresolved disagreements about the status and significance of evidence from patients, the dopamine hypothesis became the fulcrum of the commercial development of drugs marketed as antipsychotics throughout the 1960s and 1970s.

The argument about specificity of action of psychiatric drugs, and the belief in the reciprocal relation between the mode of action of the drug and the neurochemical basis of the condition, was also central to the development of antidepressants. The first, imipramine (Tofranil) was also developed from antihistamines during the early 1950s. There was little initial enthusiasm for this drug, partly because depression was not seen, at that time, as a major psychiatric problem. Tofranil was launched in 1958, to some extent inspired by the success of Thorazine and Largactil, and became established as the first 'tricyclic' antidepressant in the 1960s – so-called because of its three-ringed chemical structure. The antidepressant story is also a narrative culminating in the claim to drug specificity – the claim that the drug acts at the neuronal site of the disorder. In the early 1950s, an antitubercular drug called iproniazid was developed from left-over V-2 rocket fuel which had been bought cheaply by Hoffman-La Roche. But when it was used to treat tuberculosis it produced euphoria: newspapers reported TB patients dancing in the corridors. Psychiatrists were soon experimenting with its potential for the treatment of patients with mental disease. Iproniazid was initially considered in the same category as other stimulants. But in 1952 a series of papers were published arguing that it worked by inhibiting the action of an enzyme called monoamine oxidase, thus slowing down the depletion of these monoamines in the brain. And the substances then identified as neurotransmitters in the brain were indeed monoamines – adrenaline, norepinephrine, dopamine (the so-called catecholamines) and serotonin (an indoleamine). Researchers began to suggest that depression and elation themselves were correlated with the levels of these neurotransmitters, these monoamines, in the brain. Initially, there seemed to be one very serious anomaly – the tricyclic antidepressants such as imipramine did not inhibit monoamine oxidase. However, this turned out to be a clue to a mechanism that would be of major significance – that of reuptake. The tricyclics were shown to block the mechanism by which neurones reabsorb and hence conserve the neurotransmitters they secrete, leaving more of the active neurotransmitter present in the synapse for longer. This mode of action has become crucial to the development of the new family of selective serotonin reuptake inhibitors – SSRIs.

In 1960, there was resistance to the very idea that neurones in the brain communicated chemically, and still more to the idea that the activity of neurotransmitters could influence behaviour. Indeed, this whole way of thinking was still controversial – this was the era of European antipsychiatry on the one hand, and the psychoanalytic dominance of psychiatry in the United States on the other. But, within two decades biological psychiatry had come to define the common sense of psychiatric thought, and had established the pharmaceutical companies as key players in understanding and treating mental health problems. Pharmaceutical companies invested heavily in psychopharmacological research, in the hope that it would lead to the development of new and profitable drugs. There was only one major conceptual development over this period – attention switched from the secretion of the neurotransmitters to the actions of the receptors which 'recognized' certain amines and were activated when they were released into the synapse. It was now argued that antidepressant drugs worked because they too were 'recognized' by these receptors. When their molecules 'bound' to receptor sites they might stimulate them, or they might block their action: this became known as upregulation and downregulation of receptors. In the new images, receptors and neurotransmitters were imagined as locks and keys, the one working because it fit exactly into the other. The iconic status of Prozac (fluoxetine hydrochloride) arose less from its efficacy than from the belief that it was the first 'smart drug'. A molecule was designed with a shape that would enable it specifically to lock into identified receptor sites in the serotonin system – hence, affecting only the specific symptoms being targeted and having a low 'side-effect profile'.

Initially, each neurotransmitter was allocated to a particular 'condition': dopamine to schizophrenia, serotonin to depression. As research progressed, this simple belief was shown to be unsupportable – dopamine receptors were soon found to be of two types, D_1 and D_2, and by the end of the 1980s, the D_3 and D_4 receptors were identified. In the case of serotonin there were at least seven 'families' of 5HT receptors and most had several subtypes. But this again proved to be no obstacle to this explanatory regime – for it was argued that each of these receptors had a specific function, that anomalies in each type were related to specific psychiatric symptoms, and that they could be ameliorated by drugs designed specifically to affect them. Furthermore, many other neurotransmitters were identified, including amino acids – notably gamma aminobutyric acid or GABA: by the start of the twenty-first century, the number has grown into the hundreds. However, this did not prove a problem for this form of explanation, because it seemed that each neurotransmitter might potentially be involved in each specific form of mental disorder and hence be targeted by appropriately formulated psychotherapeutic drugs. Indeed, this linked well with the central presupposition in recent advances in the development of psychiatric drugs – perhaps more significant than any individual drug – that of *specificity*. This presupposition is actually three-sided. First, it is premised on the neuroscientific belief that these drugs could, and ideally should, have a specificity of target. Second, it is premised on the clinical belief that doctors could specifically diagnose each array of changes in mood, will, desire and affect as a discrete condition. Third, it is based on the neuroscientific belief that specific configurations in neurotransmitter systems underlay specific moods, desires and affects. The three presuppositions map onto one another. And they also meshed very well with the proliferation of disease categories in each successive edition of the American Psychiatric Association's *Diagnostic and Statistical Manual* (*DSM*), with the number of distinct diagnoses reaching in excess of 350 by 1994 (American Psychiatric Association 1952, 1968, 1980, 1994). This multiplicity of classifications provides a key marketing opportunity, as companies seek to diversify their products and niche-market them, either by making minor modifications to produce new molecules, or by licensing their existing drugs as specifics for particular *DSM-IV* diagnostic categories.

In the course of these developments, two key distinctions began to wither away. The first was the distinction between states and traits – states of illness and traits of personality – since it began to be argued that both episodes of illness such as depression, and variations in traits such as shyness or hostility, could be altered by psychiatric drugs (Knutson *et al.* 1998). The second was the distinction between mental and physical disorders themselves: as the fourth edition of the *Diagnostic and Statistical Manual* puts it: 'although this volume is titled the *Diagnostic and Statistical Manual of Mental Disorders*, the term *mental disorder* unfortunately implies a distinction between "mental" disorders and "physical" disorders that is a reductionist anachronism of mind/body dualism'.[4]

Furthermore, molecular neuropsychiatry began to 'dissect out' numerous distinct elements of neurotransmitter systems whose variations might be psychiatrically significant – receptor sites, membrane potentials, ion channels, synaptic vesicles and their migration, docking and discharge, receptor regulation, receptor blockade, receptor binding and much more. With the developments in genome mapping resulting from the Human Genome Project, these variations in elements of neurotransmitter systems were mapped onto variations in the DNA sequences thought to code for the diverse aspects of neurotransmission – variations now traced to the level of single nucleotide polymorphisms. As the twenty-first century dawned, there were significant further developments in attempts to map the apparent therapeutic profile of different psychopharmaceuticals onto the aspects of neural communication. Some researchers have focused on G-protein coupled signal transduction pathways, second messenger generating systems, and on the modulation of gene expression, partly to account for the fact that while the effect of drugs at receptor sites is almost instantaneous, therapeutic effects are delayed by days or weeks.[5] This research has also been stimulated by the wish to find molecular mechanisms underlying the mode of action of such 'mood stabilizing' drugs as lithium carbonate for the treatment of bi-polar disorder – for these drugs do not directly modulate the secretion or uptake of neurotransmitters. Others have argued for the possible role that psychopharmaceuticals play in modulating neurogenesis in the adult brain, and have suggested a role for neurogenesis in the pathophysiology and treatment of neurobiological illnesses such as depression, post-traumatic stress disorder and drug abuse.[6] These developments, and the more complex and environmentally open pathways to illness they suggest, open new links between biographical and neuronal conceptions of the aetiology and treatment of mental health problems. The details need not detain us – for the point is merely this: today, the coupling of a belief in the therapeutic efficacy of psychopharmaceuticals and theories about their neuronal mode and site of action means that, almost inescapably, it is at this molecular level that the basis for variations, normal and pathological, in human mood, will, desire and cognition are located.

Thus, by the 1990s, a fundamental shift had occurred in psychiatric thought and practice. No matter that there was little firm evidence to link variations in neurotransmitter functioning to symptoms of mental disorder in the brains of unmedicated patients – although many researchers are seeking such evidence and occasional papers announce that it has been found. And no matter that most of the new smart drugs are no more effective than their dirty predecessors – the claim is that they have fewer unpleasant 'unwanted effects'. Mental disorders are understood in ways that, in principle at least, link symptoms to anomalies in neurones, synapses, membranes, receptors, ion channels, neurotransmitters, binding, enzymes and the genes that code for them. And the fabrication and action of psychiatric drugs is conceived in these terms. Not that biographical effects are ruled out, but biography – for example, family stress, sexual abuse – has effects through its impact on the brain. Environment plays its part, but unemployment, poverty and the like have their effects only through impacting upon the brain. And experiences play their part – substance abuse, stress or trauma, for example – but once again, through their impact on the neurochemical brain. For those who develop and market psychiatric drugs, this style of thinking lent itself to a new way of presenting the specificity and effectiveness of their drug for specific psychiatric conditions, each now linked to a particular kind of anomaly in a particular aspect of a neurotransmitter system. The new age of smart psychiatric drugs had arrived.

The market for drugs

Accurate comparative and historical data on psychiatric drug prescribing since the 1950s is not readily available. The World Health Organization (WHO) has adopted one particular unit as a measure of the intensity of use of pharmaceuticals. This is the defined daily dose or DDD, and a comparative standard is emerging based on the DDD per 1000 inhabitants per day.[7] However, the compilation and publication of detailed DDD figures for psychopharmaceutical use across Europe is at an early stage and coverage is patchy. Other data is available from commercial organizations that monitor the pharmaceutical industry, notably from the leading organization, IMS Health. In this chapter, we largely draw upon studies specially commissioned from IMS Health to illustrate some general trends and patterns. The IMS measure used to assess these trends is the standard dosage unit, or SU (see Note 1 for an explanation of this measure) which is not directly convertible into DDDs.[8] While the interpretation of the detailed figures is subject to many qualifications, and actual numbers should be regarded simply as indicative, they are sufficiently robust for these purposes.

Let us begin by considering some broad regional differences. An initial overview (see Table 7.1) reveals a marked rising trend in prescription of psychiatric medication in all regions from 1990 to 2000 as measured in standard dosage units. In the more developed regions, the United States shows a growth of about 70 per cent, Europe of around 44 per cent and Japan of about 30 per cent. In the less developed regions, South America remains remarkably constant with a growth of only 1.6 per cent, South Africa shows a growth of about 13 per cent, but the use of prescription drugs in Pakistan has grown by over 33 per cent (although from a low base).[9]

This variation in the quantity of drug prescriptions is instructive, but we see a rather different pattern when we relate the number of standard doses prescribed

Table 7.1 Psychiatric drug prescribing 1990–2000 in selected regions (standard dosage units, thousands)

	1990	*1992*	*1994*	*1996*	*1998*	*2000*
EU	30,612,851	32,975,134	34,026,814	38,169,030	40,443,452	42,464,477
USA	9,965,639	11,540,978	13,830,291	16,074,244	19,001,486	18,953,979
Japan	7,817,352	8,144,026	8,398,988	8,974,334	9,243,612	10,049,994
Latin America	3,696,757	3,695,284	3,515,827	3,483,267	3,521,456	3,723,646
Pakistan	631,172	680,378	874,607	927,253	868,876	825,437
South Africa	277,579	303,834	314,972	383,234	345,159	378,434

Source: IMS Health Second Study. See Note 1.

in each region (IMS figures) to its population (our data). Figures for the year 2001 (see Table 7.2) show that the *total* annual rate of prescribing psychiatric drugs is actually remarkably similar in the more developed regions – the United States, Europe and Japan – at between 66 and 75 standard doses per 1000 persons per year. The rate of prescribing in the three less developed regions is roughly similar, although it stands at around 10 per cent of that in the more developed regions. However, within these figures, there are significant regional variations in the *proportions* of different classes of psychiatric drugs being prescribed.

In the United States, antidepressants form a much higher proportion of psychiatric drugs than any other region, at almost 45 per cent, and antipsychotics, hypnotics and sedatives are proportionally low. High proportions of tranquillizer prescribing are shown in Japan, South America and Pakistan, with correlatively low levels of antidepressant prescriptions. The United States is the only region where psychostimulants such as methylphenidate and amphetamine are a significant proportion of the psychiatric drug market, amounting to almost 10 per cent in 2000. In Europe, antidepressants amount to some 28 per cent of the total of psychiatric drugs, while tranquillizers amount to some 35 per cent, with psychostimulants amounting to around 0.5 per cent.

The most interesting comparator for Europe as a whole is Japan. While the overall rate of psychiatric drug prescribing there is broadly similar to that in Europe (and the United States), a far greater proportion of those prescriptions are for tranquillizers and antipsychotics, and less than 15 per cent are for antidepressants. Japan seems not to have had the wave of concerns over the benzodiazepines and the traditional neuroleptics that shook psychopharmacology in the West, nor does it seem to have experienced the 'epidemic' of depression and antidepressants (Healy 2001). Indeed fluoxetine hydrochloride was never marketed in Japan, and the first SSRI-type drugs (fluvoxamine and paroxetine) did not come on the market until 1999 and 2000. And attention deficit hyperactivity disorder (ADHD) is only just being 'discovered' in Japan. Let us turn to explore variations between European countries in more detail, to see if similar differences are evident even within a confined geographical region, and if so, how they may be understood.

Table 7.2 Psychiatric drug prescribing in 2001 in selected regions by drug class (standard dosage units per 1000 population)

	USA	Europe	Japan	South America	South Africa	Pakistan
Tranquillizers	20,361	22,630	28,211	4,781	2,266	3,802
Antidepressants	33,768	19,010	9,202	1,835	2,330	919
Sedatives and hypnotics	7,362	15,562	14,721	1,299	1,701	387
Antipsychotics – all	6,954	8,373	14,437	1,062	1,490	754
Psychostimulants	6,488	364	184	47	105	7
Total	74,934	65,940	66,755	9,023	7,892	5,868

Source: IMS Health Second Study. See Note 1.

The European Union

If we examine the figures for the European Union (EU-15) in more detail over the decade of the 1990s (see Table 7.3), while the overall number of SUs prescribed rose by about 19 per cent, prescribing of tranquillizers, sedatives and hypnotics remained relatively stable, showing a slight growth over the period of around 5 per cent. Prescribing of antipsychotics has risen by 17 per cent, mostly as a result of the growth in the market for the newer 'atypicals', and psychostimulants rose by almost 90 per cent from a low base. However, the major growth area was in antidepressant drugs: prescribing of antidepressants rose by almost 50 per cent across this decade.

The figures and trends are clearest if expressed as SUs per 1000 population (see Table 7.4). Once again, prescribing of tranquillizers, sedatives, hypnotics and antipsychotics remained relatively stable over the decade. The most marked rises were shown in psychostimulants – where prescribing increased tenfold – and antidepressants – where prescribing almost doubled over the period, an increase almost entirely due to the 14-fold increase in prescriptions for SSRI-type pharmaceuticals (see Table 7.5).

Table 7.3 Psychiatric drug prescribing 1990–2000 in Europe (standard dosage units, thousands)

	1990	1992	1994	1996	1998	2000
Tranquillizers	7,513,609	7,571,866	7,438,466	7,836,741	7,889,968	8,127,616
Antidepressants	3,399,914	3,855,187	4,261,443	5,237,285	5,909,638	6,451,185
Sedatives and hypnotics	5,277,560	5,472,512	5,476,647	5,782,375	5,849,562	5,626,615
Antipsychotics – all	2,486,725	2,737,709	2,728,829	2,890,676	2,921,099	3,015,128
Psychostimulants	12,069	14,785	18,412	36,656	62,605	113,005
Total	18,689,877	19,652,059	19,923,797	21,783,733	22,632,872	23,333,549

Source: IMS Health Second Study. See Note 1.

Table 7.4 Psychiatric drug prescribing 1990–2000 in Europe (standard dosage units per 1000 population)

	1990	1992	1994	1996	1998	2000
Tranquillizers	20,599	20,758	20,393	21,484	21,630	22,282
Antidepressants	9,321	10,569	11,683	14,358	16,201	17,686
Sedatives and hypnotics	14,468	15,003	15,014	15,852	16,037	15,425
Antipsychotics – all	6,817	7,505	7,481	7,925	8,008	8,266
Psychostimulants	33	41	50	100	172	310
Total	51,238	53,876	54,621	59,720	62,048	63,969

Source: IMS Health Second Study. See Note 1.

Table 7.5 Antidepressant prescribing 1990–2000 in Europe (standard dosage units per 1000 population)

	1990	1992	1994	1996	1998	2000
Non-SSRI antidepressants	8,831	9,588	9,950	11,218	11,467	10,634
SSRI antidepressants	534	1,013	1,752	3,147	4,741	7,070
Antidepressants – all	9,321	10,569	11,683	14,358	16,201	17,686

Source: IMS Health Second Study. See Note 1.

These overall figures obscure large variations in the usage of different types of psychiatric drugs between the countries of the EU. Relevant data for three classes of drugs – antidepressants, antipsychotics and psychostimulants – are presented in Tables 7.6–7.13.

No clear patterns emerge from the data, except one of national variability. France has the highest level of *antidepressant* prescribing, followed closely by Belgium and the United Kingdom, while levels in Italy and Greece are relatively low. Germany, whose level of overall antidepressant prescribing is at the low end of the EU-15 range, has moved most slowly towards the use of SSRIs. Overall, antidepressant prescribing per 1000 population doubled from 1993 to 2002, and within this rise, the use of SSRIs increased tenfold. There is great variation in the rate of prescribing of *anxiolytics*. While prescribing rates have remained relatively stable in most countries over the decade, levels have declined in France, although usage remains high. Usage in Portugal was the highest in all EU-15 countries in 1993, and has increased by about 30 per cent over the decade. Spain shows a similar increase, from a lower base. For *antipsychotics*, Finland, which is sixth highest in prescribing of antidepressants, has by far the highest level of antipsychotic prescribing per head of population, prescribing antipsychotics at a rate about ten times greater than Sweden and Germany, which make the next highest use of this class of drug. While some studies have suggested a point prevalence of schizophrenia in Finland above that in many other countries, at approximately 1.3 per cent (e.g. Hovatta *et al.* 1997), more recent evidence suggests a decline in prevalence (Suvisaari *et al.* 1999) and even the higher estimates cannot themselves account for a tenfold greater usage of antipsychotics – Finland is also sixth highest in its usage of antidepressants. The United Kingdom has a low usage of antipsychotics compared with its EU partners. There is also great variation in the usage of *psychostimulants*, with none at all being prescribed in Italy, low levels of prescribing in Ireland, France, Austria and Spain, median levels in Belgium, Germany and the United Kingdom, and high levels in the Netherlands and Luxembourg.

Overall, as the summaries in Table 7.14 and Figure 7.1 show clearly, each country seems to have a distinctive pattern of usage of the major classes of psychiatric drugs; yet it is not clear that this pattern reflects differences in the relative rates of incidence of different mental disorders.

IMS data does not give good coverage of the Nordic countries. Fortunately,

Table 7.6 Europe by drug type and country: antidepressants – all

All Antidepressants (including mood stabilisers) (SU per 1000 population)

	1993	1994	1995	1996	1997	1998	1999	2000	2001	2002
Austria	8,179	9,037	9,425	10,160	11,334	12,568	14,863	16,584	17,460	18,639
Belgium	14,277	15,106	16,495	17,860	19,221	20,931	22,683	24,199	25,178	26,691
Denmark*	–	–	–	–	–	–	–	–	–	–
Finland	10,544	11,820	13,092	14,255	14,825	15,672	17,084	18,295	19,471	20,759
France	20,098	20,375	20,659	20,306	21,144	22,121	22,680	23,856	25,954	26,893
Germany	10,708	12,401	15,064	17,266	17,544	19,205	18,739	17,932	17,523	17,438
Greece***	5,206	5,086	5,014	5,781	5,922	6,638	7,671	8,433	9,751	11,656
Ireland***	9,729	10,672	11,599	12,590	13,442	14,255	15,570	17,938	19,625	20,906
Italy	6,727	6,718	6,875	7,058	7,200	7,249	7,838	8,773	10,589	11,155
Luxembourg***	8,921	9,307	10,420	11,932	12,876	14,917	16,113	16,220	16,817	17,786
Netherlands**	–	–	–	–	–	–	–	3,901	15,983	16,754
Portugal***	10,254	11,743	12,825	14,119	15,120	16,140	17,186	19,018	20,903	22,659
Spain**	6,922	7,737	8,775	9,922	11,036	12,267	13,909	15,379	16,902	18,673
Sweden*	–	–	–	–	–	–	–	–	–	–
United Kingdom	12,705	13,444	15,446	17,242	18,915	20,247	21,415	22,234	24,167	25,623

* No IMS data available.
** No data available for Spain (hospital) until 1999 and from Netherlands (retail) until 2000.
*** Data from retail panels only.

Source: IMS Health Third Study. See Note 1.

Table 7.7 Europe by drug type and country: antidepressants – conventional

Non-SSRI antidepressants (SU per 1000 population)

	1993	1994	1995	1996	1997	1998	1999	2000	2001	2002
Austria	7,071	7,322	6,981	7,008	7,128	7,373	8,568	9,383	9,525	9,865
Belgium	11,818	11,339	11,481	11,648	12,044	13,252	13,945	14,452	14,711	15,218
Denmark*	–	–	–	–	–	–	–	–	–	–
Finland	8,780	9,116	8,957	8,983	8,935	9,127	9,584	9,864	10,154	10,552
France	17,050	16,720	16,080	14,852	14,655	14,452	14,208	14,708	15,528	15,869
Germany	10,509	12,131	14,714	16,811	16,872	18,289	17,592	16,493	15,683	15,087
Greece***	4,900	4,560	4,229	4,583	4,529	4,768	5,095	5,063	5,260	5,939
Ireland***	8,964	9,320	9,636	9,962	10,077	10,081	10,287	11,131	11,920	12,456
Italy	5,866	5,827	5,728	5,763	5,713	5,603	5,403	5,392	5,576	5,363
Luxembourg***	7,899	7,471	7,652	8,007	8,288	9,486	9,313	9,076	9,228	9,389
Netherlands**	–	–	–	–	–	–	–	2,027	8,165	8,415
Portugal***	9,353	9,820	10,156	10,840	11,231	11,486	11,158	11,511	11,985	12,274
Spain**	5,499	5,528	5,660	5,990	6,118	6,355	6,656	6,887	7,288	7,750
Sweden*	–	–	–	–	–	–	–	–	–	–
United Kingdom	11,203	11,334	12,430	13,106	13,716	14,240	14,443	14,180	14,846	15,454

* No IMS data available.
** No data available for Spain (hospital) until 1999 and from Netherlands (retail) until 2000.
*** Data from retail panels only.

Source: IMS Health Third Study. See Note 1.

Table 7.8 Europe by drug type and country: antidepressants – SSRI

SSRI (SU per 1000 population)

	1993	1994	1995	1996	1997	1998	1999	2000	2001	2002
Austria	1,107	1,716	2,445	3,152	4,206	5,195	6,294	7,201	7,935	8,774
Belgium	2,459	3,766	5,014	6,212	7,177	7,679	8,738	9,747	10,468	11,473
Denmark*	–	–	–	–	–	–	–	–	–	–
Finland	1,764	2,704	4,136	5,272	5,890	6,545	7,500	8,432	9,317	10,207
France	3,048	3,655	4,579	5,455	6,489	7,669	8,472	9,148	10,425	11,024
Germany	199	271	350	454	672	916	1,147	1,439	1,840	2,351
Greece***	306	526	785	1,198	1,394	1,870	2,576	3,370	4,491	5,717
Ireland***	765	1,352	1,964	2,628	3,364	4,174	5,283	6,807	7,704	8,450
Italy	861	890	1,147	1,295	1,487	1,645	2,434	3,381	5,013	5,792
Luxembourg***	1,022	1,836	2,768	3,925	4,587	5,431	6,800	7,144	7,589	8,397
Netherlands**	–	–	–	–	–	–	–	1,874	7,818	8,339
Portugal***	901	1,923	2,669	3,279	3,890	4,653	6,028	7,507	8,918	10,384
Spain**	1,423	2,209	3,115	3,933	4,918	5,912	7,253	8,492	9,615	10,923
Sweden*	–	–	–	–	–	–	–	–	–	–
United Kingdom	1,502	2,110	3,016	4,137	5,199	6,007	6,972	8,054	9,322	10,169

* No IMS data available.
** No data available for Spain (hospital) until 1999 and from Netherlands (retail) until 2000.
*** Data from retail panels only.

Source: IMS Health Third Study. See Note 1.

Table 7.9 Europe by drug type and country: antipsychotics – all

All antipsychotics (SU per 1000 population)

	1993	1994	1995	1996	1997	1998	1999	2000	2001	2002
Austria	6,799	6,756	7,008	7,239	7,262	7,298	7,430	7,518	7,759	8,165
Belgium	8,954	8,726	8,768	8,752	9,034	9,031	9,098	8,774	8,868	9,040
Denmark*	–	–	–	–	–	–	–	–	–	–
Finland	19,277	19,744	19,741	19,749	19,343	19,016	18,900	18,617	18,273	17,975
France	11,099	11,026	10,535	10,687	10,493	10,155	10,074	10,073	10,071	9,868
Germany	9,236	9,261	9,492	9,670	9,761	9,791	9,740	9,726	9,951	10,310
Greece***	5,986	5,721	5,519	6,165	5,946	6,058	6,705	7,102	7,563	8,466
Ireland***	5,279	5,587	5,816	6,198	6,412	6,476	6,613	6,854	6,600	6,768
Italy	4,292	4,296	4,506	4,600	4,638	4,696	4,888	5,302	5,697	5,558
Luxembourg***	5,017	5,101	5,575	5,606	5,537	5,994	5,964	5,731	5,748	5,861
Netherlands**	–	–	–	–	–	–	–	2,076	4,228	4,275
Portugal***	6,145	6,525	7,078	7,650	7,826	8,039	8,460	9,268	9,600	9,881
Spain**	6,284	6,587	6,902	7,277	7,657	7,907	8,640	8,996	9,367	9,615
Sweden*	–	–	–	–	–	–	–	–	–	–
United Kingdom	4,160	4,162	4,504	4,231	4,163	3,938	3,712	3,379	4,045	3,838

* No IMS data available.
** No IMS data available for Spain (hospital) until 1999 and from Netherlands (retail) until 2000.
*** Data from retail panels only.

Source: IMS Health Third Study. See Note 1.

Table 7.10 Europe by drug type and country: antipsychotics – typical

Typical antipsychotics (SU per 1000 population)

	1993	1994	1995	1996	1997	1998	1999	2000	2001	2002
Austria	6,388	6,292	6,477	6,606	6,444	6,162	5,825	5,541	5,375	5,294
Belgium	8,954	8,726	8,768	8,620	8,577	8,380	8,096	7,337	6,969	6,511
Denmark*	–	–	–	–	–	–	–	–	–	–
Finland	18,475	18,776	18,448	18,195	17,383	16,685	15,877	14,800	13,472	12,118
France	10,546	10,376	9,829	9,780	9,406	8,891	8,637	8,519	8,231	7,756
Germany	8,808	8,768	8,945	9,034	9,012	8,882	8,624	8,384	8,150	8,040
Greece***	5,948	5,517	5,201	5,701	5,310	5,132	5,341	5,186	4,915	4,773
Ireland***	5,279	5,556	5,727	6,015	6,050	5,848	5,679	5,488	4,212	3,663
Italy	4,288	4,196	4,241	4,086	3,857	3,665	3,570	3,611	3,360	3,055
Luxembourg***	4,990	5,060	5,478	5,410	5,267	5,490	5,176	4,590	4,297	3,991
Netherlands**	–	–	–	–	–	–	–	1,406	2,726	2,564
Portugal***	5,500	5,781	6,180	6,680	6,756	6,876	7,113	7,374	7,153	6,845
Spain**	6,269	6,454	6,606	6,861	6,970	6,761	7,035	6,943	6,772	6,466
Sweden*	–	–	–	–	–	–	–	–	–	–
United Kingdom	4,160	4,162	4,504	4,231	4,163	3,905	3,612	3,226	3,858	3,620

* No IMS data available.
** No IMS data available for Spain (hospital) until 1999 and from Netherlands (retail) until 2000.
*** Data from retail panels only.

Source: IMS Health Third Study. See Note 1.

Table 7.11 Europe by drug type and country: antipsychotics – atypical

Atypicals (amisulpride, clozapine, olanzapine, quietapine, risperadone, sertindole, zotepine) (SU per 1000 population)

	1993	1994	1995	1996	1997	1998	1999	2000	2001	2002
Austria	411	464	532	633	818	1,136	1,605	1,977	2,384	2,871
Belgium	0	0	0	133	457	651	1,002	1,437	1,899	2,529
Denmark*	–	–	–	–	–	–	–	–	–	–
Finland	802	967	1,293	1,554	1,960	2,332	3,023	3,817	4,801	5,857
France	553	650	706	908	1,088	1,264	1,437	1,554	1,840	2,112
Germany	428	493	547	635	749	910	1,117	1,342	1,801	2,270
Greece***	38	204	319	464	636	926	1,364	1,916	2,648	3,693
Ireland***	0	31	89	183	362	628	934	1,366	2,389	3,105
Italy	4	100	265	514	781	1,031	1,318	1,691	2,337	2,503
Luxembourg***	27	41	97	196	270	504	787	1,141	1,451	1,870
Netherlands**	–	–	–	–	–	–	–	671	1,501	1,711
Portugal***	645	744	898	970	1,070	1,164	1,346	1,895	2,447	3,035
Spain**	15	132	296	415	687	1,146	1,605	2,053	2,595	3,149
Sweden*	–	–	–	–	–	–	–	–	–	–
United Kingdom	–	–	–	–	–	33	100	153	187	218

* No IMS data available.
** No IMS data available for Spain (hospital) until 1999 and from Netherlands (retail) until 2000.
*** Data from retail panels only.

Source: IMS Health Third Study. See Note 1.

Table 7.12 Europe by drug type and country: anxiolytics

Anxiolytics (SU per 1000 population)

	1993	1994	1995	1996	1997	1998	1999	2000	2001	2002
Austria	12,140	11,792	11,514	11,540	12,087	12,292	12,422	12,429	12,451	12,411
Belgium	38,609	37,337	36,965	37,484	38,391	38,830	39,035	39,034	38,778	38,583
Denmark*	–	–	–	–	–	–	–	–	–	–
Finland	19,927	20,258	20,350	20,457	20,631	21,006	20,972	21,297	21,656	22,201
France	46,599	45,363	43,801	42,559	41,513	41,067	39,957	40,460	41,101	39,960
Germany	9,583	9,312	9,205	9,065	8,801	8,703	8,534	8,868	8,609	7,719
Greece***	17,380	16,684	16,484	18,118	16,833	17,416	18,739	18,862	19,299	21,682
Ireland***	12,284	12,815	13,276	14,065	14,337	14,788	14,434	15,813	16,237	16,400
Italy	22,549	22,457	23,444	24,172	23,844	23,758	23,841	24,002	24,044	23,416
Luxembourg***	26,663	26,367	28,375	29,531	30,862	32,506	32,119	31,156	31,265	31,530
Netherlands**	–	–	–	–	–	–	–	–	16,862	16,643
Portugal***	44,938	48,532	49,823	52,499	52,274	53,551	56,073	58,210	59,414	59,131
Spain**	21,657	22,974	24,726	26,498	28,674	30,363	32,891	34,756	36,403	37,824
Sweden*	–	–	–	–	–	–	–	–	–	–
United Kingdom	6,848	6,545	6,706	6,973	7,174	7,406	7,496	6,887	7,031	6,960

* No IMS data available.
** No IMS data available for Spain (hospital) until 1999 and from Netherlands (retail) until 2000.
*** Data from retail panels only.

Source: IMS Health Third Study. See Note 1.

Table 7.13 Europe by drug type and country: psychostimulants (methylphenidate and dexamphetamine)

Psychostimulants (SU per 1000 population)

	1993	1994	1995	1996	1997	1998	1999	2000	2001	2002
Austria	0	2	4	3	6	20	36	56	85	109
Belgium	107	125	153	193	265	333	455	582	699	885
Denmark**	–	–	–	–	–	–	–	–	–	–
Finland**	–	–	–	–	–	–	–	–	–	–
France	3	4	4	9	15	19	25	39	53	77
Germany	47	59	82	123	167	241	351	521	665	681
Greece*	–	–	–	51	4	–	–	–	–	8
Ireland	–	–	–	138	12	–	–	–	–	23
Italy**	–	–	–	–	–	–	–	–	–	–
Luxembourg	32	38	41	86	138	225	372	726	999	1,191
Netherlands	–	–	–	–	–	–	–	568	1,257	1,423
Portugal**	–	–	–	–	–	–	–	–	–	–
Spain	250	187	71	77	86	106	128	170	211	262
Sweden**	–	–	–	–	–	–	–	–	–	–
United Kingdom	114	124	166	247	337	419	507	602	646	667

* Data from retail panels only.
** No IMS data available.

Source: IMS Health Third Study. See Note 1.

there is good data on these countries, although it uses the WHO index of the DDD. These data are presented in Tables 7.15 to 7.18.[10]

Using Finland (for which we also have IMS data) as a comparator, we can see that all the Nordic countries are at the higher end of European antidepressant usage. However, Finland remains remarkable, even among the Nordic countries, for its very high use of antipsychotics (see Table 7.16) together with the highest levels of the Nordic countries in the use of sedative and tranquillizing drugs, anxiolytics and hypnotics.

Psychopharmaceuticals and the health care system

These shifts have to be placed in the context of the general transformation of mental health practice in Europe over this period, notably the move away from inpatient care to 'care in the community'. In the 1980s, most of those who wrote on changes in mental health policy linked the move from inpatient treatment to treatment in the community to the rising use of psychiatric drugs,

Table 7.14 Europe comparative prescribing of major drug classes by country (2002) (SU per 1000 population)

	All antidepressants	SSRIs	Anxiolytics	Antipsychotics	Psychostimulants
Austria	18,639	8,774	12,411	8,165	109
Belgium	26,691	11,473	38,583	9,040	885
Denmark*	–	–	–	17,661	–
Finland	20,759	10,207	22,201	112,259	–
France	26,893	11,024	39,960	9,868	77
Germany	17,438	2,351	7,719	10,310	681
Greece***	11,656	5,717	21,682	8,466	8
Ireland***	20,906	8,450	16,400	6,768	23
Italy	11,155	5,792	23,416	5,558	–
Luxembourg***	17,786	8,397	31,530	5,861	1,191
Netherlands**	16,754	8,339	16,643	4,275	1,423
Portugal***	22,659	10,384	59,131	9,881	–
Spain**	18,673	10,923	37,824	9,615	262
Sweden*	–	–	–	10,710	–
United Kingdom	25,623	10,169	6,960	3,838	667

* No IMS date available.
** No data available for Spain (hospital) until 1999 and from Netherlands (retail) until 2000.
*** Data from retail panels only.

Source: IMS Health Third Study. See Note 1.

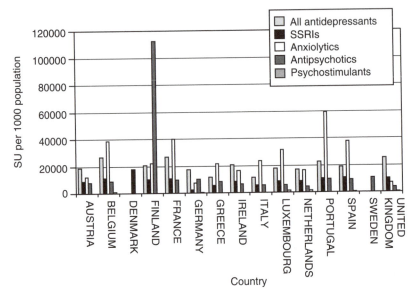

Figure 7.1   EU comparative prescribing of main drug classes, 2002 (SU per 1000 population)

Source: IMS Health Third Study. See Note 1.

Table 7.15 Antidepressant prescribing 1996–2001 in the Nordic countries in DDD per 1000 inhabitants

	1996	1997	1998	1999	2000	2001
Denmark	20.5	24.1	27.1	30.3	33.5	–
Finland	23.5	25.4	27.4	31.8	35.5	39.4
Norway	30.9	31.5	31.8	36.1	41.4	–
Sweden	34.8	32.0	37.5	41.7	48.8	–

Table 7.16 Antipsychotic prescribing 1996–2001 in the Nordic countries in DDD per 1000 inhabitants

	1996	1997	1998	1999	2000	2001
Denmark	8.1	8.3	8.3	8.3	8.9	–
Finland	15.2	15.0	14.7	15.2	15.3	15.7
Norway	8.5	8.5	8.5	8.7	9.0	–
Sweden	9.3	7.8	8.3	8.5	8.6	–

although the direction of causality was disputed. Comparative data on the decline in psychiatric inpatient beds is available from the WHO's 'European Health for All' database. These data give a picture of a common direction of

Table 7.17 Anxiolytic prescribing 1996–2001 in the Nordic countries in DDD per 1000 inhabitants

	1996	1997	1998	1999	2000	2001
Denmark	25.7	24.2	23.4	22.6	22.0	–
Finland	29.0	29.1	28.9	29.8	30.1	31.0
Norway	18.0	18.0	18.5	18.8	19.0	–
Sweden	17.4	16.0	16.4	16.8	17.1	–

Table 7.18 Hypnotic prescribing 1996–2001 in the Nordic countries in DDD per 1000 inhabitants

	1996	1997	1998	1999	2000	2001
Denmark	38.9	35.1	33.2	32.0	31.1	–
Finland	40.8	42.9	43.7	47.3	49.0	51.6
Norway	26.8	28.4	29.4	30.3	31.8	–
Sweden	44.3	42.3	44.3	45.5	47.2	–

change across all European countries, but show that the nature and pace of the changes, as well as the politics and organization, varies greatly from country to country (see Tables 7.19 and 7.20).

According to these WHO data, in 2000, the number of inpatient beds per 100,000 of the population, within the EU-15, varied from 14.1 in Italy to 186.3 in Belgium, and the decline from 1986 to 2000 varied from 85.9 per cent in Italy to as low as 7.1 per cent in the Netherlands. There is reason to be sceptical about the accuracy of these figures, which are not always confirmed by other research, especially when non-hospital psychiatric residential facilities are included. This is particularly notable in the case of Italy where, as we shall see presently, the issue of bed numbers has a particular salience given the debate over the consequences of Law 180, passed in 1978, which was intended to initiate the phasing-out of mental hospitals. In 1978 there were 78,538 beds in public mental hospitals; the PROGRES study, funded by the Italian National Institute of Health, found that on 31 May 2000, 1370 non-hospital residential facilities provided a total of 17,138 beds, and recommended an additional 4500 acute beds in public wards, and 5500 in private facilities: a total of 27,138 beds or 47.6 per 100,000 – a figure that is still low by European standards but is over three times that given in the WHO database (De Girolamo *et al.* 2002).

Indeed, overall, the inpatient bed figures given by WHO are not a good indicator of actual bed use. For example, in the United Kingdom, inpatient numbers in public hospitals for those with a mental illness (expressed as available hospital beds for the year from 1984) declined from a peak of over 150,000 in 1954 to under 40,000 in 1998, and the rate declined from almost 3.5 persons detained per 1000 population in 1954, to less than 0.8 per 1000 at the end of the century. But a different picture is given if one considers the number of occupied bed days

Table 7.19 Psychiatric inpatient beds 1986–2001 in Europe per 100,000 population

Country	1986	1991	1995	1996	1997	1999	2000
Albania	. . .	39.85	30.07	29.76	28.22	27.72	29.38
Armenia	80.05	63.13	55.45	46.38	46.36	47.23	42.21
Austria	101.83	95.71	80.69	74.17	71.54	62.75	61.27
Belgium	215.04	179.31	165.47	164.26	164.04	186.99	186.36
Bulgaria	86.37	87.94	88.96	87.79	88.69	64.85	63.93
Croatia	140.96	117.05	100.73	105.93	103.29	100.22	104.19
Czech Republic	148.11	132.79	113.87	113.22	112.13	110.86	113.01
Denmark	170.75	91.81	80.42	80	78.74	77.98	. . .
Estonia	188.32	184.14	106.29	99.82	97.25	82	79.08
Finland	318.35	216.21	126.24	120.34	113.82	106.07	103.45
France	199.91	154.2	128.82	120.02	119.54	111.59	107.07
Germany	. . .	153.82	131.64	127.94	126.95	127.03	127.68
Greece	120.3	113.93	110.29	106.96	107.02	92.12	90
Hungary	127.12	128.47	48.9	48.39	47.87	44.35	43.42
Iceland	180.51	142.25	117.85	. . .	. . .	. . .	. . .
Ireland	326.46	216.64	161.39	149.11	136.56	123.21	122.82
Israel	178.42	144.07	122.42	118.08	108.19	98.04	88.87
Italy	100	62.79	42.34	38.68	28.65	16.16	14.14
Kazakhstan	77.39	88.03	78.57	76.04	68.85	65.61	66.05
Kyrgyzstan	89.14	84.83	66.83	66.03	62.98	55.41	56.49
Latvia	210.39	191.47	198.91	177.88	179.38	166.83	168.65
Lithuania	186.65	159.82	133.83	133.47	128.78	127.04	127.73
Luxembourg	272.88	205.89	101.05	99.62	98.34	. . .	. . .
Netherlands	167.52	176.56	170.88	171.76	170.76	158	155.68
Norway	123.48	81.35	68.5	68.18	67.78	66.14	66.31
Poland	95.45	88.96	80.04	79.31	76.9	68.65	67.44
Portugal	90.75	86.74	72.52	73.73	71.56	. . .	. . .
Republic of Moldova	94.03	101.25	94.73	93.88	91.64	73.86	69.24
Romania	81.27	79.4	76.53	76.1	76.12	75.23	75.89
Russian Federation	133.66	132.19	126.86	124.82	123.23	119.5	119.3
Slovakia	90.74	99.63	91.65	91.57	92.42	90.15	89.43
Slovenia	81.29	80.74	80.38	80.3	79.95	77.77	77.13
Spain	85.64	67.65	60.29	58.75	56.65	. . .	. . .
Sweden	229.26	150.46	94.85	82.3	70.84	65.32	62.72
Switzerland	185.04	161.08	137.57	128.62	113.44	113.75	115.56
The former Yugoslav Republic of Macedonia	66.85	84.78	77.57	75.13	70.61	72.83	70.77
Turkey	10.93	14.96	13.34	13.04	13.07	12.8	12.65
Ukraine	131.82	132.17	120.99	110.78	100.8	98.2	97.72
United Kingdom	235.1	164.03	88.5	84.76	81.87	. . .	. . .

Source: WHO European Health For All Database at http://www.euro.who.int/hfadb.

NOTE: These data do not always match country data collected by other means and should be treated with caution.

Table 7.20 Decline in psychiatric inpatient beds 1986–2001 in EU-15 and Nordic Countries (figures are beds per 100,000)

Country	1986	1991	1995	1996	1997	1999	2000	Percentage decline 1986–2000
Austria	101.83	95.71	80.69	74.17	71.54	62.75	61.27	39.8
Belgium	215.04	179.31	165.47	164.26	164.04	186.99	186.36	13.3
Denmark	170.75	91.81	80.42	80	78.74	77.98	…	54.3*
Finland	318.35	216.21	126.24	120.34	113.82	106.07	103.45	67.5
France	199.91	154.2	128.82	120.02	119.54	111.59	107.07	46.4
Germany	…	153.82	131.64	127.94	126.95	127.03	127.68	16.8**
Greece	120.3	113.93	110.29	106.96	107.02	92.12	90	25.2
Iceland	180.51	142.25	117.85	…	…	…	…	…
Ireland	326.46	216.64	161.39	149.11	136.56	123.21	122.82	62.4
Italy	100	62.79	42.34	38.68	28.65	16.16	14.14	85.9****
Luxembourg	272.88	205.89	101.05	99.62	98.34	…	…	64.0***
Netherlands	167.52	176.56	170.88	171.76	170.76	158	155.68	7.1
Norway	123.48	81.35	68.5	68.18	67.78	66.14	66.31	46.3
Portugal	90.75	86.74	72.52	73.73	71.56	…	…	21.1***
Spain	85.64	67.65	60.29	58.75	56.65	…	…	33.9***
Sweden	229.26	150.46	94.85	82.3	70.84	65.32	62.72	72.5
United Kingdom	235.1	164.03	88.5	84.76	81.87	…	…	65.2

* 1986–1999
** 1991–2000
*** 1986–1997
**** Note the reservations expressed in the text. If all beds are taken into account, the decline in Italy is closer to 50%

Source: WHO European Health For All Database at http://www.euro.who.int/hfadb.

NOTE: These data do not always match country data collected by other means and should be treated with caution.

which were commissioned by public health providers for people with a mental illness. In the five years from 1991 to 1992 and 1997 to 1998, this fell by 21 per cent to 11.5 million, while, over the same period, bed days commissioned 'in the community' – that is to say in nursing homes and residential homes – rose by 86 per cent to 4.2 million, the number of *admissions* to National Health Service (NHS) hospitals under mental illness specialities actually increased from 4.2 to 4.4 million, and the number of first attendances at outpatients clinics, clinical psychology services, community psychiatric nursing and at psychiatric day care facilities all rose (Government Statistical Service 1998: Tables B22–7). To this picture of short stays, multiple admissions and the increasing role of supervision by non-medical professionals that are familiar to most countries that have seen a large decline in inpatient beds, we need to add those who receive treatment for mental health problems from general practitioners (GPs).

Thus, we should not treat a decline in bed numbers as equating, in any simple way, to a decline in the use of psychiatric inpatient treatment for individual patients. It is also clear from Table 7.21 that there is no simple relationship between the number of psychiatric beds per 100,000 population and the rate of psychiatric drug prescribing; nor is there a relationship, at least over the years when comparative data is available, between rates of decline of inpatient beds and rates of increase in the use of antidepressants or other types of psychiatric medication. Explanations of variations in rates of drug use must, therefore, lie elsewhere.

Table 7.21 Relation of inpatient bed numbers per 100,000 (1997) to rates of prescribing antidepressants and antipsychotics (SU per 1000) (1997 chosen for most complete year of bed statistics)

	Inpatient bed numbers per 100,000 population	Antidepressants	Antipsychotics
Portugal	170.76	15,120	7,826
Belgium	164.04	19,221	9,034
Italy	136.56	7,200	4,638
Germany	126.95	17,544	9,761
France	119.54	21,144	10,493
Finland	113.82	14,825	19,343
Greece	107.02	5,922	5,946
Netherlands	98.34	–	–
Denmark	78.74	–	–
Sweden	71.56	–	–
Austria	71.54	11,334	7,262
Spain	67.78	11,036	7,657
United Kingdom	56.65	18,915	4,163
Luxembourg	28.65	12,876	5,537
Ireland	. . .	13,442	6,412

Source: IMS data and European Health for All Database at http://www.euro.who.int/hfadb.

Note: Inpatient bed data used here do not always match country data collected by other means and should be treated with caution.

It might be thought that the best predictor of the usage of psychiatric drugs would be the prevalence of mental disorder. Unfortunately, the data in the European Health for All database on the incidence and prevalence of mental disorders by European country is very patchy, and not available for most of the newer member states and pre-accession countries of the EU – that is to say, for those countries where we have the best data on the use of psychiatric drugs. The information that is available, which is based on the existing national systems of reporting from health facilities, does not support the belief that there is some simple relationship of this type. For example, at the start of the 1990s, the recorded prevalence of mental disorders in Austria and France was almost identical, at around 0.95 per cent, yet prescribing rates in France for antidepressants and antipsychotics were twice as high as those in Austria. The recorded prevalence rates in the United Kingdom and Finland were also roughly equivalent, at around 1.5 per cent, but while these two countries had roughly equivalent levels of antidepressant prescribing, the rate of prescription of antipsychotics in Finland was over four times higher than that in the United Kingdom. While the data on prevalence is certainly not robust, it gives little support to the suggestion that we can, in any simple way, look to differences in the prevalence of diagnosed disorders to account for variations in prescribing rates.

The database contains information on another factor that might be anticipated to be related to use of psychiatric drugs – the proportion of total health expenditure spent on pharmaceuticals. One might have predicted that psychiatric drug prescribing rates would be linked to the general propensity of the health system and practitioners in any county to use drug-based treatments. However, as shown in Table 7.22, there is no clear relationship between these indices.

We have little option, then, but to conclude that rates of prescribing of psychiatric drugs have more to do with divergences in the prescribing beliefs and habits of physicians in different countries, no doubt linked also to the demands and expectations of the actual and potential patient population, than with the overall characteristics of health care systems, or the general propensity of such systems to depend on inpatient treatment. Let us turn to a limited exploration of data on individual countries within the EU.

The United Kingdom

Data on psychiatric drug prescribing in the early part of the period under consideration is hard to obtain. Data from the United Kingdom presented by Ghodse and Khan (1988) covering 1960–85 (see Figure 7.2) show a rising trend in prescriptions of tranquillizers and antidepressants over this period, and a decline in prescriptions for stimulants (which may arise from their reclassification as appetite suppressants).[11] While, in the 1980s, there was a public debate about the extent to which minor tranquillizers were being prescribed for everyday unhappiness and stress, about the possible long-term consequences of such drugs, and about problems of dependence, this debate did not extend to the use of other psychiatric drugs in the growing community-psychiatric sector. Or rather, it did so obliquely, in terms of the problems caused by patients in the

Table 7.22 Relation of psychiatric drug prescribing and proportion of health budget spent on pharmaceuticals

Countries ranked by proportion of total health expenditure spent on pharmaceuticals	Total pharmaceutical expenditure as % of total health expenditure both sexes (2001 except where specified)	Antidepressant prescribing (SU per 1000 population) (2001)	Antipsychotic prescribing (SU per 1000 population) (2001)
Portugal	*22.8	20,983	9,600
Italy	22.3	10,589	5,697
France	21.0	25,954	10,071
Spain	**17.8	16,902	9,367
Belgium	***16.3	25,178	8,868
United Kingdom	***15.8	24,167	4,045
Finland	15.7	19,471	18,273
Austria	15.1	17,460	7,759
Germany	14.3	17,523	9,951
Greece	14.0	9,751	7,563
Sweden	13.5	–	–
Luxembourg	****12.1	16,817	5,748
Ireland	10.3	19,625	6,600
Netherlands	10.1	15,983	4,228
Denmark	8.9	–	–

* 1998 ** 1990 *** 1997 **** 2000

Source: IMS data and European Health for All Database at http://www.euro.who.int/hfadb.

community being inadequately supervised, and discontinuing their medication to the detriment of their own capacity to function and with undesirable consequences for their family and the community. The debate was largely between those who thought that 'care in the community' was inherently more humane because it was less restrictive of freedom and who were concerned about its partial and slow implementation, and those who suggested that the problem lay in the 'abandonment' of the mentally ill under the dangerous illusion that they could survive in the harsh world outside the hospital. It did not dwell much on the possibility that there might be a simple substitution of psychopharmacological restraints for physical ones. In this debate, whatever their differences, most people took the view that progress lay in emphasizing the similarity of mental illness and physical illness, which would remove or reduce stigma and facilitate prompt treatment, and also in emphasizing the availability of effective and appropriate pharmacological treatments for mental illness. Objections to the rise of pharmacological psychiatry were left to a few maverick psychiatrists, displaced and defensive psychoanalysts and psychodynamic therapists, and the residual elements of the antipsychiatric movements of the 1960s. And as the focus of political concern shifted in the 1980s to the management of the risk apparently posed to 'the general public' by 'community psychiatric patients', a key role, once again, was accorded to drugs; it was, apparently, lack of compliance with drug regimes that was a major cause of the relapse of these

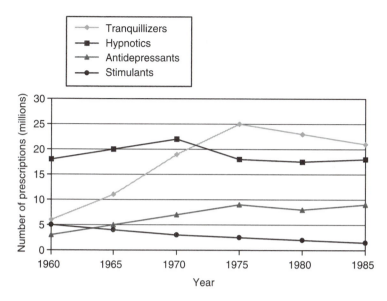

Figure 7.2 Prescriptions for psychoactive drugs (millions) in the United Kingdom 1960–1982

Source: Approximate figures, redrawn from Ghodse and Khan, 1988, Figure 1, derived mainly from the Office of Health Economics, London.

individuals, and in extreme cases, the cause of their homicidal conduct. It seemed that from this time on, an open psychiatric system would be fundamentally dependent on the belief in the therapeutic and management possibilities of psychopharmacology.

Trend data from 1980 to 2000 (see Table 7.23) show that over the 20 years from 1980, the total number of prescription items dispensed in the four main classes of drugs used for psychiatric conditions – hypnotics and anxiolytics, antipsychotics, antidepressants and stimulants, rose from about 34.5 million items to about 44.5 million – a growth of almost 30 per cent. However, this overall growth disguises the fact that, from 1980 to 1994, the number of prescription items actually declined, largely as a result of a reduction in prescribing for hypnotics and anxiolytics – the minor tranquillizers and sleeping pills whose use had caused concern. The figures show a decline in prescriptions for hypnotics and anxiolytics of about 32 per cent (from about 24.5 million prescription items to about 16.5 million prescription items per year) matched by a rise in prescriptions for antidepressants of about 200 per cent (from about 7.5 million prescription items to around 22 million prescription items per year).[12] These figures show a relatively small increase in the number of prescription items dispensed for the two drugs used to tread ADHD – dexamphetamine and methylphenidate – from just over 111,000 items in 1980 to just over 260,000 in 2000. However, this figure is misleading. In terms of quantity, the rise has been almost fivefold, from 6,280,790 standard units in 1980 to 29,358,340 in 2000, and almost two-thirds of this growth is accounted for by Ritalin which has grown at a great rate since its introduction in 1991. The net ingredient cost of

Table 7.23 Psychiatric drug prescribing in England 1980–2000 (millions of prescription items dispensed)

Drug class	1980	1982	1984	1986	1988	1990	1992	1994	1996	1998	2000
Hypnotics and anxiolytics	24,459	24,373	22,035	21,870	19,642	17,471	16,850	15,970	15,882	16,244	16,464
Drugs used in psychoses & related disorders	2,438	2,350	2,342	2,508	2,771	3,039	3,793	4,273	4,826	5,396	5,874
Antidepressant drugs	7,369	7,312	6,886	7,029	7,348	8,027	9,914	11,816	14,962	18,424	22,022
Central nervous system stimulants	213	135	80	75	62	64	76	97	154	224	269
Total*	34,480	34,171	31,343	31,481	29,824	28,601	30,633	32,156	35,822	40,284	44,629

* May not precisely match figures quoted because of rounding.

Source: Government Statistical Service. See Note 1.

these ADHD-related drugs rose from GBP£72,970 in 1980 to a staggering GBP£29,358,340 in the year 2000. However, although the cost of all these classes of psychiatric drugs had risen tenfold, from around GBP£50 million per annum in 1980 to around GBP£530 million in 2000, this was broadly consistent with the rising cost of the drug bill generally, and expenditure on psychiatric drugs remains at about 8 per cent of NHS drug expenditure.

Italy

It is interesting to compare these data with the case of Italy, where the move to community psychiatry was spearheaded by the work of a group of politically committed young psychiatrists who gathered around Franco Basaglia from the early 1960s up to his early death in 1980 (Scheper-Hughes *et al.* 1987). Under the banner of 'democratic psychiatry', they tried to combat what they thought of as the scientific criminalization of otherness and deviance, which was manifested in the segregation of the mentally ill in the closed asylum. In Italy, this was invariably a result of a legal commitment process. Their campaign culminated in Law 180, enacted in 1978, which put severe legal constraints on any new compulsory admissions to asylums, and provided for their gradual phasing-out by the resocialization of their inmates, and the provision of a network of outpatient services, general hospital provision and community mental health centres.

According to Michael Donnelly, mental hospital beds in Italy increased consistently in the post-war period until the mid-1960s to a peak of over 98,000 beds, or 173 beds per 100,000 of the adult population (Donnelly 1992). From that point on they began to decline by about 1390 beds per year, and the decline accelerated from 1973 to 1978 to a loss of over 3000 beds per year, and accelerated even further from 1978 to 1983, to a loss of over 4000 beds per year. The actual number of hospital *residents* (as opposed to available beds) reached its peak in 1993 at almost 92,000 patients, a figure which had declined to about 38,000 by 1981.

There was much debate in the succeeding period as to whether these reforms had been fully implemented, with their proponents arguing that they had been blocked and betrayed, while their opponents argued that they had simply led to a transfer of institutional care to the private sector for those who could afford it, and to abandonment on the streets of those who could not.[13] Much less debated was the extent to which this new 'open' psychiatric system might be dependent on the prescription of psychiatric drugs to maintain patients 'in the community'. Data on prescribing for the early period is hard to obtain. However, from 1990 to 2000, the data do not support the view that the decline in hospital beds in Italy is linked to a higher than average level of prescription of psychiatric drugs: despite a higher level of psychiatric hospital bed provision in France (even taking the higher Italian figures from the PROGRES study), the figures in all classes in France run at about twice the rate of that in Italy (see Table 7.24). In both countries, the increase in prescribing of antidepressants over this period is entirely produced by the SSRIs: these have risen sixfold in France over this period from 207 to 1323 SUs per

Table 7.24 Psychiatric drug prescribing (retail sales) 1990–2001 in Italy and France in standard dosage units per 1000 population

	1990	1992	1994	1996	1998	2000	2001
Italy: tranquillizers	2,118	2,085	2,146	2,318	2,280	2,269	2,279
France: tranquillizers	4,998	4,821	4,584	4,301	4,150	4,089	4,192
Italy: antidepressants	640	633	644	691	711	852	1,036
France: antidepressants	1,952	1,998	2,059	2,052	2,236	2,411	2,653
Italy: sedatives + hypnotics	956	862	857	908	863	868	885
France: sedatives + hypnotics	2,870	2,924	3,136	3,211	3,524	3,369	3,482
Italy: antipsychotics	337	322	339	382	410	442	475
France: antipsychotics	1,204	1,147	1,114	1,080	1,026	1,018	1,018
Italy: psychostimulants	0	0	0	0	0	0	0
France: psychostimulants	0	0	0	1	2	4	5
Italy: psycholeptics/psychoanaleptics	113	106	104	98	90	78	74
Italy: total	4,164	4,007	4,089	4,397	4,354	4,508	4,749
France: total	11,025	10,891	10,894	10,645	10,938	10,891	11,350

Source: IMS Health Second Study. See Note 2.

1000 population, and 13-fold in Italy from 43 to 583 SUs per 1000 population.[14] A second striking feature is the low level of use of psychostimulants – none are prescribed in Italy, and the rate of prescribing in France, while increasing, remains low. Tranquillizer prescribing remains relatively stable across this period, but here, as in other categories, the rate of prescription in France is about twice that in Italy.

France

We have seen that, among EU countries, while France is about average in its use of antipsychotics, it has a very high rate of prescribing of antidepressants and tranquillizers. This may, in part, arise from the fact that France spends the third highest proportion of its overall health budget on pharmaceuticals at 21 per cent. However, Italy, despite its low usage of psychopharmaceuticals, spends an even greater proportion (22.3 per cent) on pharmaceuticals. There must, therefore, be particular national cultural, patient or practitioner characteristics involved.

This certainly appears to be the view of French commentators. A report published in November 2003, described in the English newspaper, *The Guardian*, estimated that nearly one in four French people are on tranquillizers, antidepressants, antipsychotics or other mood-altering prescription drugs. According to *The Guardian*, the report revealed that an average of 40 per cent of men and women aged over 70 in France were routinely prescribed at least one of this class of dependence-creating drug, as well as some 4 per cent of all children under nine. Commentators linked this to the fact that the French are keen consumers of medication, and pointed to recent attempts by the health minister to remove some 900 medicines out of the total of 4300 prescribed in France, from the list of those that would be reimbursed by the health service. Edouard Zarifian, a professor of medical psychology, was reported as saying that the rate of use of these drugs arose from both doctors and patients – patients not being happy unless they walk out of a consultation with a prescription, and doctors because they are happy to write them. He is quoted as remarking that 'French doctors have become merchants of false happiness. They are unable to resist the pressures of either the patients or the big drugs companies. They are the ones who really need educating'.[15] This comment exemplifies the most common way in which the rise of psychopharmaceuticals has been understood by critical psychiatrists and social scientists – as the influence of the pharmaceutical companies and their marketing strategies on the beliefs and prescribing habits of doctors, both psychiatric specialists and GPs. In December 2004, the French Minister of Health raised the possibility of a complete ban on prescriptions of antidepressants for under-18s, joining a growing number of those who have expressed concern about the use of such drugs for children.

Accounting for psychopharmacology

While prescribing patterns vary considerably across Europe, there has been a steady increase in the prescription of antidepressants in almost all countries. Perhaps, then, a focus on this class of drug might help us understand the factors influencing the prescribing of psychopharmaceuticals more generally. Of course, the simplest explanation for the remarkable rise in the prescription of antidepressants over the last decade is, firstly, that depression is more common than has previously been realized, and secondly, that we now have powerful and effective new drug therapies to treat it. The first proposition represents the view, for example, of the WHO, whose 2001 report claimed depression affects over 340 million people worldwide, argued that it is exacerbated by social factors such as an ageing population, poverty, unemployment and similar stressors, and predicted that:

> By the year 2020, if current trends for demographic and epidemiological transition continue, the burden of depression will increase to 5.7 per cent of the total burden of disease, becoming the second leading cause of DALYs (disability adjusted life years) lost. Worldwide it will be second only to ischemic heart disease for DALYs lost for both sexes. In the developed regions, depression will then be the highest ranking cause of burden of disease.
>
> (World Health Organization 2001: 30)

The proposition that we now have powerful and effective drug therapies is certainly the view, not just of the drug companies and some psychiatrists, but also of some key campaigning groups, especially in the United States. Thus, by 2001 the National Alliance for the Mentally Ill in America proclaimed mental illness a biological brain disorder, linked to a chemical imbalance in the neurotransmitters norepinephrine, serotonin and dopamine, sometimes arising from a genetic predisposition triggered by life events, and treatable with medication that increases the availability of neurotransmitters, just like diabetes is treated with insulin (Styron 1991).[16] In both the United Kingdom and the United States, campaigns to 'recognize depression' operate in these terms: arguing that depression is an illness, often inherited in the form of increased susceptibility and triggered by life events, that it is often untreated, and that drugs form the first line of treatment – for example, in the recent Defeat Depression campaign in the United Kingdom. This view of the biochemical basis of, and treatability of, depression has also been popularized in a number of autobiographical accounts by well-known public figures: for example, *Darkness Visible* by William Styron (1991), or *The Noonday Demon* by Andrew Solomon (2001).

Most social scientists who have explored the rise in depression and its treatment are not satisfied with such a 'realist' account. There is certainly convincing epidemiological evidence that such factors as poor housing, poverty, unemployment or precarious and stressful working conditions are associated with increased levels of psychiatric morbidity. But these factors do not seem sufficient to account for such a rapid increase in diagnosis and prescription, even if it was accepted that contemporary social conditions were more pathogenic than those that preceded them. Older sociological explanations that linked the rise of mental disorders to general features of social organization have fallen out of fashion; for example, the suggestion that urban life generates neurasthenia or that capitalism isolates individuals and hence places strains on them that lead to mental breakdown – with the possible exception of feminist accounts in terms of patriarchy. Alain Ehrenberg has recently suggested that the very shape of depression is the reciprocal of the new conceptions of individuality that have emerged in modern societies (2000). At the start of the twentieth century, he argues, the norm of individuality was founded on guilt, and hence the exemplary experience of pathology was neurosis. But in societies that celebrate individual responsibility and personal initiative, the pathological other side of that norm of active self-fulfilment is depression. While such a global cultural account is probably insufficient, it is plausible to suggest that experience coded as depression – by individuals and their doctors – does so in relation to a cultural norm of the active, responsible, choosing self, realizing his or her potential in the world through shaping a lifestyle. The continual incitements to action, to choice, to self-realization and self-improvement generate an image of the normal person which individuals and others use to judge themselves, and to code differences as pathologies. And this norm, and the individual and social expectations to which it gives rise, seems linked to the recent emergence to prominence of the anxiety disorders – in particular, generalized anxiety disorder, social anxiety disorder, panic disorder, obsessive compulsive disorder and post-traumatic stress disorder.[17]

But other factors also need to be addressed. Firstly, no doubt, these developments are related to the increasing salience of health to the aspirations and ethics of the wealthy West, the readiness of those who live in such cultures to define their problems and their solutions in terms of health and illness, and the tendency for contemporary understandings of health and illness to be posed largely in terms of treatable bodily malfunctions. Secondly, they are undoubtedly linked to a more profound transformation in personhood. The sense of ourselves as 'psychological' individuals that developed across the twentieth century – beings inhabited by a deep internal space shaped by biography and experience, the source of our individuality and the locus of our discontents – is being supplemented by the tendency to define key aspects of one's individuality in bodily terms; that is to say, to think of oneself as 'embodied', and to understand that body in the language of contemporary biomedicine (Novas and Rose 2000). While discontents might previously have been mapped onto a psychological space – the space of neurosis, repression, psychological trauma – they are now mapped upon the body itself, or one particular organ of the body – the brain. Perhaps, however, the key dimension here is the shaping of the gaze of clinical practitioners, their understandings of illness, diagnosis and appropriate treatment.

In countries that do not permit direct-to-consumer advertising of psychiatric drugs, marketing first of all targets these professionals. The earliest (and most quoted) example of this co-production of disorder and treatment concerns depression. Frank Ayd had undertaken one of the key clinical trials for Merck, which filed the first patent for the use of amitryptiline as an antidepressant. Ayd's book of 1961, *Recognizing the Depressed Patient*, argued that much depression was unrecognized, but that it did not require a psychiatrist for its diagnosis – it 'could be diagnosed on general medical wards and in primary care offices' (Healy 1997). Merck bought up 50,000 copies of Frank Ayd's book and distributed it worldwide. As Healy argues, Merck not only sold amitryptiline, it sold a new idea of what depression was and how it could be diagnosed and treated. From this point on, it appeared that there was an untapped market for antidepressant drugs outside hospitals. There was also an audience for the idea that certain drugs specifically targeted the neurochemical basis of depression, and pharmaceutical companies invested funds in research to develop anti-depressants. Rating scales to identify depression were developed (notably the Hamilton depression scale); these generated new norms of depression which were not only used to test the efficacy of drugs, but also changed the shape of the disorder itself. The serotonin hypothesis of depression was formulated, and despite its obvious scientific inadequacies, it became the basis of drug devel-opment leading to the SSRIs and the basis of a new way of thinking about variations in mood in terms of levels of brain chemicals that penetrated deeply into the imagination of medical practitioners and into popular accounts of depression.

Co-production

However, the developments that we have described require more than the transformation of the professional gaze – they involve a more complex co-production of the disease, the treatment and the demand. The best example here concerns the anxiety disorders – social anxiety disorder, panic disorder and generalized anxiety disorder (GAD) – and their relation, in the first instance, with one particular brand – Paxil (paroxetine, known as Seroxat in Europe), owned by GlaxoSmithKline.

As recently as 1987, the section on prevalence of this disorder (coded 300.02) in the third, revised edition of the *Diagnostic and Statistical Manual* said 'When other disorders that could account for the anxiety symptoms are ruled out [they previously stipulated that the disorder should not be diagnosed if the worry and anxiety occurs during a mood disorder or a psychotic disorder, for example], the disorder is not commonly diagnosed in clinical samples' (American Psychiatric Association 1987). By the publication of the fourth edition, in 1994, the same section read 'In a community sample, the lifelong prevalence rate for General-ized Anxiety Disorder was approximately 3 per cent, and the lifetime prevalence rate was 5 per cent. In anxiety disorder clinics, approximately 12 per cent of the individuals present with Generalized Anxiety Disorder' (American Psychiatric Association 1994). In this move, GAD was reframed: the diagnosis could now co-exist with mood disorders, and could be separated out from the general class of mood disorders. The clinical trials of Paxil in the treatment of GAD thus enabled it to be advertised as a specific treatment for this condition, and hence the disorder could be freed, in its public representations at least, from depres-sion. And once it could stand as a diagnosis without subsumption into the class of depression, its prevalence could be recalculated. By April 2001, when Glaxo-SmithKline announced that the US Food and Drug Administration (FDA) had approved Paxil for the treatment of GAD – the first SSRI approved for this disorder in the United States – it was widely being claimed that GAD affected 'more than 10 million Americans, 60 per cent of whom are women'.[18]

The links and relays between classification of disorders, marketing disorders and testing, licensing and promoting psychopharmaceuticals have recently come in for much criticism. Many leading figures in American – and worldwide – psychiatry act as consultants for the pharmaceutical companies, rely upon them for funds for their research, are involved in trialling, testing and evaluating their products, are on the committees responsible for revising and updating diagnostic criteria, advise the licensing authorities on the acceptability and risk of drugs, and indeed have financial interests and shares in the companies themselves.[19] It is certainly the case that as soon as the FDA licence for Paxil was issued in the spring of 2001, GlaxoSmithKline engaged in a marketing campaign in the United States. What was characteristic about this campaign is that it marketed, not so much the drug, Paxil, as the disease, GAD. GlaxoSmithKline argued in advertisements, especially the direct-to-consumer advertisements permitted in the United States, that GAD was a condition affecting many millions of people, that it was distinct from ordinary worrying and a genuine medical condition, that it was caused by anomalies in the neurotransmitter system in the brain, and that these could be treated effectively with Paxil. As an SSRI drug for the treatment of depression, Paxil had arrived relatively late on the scene. But nonetheless, the rate of increase in prescribing in the United States kept pace with the brand leaders, and by 2001, as it succeeded in linking itself to the treatment of anxiety disorders, it achieved a market share about equal to Pfizer's Zoloft and Lilley's Prozac. Other drug manufacturers rushed to trial and re-license their own antidepressants so that they could promote them as treatments for GAD and the other related anxiety disorders – Wyeth with Venlafaxine XF, Pfizer with Zoloft – or to patent and license new molecules specifically for this diagnosis. Pfizer bought the rights to Pagoclone from Indevus Pharmaceuticals, but returned them in June 2002 when the results of its clinical trials failed to show levels of efficacy significantly above placebo; Indevus stocks dropped by 65 per cent on the day of the announcement and Pfizer concentrated their efforts on their own drug, Pregabalin.[20] Shareholder value and clinical value appear inextricably entangled.

Direct-to-consumer advertising of prescription drugs in the United States has grown into a US$2.5 billion a year industry since drug advertising legislation was relaxed in 1997. But the USA is not the only country where 'disease mongering' has become a key marketing tactic.[21] As Ray Moynihan and others have pointed out, this process involves alliances being formed between drug companies anxious to market a product for a particular condition, biosocial groups organized by and for those who suffer from a condition thought to be of that type, and doctors eager to diagnose underdiagnosed problems (Moynihan *et al.* 2002; Moynihan 2003a, 2003b). Disease awareness campaigns, directly or indirectly funded by the pharmaceutical company which has the patent for the treatment, point to the misery caused by the apparent symptoms of this undiagnosed or untreated condition, and interpret available data so as to maximize beliefs about prevalence. They aim to draw the attention of lay persons and medical practitioners to the existence of the disease and the availability of treatment, shaping their fears and anxieties into a clinical form. These campaigns often involve the use of public relations firms to place stories in the media, providing victims who will tell their stories and supplying experts who will explain them in terms of the new disorder. Among the examples given by Moynihan *et al.* (2002) – which include baldness and Propecia, erectile dysfunction and Viagra, irritable bowel syndrome and Lotronex, and Pfizer's promotion of the new disease entity of 'female sexual dysfunction' – is the promotion by Roche of its antidepressant Auroxix (moclobemide) for the treatment of social phobia in Australia in 1997. This involved the use of a public relations company to place stories in the press, an alliance with a patients' group called the Obsessive Compulsive and Anxiety Disorders Federation of Victoria, funding a large conference on social phobia, and promoting maximal estimates of prevalence. These are not covert tactics – as a quick glance at the practical guides published on the web by the magazine *Pharmaceutical Marketing* will show.[22]

Mood swings

Over the past few years, however, these bright promises have become clouded. A series of well-publicized court cases involving homicides and suicides have inculpated, not so much the individuals concerned, but the drugs they were taking. In autumn 1994, the first lawsuit against Prozac reached the courtroom in Louisville (USA), concerning Joseph Wesbecker who some five years earlier, shortly after being prescribed Prozac, had shot 28 people at the printing plant where he worked, killing 8 before shooting himself. This case brought long-standing concerns about the adverse effects of these drugs into the public domain – concerns about increases in agitation (akathesia) and suicidal ideation in a small but significant number of those administered Prozac, which had led the German licensing authorities to insist upon a product warning in 1984 before they would issue a licence. As the first generation of the drugs goes out of patent, the manufacturers have found themselves fighting against a shoal of analogous cases. In the United States, in June 2001, a court in Cheyenne ordered GlaxoSmithKline to pay US$6.4 million to the family of Donald Schell who shot his wife, daughter and grand-daughter and then killed himself two days after his GP prescribed Paxil for depression. The jury decided that the drug was 80 per cent responsible for the deaths. And two weeks earlier, in May 2001, an Australian judge ruled that having been prescribed sertraline – Zoloft – which is Australia's most widely used antidepressant – caused David Hawkins to murder his wife and attempt to kill himself: 'I am satisfied that but for the Zoloft he had taken he would not have strangled his wife' (Justice Barry O'Keefe).[23] In 2003, the United Kingdom's Committee on Safety in Medicine issued a number of guidance notices to the effect that particular SSRI antidepressants had not demonstrated efficacy in children and adolescents under 18, and should not be used to treat depressive illness in such cases.

In December 2004, at the same time as the French Minister of Health was expressing concern about the prescription of antidepressants to children, the UK Medicine and Health Products Regulation Agency concluded its review of SSRIs, advising that in the majority of cases for adults, the lowest dosage should be used, and that certain of these drugs should be prescribed only by specialists and not by GPs. At the same time the UK's National Institute for Clinical Excellence (NICE) advised that while those adults diagnosed with moderate depression in primary care should be offered generic forms of SSRI antidepressants, the risks had to be carefully explained and monitored, and that those with mild depression should be treated initially with 'watchful waiting', perhaps advising exercise, self-help and cognitive-behavioural therapy, but not the use of an antidepressant, as the risk-benefit ratio was considered to be poor (National Institute for Clinical Excellence 2004). By that time, criticisms were mounting, not only of the reliability of published evidence of risk-benefit ratios for SSRIs, but of the difficulties of withdrawing from this medication – not dependency as is often suggested, but the severe and unpleasant physical effects – pains, sweating, nausea and much more – which occur when patients who have been taking these drugs for a while cease to take them, no doubt caused by the fact that the molecules act very widely in the body, and the artificial raising of the levels by the drugs leads to a down-regulation of the body's own production of, or sensitivity to, the molecules in question.[24] These cycles of enthusiasm, doubt, scandal and warning are familiar from the history of the introduction of other psychiatric drugs, notably the minor tranquillizers. They are usually followed by routinization of the uses of these drugs at lower but stable levels, out of the glare of publicity. And, while such public controversies may reshape the details of prescribing practices and the populations to which different drugs are directed, they are unlikely to challenge the basic presuppositions of biological psychiatry, its rise to dominance, and the value, both cognitive and therapeutic, that it accords to neurochemical explanations and pharmaceutical treatment of mental health problems.

Conclusions

In one sense, developments in psychiatric drug use are merely one dimension of a new set of relations between ideas of health and illness, practices of treatment and prevention of bodily malfunctions, and commercially driven innovation, marketing and competition for profits and shareholder value. But they take a specific character in relation to mental health. As we all know, in the second half of the twentieth century, psychotherapy and counselling became big business. But psychiatry itself – in the mental hospitals, the clinics, the GP surgeries and the private psychiatric consulting room – also became a huge and profitable market for the pharmaceutical industry. These developments have continued into the present century. It would be misleading to claim that all ways of understanding mental health problems are 'biological' in the way I have described in this chapter. Indeed, recent developments suggest some reconciliations between bio-medical and social frameworks for understanding mental health problems, notably through the mediation of the versatile idea of 'stress'. But even where practitioners adopt different understandings of the aetiology of such problems, in almost all cases treatment involves the use of drugs.

Because contemporary psychiatry is so much the outcome of developments in psychopharmacology, commercial decisions are actually shaping the patterns of psychiatric thought at a very fundamental level. Most pharmaceutical companies make a considerable proportion of their income from the marketing of psychiatric drugs, and their success, or failure, in attracting market share is key to maintaining the shareholder value of the company. The factories of the pharmaceutical companies are the key laboratories for psychiatric innovation, and the psychiatric laboratory has, in a very real sense, become part of the psychopharmacological factory. Paul Rabinow's assessment of the new life sciences is especially apt for psychiatry – the quest for truth is no longer sufficient to mobilize the production of psychiatric knowledge – health – or rather, the profit to be made from promising health – has become the prime motive force in generating what counts for our knowledge of mental ill health (Rabinow 1996). It may well be the case that the newer psychiatric drugs – the SSRIs and their lineage, the atypical antipsychotics – are more effective and/or have less adverse effects than those they displace. But it is also the case that the shift that this implies, from cheap generic medications to more expensive patented drugs, will have major consequences for health systems and health economics, in a context where drugs are the first line of treatment. This might be especially consequential for the countries that acceded to the EU in 2004 where western pharmaceutical companies see potential new markets despite severe limitations on available funding for mental health care. We can anticipate considerable implications across Europe of this intertwining of the rise of bio-medical understandings of mental health problems amongst psychiatric practitioners, the eastward expansion of market opportunities for western pharmaceutical companies, the move to expensive 'targeted' medication, and the co-production of disease and therapy leading to a recoding of patients' understanding of their sub-optimal conditions as amenable to treatment with psychiatric drugs.

Hence, the consequences of many of the developments I have charted here cannot be reduced to a debate about efficacy, as if illness, treatment and cure were independent of one another. The most widely prescribed of the new generation of psychiatric drugs treat conditions whose borders are fuzzy, whose coherence and very existence as illness or disorders are matters of dispute, and are not so much intended to 'cure' a specific transformation from a normal to a pathological state as to modify the ways in which vicissitudes in the life of the recipient are experienced, lived and understood. Outside psychiatry, the best-selling drugs are not those that treat acute illnesses, but those that are prescribed chronically for conditions that a previous age might have thought of as endemic in life itself – statins for the lowering of blood lipid levels thought to predispose to heart attack and stroke; hormone replacement treatments to minimize the effects of the menopause, in particular its effects on sexuality; drugs for the long-term management of high blood pressure, and for the treatment of gastroesophageal reflux disease and heartburn. The best-selling psychiatric drugs are of this sort, notably those now being heavily marketed and prescribed for the treatment of anxiety and/or depression, in its many new varieties. These are the drugs most amenable to the extension and reshaping of the boundaries of disease and 'treatability'. They promise a power to reshape life pharmaceutically that extends way beyond what we previously understood as illness, to features once understood as endemic in living.

The significance of the widespread use of pharmaceutical treatments for mental ill health lies not only in their specific effects, but also in the way in which they reshape the ways in which both experts and lay people see, interpret, speak about and understand their world. Psychoanalysis brought into existence a whole new way of understanding ourselves – in terms of the unconscious, repression, neuroses, the Oedipus complex, and, of course, the theme of the centrality of sexuality to our psychic life. So it makes sense to ask whether GPs, psychiatrists and other mental health practitioners are beginning to see the problems their clients and patients experience in terms of this simplistic model of mental ill health as a disorder of neurotransmitters. To see in this way is to imagine the disorder as residing within the individual brain and its processes, and to see psychiatric drugs as a first line of intervention, not merely for symptom relief but as specific treatments for these neurochemical anomalies. If we are experiencing a 'neurochemical' reshaping of personhood, the social and ethical implications for the twenty-first century will be profound. For these drugs are becoming central to the ways in which our conduct is problematized and governed – by others, and by ourselves.

Acknowledgements

In this chapter, I draw upon data collected by myself and Mariam Fraser for our study 'The Age of Serotonin', funded by the Wellcome Trust Programme in Biomedical Ethics based in the Department of Sociology at Goldsmiths College, University of London. Thanks to our researcher, Angelique Praat, for her work on the collection and analysis of some of this material. Like all who investigate this area, my work follows lines of enquiry first opened up by David Healy, and my argument is indebted to his work. I also draw upon a survey commissioned for that study from IMS Health, detailed in Note 1, and would like to thank Robin Keat, Pete Stephens and Ian Webster of IMS in particular for their help and advice on data, and Pete Stephens in particular for the data in the IMS Third Study. Thanks to Reinhold Killian and others who commented on an early draft of this chapter, presented first as a paper at the European Observatory on Health Systems and Policies Workshop on Mental Health Policy and Practice Across Europe held in Oslo in September 2003.

Notes

1   Data on prices and market sizes for pharmaceuticals are not readily available for many countries. For the UK, it is possible to obtain roughly consistent figures for the period commencing in 1980 by the *Government Statistical Service* and they kindly provided us with a breakdown of their data, which we use in this analysis.

   For drugs that are listed in the schedules of the UN Convention on Psychotropic Substances of 1971 – hallucinogens, stimulants, depressants and some analgesics that have medical and scientific uses but can also be drugs of abuse – international comparative data is published annually in the reports on psychotropic substances of the International Narcotics Control Board, now available on line at www.incb.org/. However, these data do not include most antidepressants or antipsychotic drugs: for that, one has to go to commercial organizations providing data to the drug companies themselves.

To access this data, we commissioned three customized studies from IMS Health based on the data that they compile from over 120 countries, which includes, for the countries chosen, drugs prescribed in hospital and sold through retail outlets. These data provided the basis for calculations made by our team, and IMS has no responsibility for these or our interpretations. The first two studies examined the situation in a number of broad geographical regions in the decade from 1990 to 2000. The regions selected were USA, Japan, the EU, South America (Argentina, Brazil, Mexico, Colombia, Peru, Uruguay, Venezuela), South Africa (data for other countries in Sub-Saharan Africa were not available) and Pakistan (12-year data for India were not available). The third study examined the situation in the 15 countries which were member states of the EU from 1993 to 2002. Unless otherwise stated, reference to 'Europe' in this chapter is to the EU-15 data.

The first study contained data on market size in US dollars at ex-manufacturers prices, adjusted according to the prevailing rates of exchange. The second contained detailed breakdowns by molecules of the volume of drugs prescribed. The third study provided country breakdowns of data for selected drug types in the countries of the EU.

The principal comparative measure used is the SU. SUs are determined by taking the number of counting units sold, divided by the standard unit factor which is the smallest common dose of a product form as defined by IMS Health. For example, for oral solid forms the standard unit factor is one tablet or capsule whereas for syrup forms the standard unit factor is one teaspoon (5 ml) and injectable forms it is one ampoule or vial. This is the best available measure for comparative purposes, but it is far from perfect. For example, a 30-day pack of a product given four times a day will contribute 120 SUs for each pack sold whereas a similar pack of a once daily product will contribute only 30 SUs. Many more products now have once daily dosing regimes than in the past. In such circumstances SU analyses can make it appear that the market has collapsed even though the days of treatment will have remained constant or increased. Therefore, there are some risks to using SUs for comparative purposes over the time periods and the regions reported here, and where these are of particular relevance we have tried to supplement SUs with other measures. Dates shown are calendar years. Prices refer to total sales ex-manufacturer (not retail prices) in US dollars at the exchange rate at the date in question. Figures credited to IMS Health are based on that report, but the analysis, tables and figures are our own. Some drugs used to treat psychiatric conditions, such as the anti-convulsants, are not included, as most prescriptions for such drugs are for non-psychiatric conditions.

Wherever appropriate, the data is standardized to population size and expressed as SU per 1000 population in the year in question. 2001 population data was used in the calculations for the IMS Second Study, derived from the CIA *World Factbook* 2001, and 2003 population data was used for the IMS Second Study, derived from the CIA *World Factbook* 2003, available at www.cia.gov/cia/publications/factbook/.

2 IMS Health: First Study.

3 The best historical work on the development of psychopharmacology has been done by David Healy, and I draw extensively on this here: notably Healy (1997, 2001).

4 American Psychiatric Association (1994).

5 Notably by Husseini Manji and his team at the Laboratory of Molecular Pathophysiology at the US National Institute of Mental Health, e.g. Manji *et al.* (2001).

6 Notably Duman and his team, e.g. Duman *et al.* (1997, 2001).

7 The DDD is the assumed average maintenance dose per day for a drug used for its main indication in adults, and DDDs are assigned by the WHO Collaborating Centre for Drug Statistics Methodology in Norway (www.whocc.no/atcddd/).

8 It is possible to calculate the conversion between SUs and DDDs, but this has to be

done for each drug individually, by transforming SUs into measures of weight, and then converting these to DDDs, which are also specified in weight.

9   Of course, even these data are affected by national policies, as they refer to drugs obtained on prescription, not those available over-the-counter (OTC) – hence if a drug or group of drugs moves from prescription status to OTC status, it ceases to appear in the figures.

10 These data were compiled by Ville Lentinen.

11 Oddly, Ghodse and Khan do not include data for neuroleptic drugs in this table, presumably because their main concern is inappropriate prescription of drugs that may lead to dependence or have the liability for abuse.

12 Earlier comparable figures are not available. Note that the data up to 1990 are not consistent with data from 1991 onwards. Figures for 1980–90 are based on fees and on a sample of 1 in 200 prescriptions dispensed by community pharmacists and appliance contractors only. Figures for 1991 onwards are based on items and cover all prescriptions dispensed by community pharmacists, appliance contractors dispensing doctors and prescriptions submitted by prescribing doctors for items personally administered.

13 Note that Donnelly's data do not support this argument about the transfer of patients to private institutional confinement.

14 Studies by Barbui and his collaborators, using various national databases, also estimate an increase in sales of antidepressants of 53 per cent from 1988 to 1996, and that by 1996, SSRI antidepressants accounted for 30 per cent of sales. See Barbui *et al.* (1999, 2003); Pietraru *et al.* (2001).

15 All quoted from *The Guardian*, 8.11.2003, available at www.guardian.co.uk/france/story/0,11882,1080507,00.html.

16 http://www.nami.org/illness/whatis.html, 12.8.02.

17 We have already seen that anxiety, not depression, has been until recently the exemplary pathology in Japan. *DSM IV* distinguishes mood disorders, which include the major depressive disorders, from anxiety disorders. Of course, the SSRI drugs were not marketed in the first instance for major depression or bipolar disorder, but for mild to moderate depression, and it is in this fuzzy area that the new links between depression and anxiety are being established. While marketing strategies tend to avoid coding the anxiety disorders as forms of depression, psychiatrists themselves tend to see them as closely linked conditions.

18 On the *Doctor's Guide* website, www.pslgroup.com/dg/1f8182.htm, 12.8.02.

19 Healy (1997); see also the resignation letter of leading American social psychiatrist from 'The American Psychopharmaceutical Association: Lauren Mosher, Resignation letter to APA, 1998: at www.oikos.org/mosher.htm, 12.8.02.

20 http://biz.yahoo.com/bw/020607/72033_2.html: 15.8.02; www.biospace.com/ccis/news_story.cfm?StoryID=8819419&full=1: 15.8.02.

21 See Cassels, Alan (2002) The drug companies' latest marketing tactic: 'disease awareness' pitch – a new licence to expand drug sales, at www.policyalternatives.ca/publications/articles/article315.html, 12.8.02.

22 www.pmlive.com/pharm_market/prac_guides.cfm, 12.8.02.

23 Quoted at http://www.antidepressantsfacts.com/David-John-Hawkins.htm.

24 A 1997 review of these effects can be found on the website of the American Society of Consultant Pharmacists http://www.ascp.com/public/pubs/tcp/1997/oct/ssri.html, 12.8.02.

References

American Psychiatric Association (1952) *Diagnostic And Statistical Manual For Mental Disorders: With Special Supplement On Plans For Revision. Prepared by the Committee on Nomenclature and Statistics of The American Psychiatric Association.* Washington, DC: American Psychiatric Association.

American Psychiatric Association (1968) *DSM II Diagnostic and Statistical Manual of Mental Disorders.* Washington, DC: American Psychiatric Association.

American Psychiatric Association (1980) *Diagnostic and Statistical Manual of Mental Disorders.* Washington, DC: American Psychiatric Association.

American Psychiatric Association (1987) *Diagnostic and Statistical Manual of Mental Disorders: DSM-111-R.* Washington, DC: American Psychiatric Association.

American Psychiatric Association (1994) *Diagnostic and Statistical Manual of Mental Disorders: DSM-IV. Prepared by the Task Force on DSM-IV and Other Committees and Work Groups of The American Psychiatric Association.* Washington, DC: American Psychiatric Association.

Ayd, F.J. (1961) *Recognizing the Depressed Patient: With Essentials of Management and Treatment.* New York: Grune & Stratton.

Barbui, C., Broglio, E., Laia, A.C., D'agostino, S., Enrico, F., Ferraro, L., Fiorio, E., Miletti, F., Pietraru, C., Poggio, L. and Tognoni, G. (2003) Cross-sectional database analysis of antidepressant prescribing in Italy, *Journal of Clinical Psychopharmacology*, 23(1):1–34.

Barbui, C., Campomori, A., D'avanzo, B., Negri, E. and Garattini, S. (1999) Antidepressant drug use in Italy since the introduction of SSRI: national trends, regional differences and impact on suicide rates, *Social Psychiatry and Psychiatric Epidemiology*, 34(3): 152–6.

Donnelly, M. (1992) *The Politics of Mental Health in Italy.* London: Routledge.

Duman, R.S., Heninger, G.R. and Nestler, E.J. (1997) A molecular and cellular theory of depression, *Archives of General Psychiatry*, 54(7): 597–606.

Duman, R.S., Malberg, J. and Nakagawa, S. (2001) Regulation of adult neurogenesis by psychotropic drugs and stress, *Journal of Pharmacology and Experimental Therapeutics*, 299(2): 401–7.

Ehrenberg, A. (2000) *La Fatigue d'Etre Soi.* Paris: Odile Jacob.

Gelman, S. (1999) *Medicating Schizophrenia: A History.* New Brunswick, NJ: Rutgers University Press.

Ghodse, H. and Khan, I. (eds) (1988) *Psychoactive Drugs: Improving Prescribing Practices – Meeting on the Training of Health Care Professionals in Rational Prescribing.* Geneva: World Health Organization.

Government Statistical Service (1998) *Health and Personal Social Statistics: England.* London: Government Statistical Service.

Healy, D. (1997) *The Antidepressant Era.* Cambridge, MA: Harvard University Press.

Healy, D. (2001) *The Creation of Psychopharmacology.* Cambridge, MA: Harvard University Press.

Hovatta, I., Terwilliger, J.D., Lichtermann, D., Makikyro, T., Suvisaari, J., Peltonen, L. and Lonnqvist, J. (1997) Schizophrenia in the genetic isolate of Finland, *American Journal of Medical Genetics*, 74(4): 353–60.

Knutson, B., Wolkowitz, O.M., Cole, S.W., Chan, T., Moore, E.A., Johnson, R.C., Terpstra, J., Turner, R.A. and Reus, V.I. (1998) Selective alteration of personality and social behavior by serotonergic intervention, *American Journal of Psychiatry*, 155(3): 373–9.

Manji, H.K., Moore, G.J. and Chen, G. (2001) Bipolar disorder: leads from the molecular and cellular mechanisms of action of mood stabilisers, *British Journal of Psychiatry*, 178: S107–19.

Moynihan, R. (2003a) Who pays for the pizza? Redefining the relationships between doctors and drug companies. 1: Entanglement, *British Medical Journal*, 326: 1189–92.

Moynihan, R. (2003b) Who pays for the pizza? Redefining the relationships between doctors and drug companies. 2: Disentanglement, *British Medical Journal*, 326: 1193–6.

Moynihan, R., Heath, I. and Henry, D. (2002) Selling sickness: the pharmaceutical industry and disease mongering, *British Medical Journal*, 324: 886–91.

National Institute For Clinical Excellence (2004) *Depression: Management of Depression in Primary and Secondary Care*. London: National Institute For Clinical Excellence.

Novas, C. and Rose, N. (2000) Genetic risk and the birth of the somatic individual, *Economy And Society*, 29(4): 485–513.

Pietraru, C., Barbui, C., Poggio, L. and Tognoni, G. (2001) Antidepressant drug prescribing in Italy, 2000: analysis of a general practice database, *European Journal of Clinical Pharmacology*, 57(8): 605–9.

Rabinow, P. (1996) *Essays on the Anthropology of Reason*. Princeton, NJ: Princeton University Press.

Scheper-Hughes, N., Lovell Anne, M. and Basaglia, F. (1987) *Psychiatry Inside Out: Selected Writings of Franco Basaglia*. New York: Columbia University Press.

Solomon, A. (2001) *The Noonday Demon: An Anatomy of Depression*. London: Chatto & Windus.

Styron, W. (1991) *Darkness Visible: A Memoir of Madness*. London: Cape.

Suvisaari, J.M., Haukka, J.K., Tanskanen, A.J. and Lonnqvist, J.K. (1999) Decline in the incidence of schizophrenia in Finnish cohorts born from 1954 to 1965, *Archives of General Psychiatry*, 56(8): 733–40.

World Health Organization (2001) *The World Health Report 2001. Mental Health: New Understanding, New Hope*. Geneva: WHO.

chapter eight

A policy framework for the promotion of mental health and the prevention of mental disorders

Eva Jané-Llopis and Peter Anderson

The burden of mental disorders

Mental and behavioural disorders are found in people of all ages, regions, countries and societies, being present at any point in time in 10 per cent of the adult population (WHO 2001). More than one person in four will develop one or more mental or behavioural disorders during their life. Five of the ten leading causes of disability and premature death worldwide are mental and behavioural disorders, including depression, harmful alcohol use, schizophrenia and compulsive disorder (Murray and Lopez 1996). In 1990 mental and neurological disorders accounted for 10 per cent of global disability and premature death. In 2002 this increased to 12.9 per cent. In 2020, it is estimated that this will increase to 15 per cent, with unipolar depression alone accounting for 5.7 per cent of worldwide disability (Murray and Lopez 1996).

In addition to the health burden, the social and economic costs of mental ill health for societies are wide ranging, long lasting and enormous. Besides the health and social service costs, lost employment and reduced productivity, the impact on families and caregivers, levels of crime and public safety, and the negative impact of premature mortality, there are many other immeasurable costs that have not been taken into account, such as lost opportunity costs to individuals and families (WHO 2001).

Mental health promotion and mental disorder prevention

Different reviews and publications have defined the differences and overlaps between prevention and promotion in mental health. Some definitions are presented in Box 8.1.

Box 8.1 Definitions of mental health promotion and mental disorder prevention

Mental health promotion aims to protect, support and sustain emotional and social well-being and create individual, social and environmental conditions that enable optimal psychological and psychophysiological functioning, enhance mental health while showing respect for culture, equity, social justice and personal dignity. Initiatives, developed in an empowering manner, involve individuals who are not at risk as well as those who are suffering or recovering from mental health problems, in the process of achieving positive mental health, enhancing quality of life and narrowing the gap in health expectancy between countries and groups.

To 'prevent' literally means 'to intervene or to take steps in advance to stop something from happening'. Mental disorder prevention focuses on reducing risk factors and enhancing protective factors associated with mental ill health, with the aim to reduce risk, incidence, prevalence and recurrence of mental disorders, the time spent with symptoms, or the risk condition for a mental illness, preventing or delaying recurrences and also decreasing the impact of illness in the affected person, their families and society.

Definitions derived from: Mrazek and Haggerty (1994); Hosman and Jané-Llopis (1999); Detels *et al.* (2002); WHO (2004b, 2004c).

As the definitions suggest, it has been argued that prevention and promotion are distinct but overlapping strategies (WHO 2004a, 2004b), where mental health promotion, focusing on the determinants of health, is more than the prevention of mental disorders, which is often considered as part of the broader mental health promotion concept (Herrman and Jané-Llopis 2005).

The efficacy of promotion and prevention in mental health

In addition to the advantages that treatment can have for mental disorders, two recent summary reports by the World Health Organization (WHO) (WHO 2004b, 2004c) and their accompanying publications, present the evidence that mental health promotion (Herrman *et al.* 2005) and mental disorder prevention (Hosman *et al.* 2006a) can be effective and lead to important health, social and economic gains.

Although many remain unconvinced that promotion and prevention can contribute to reducing the increasing burden and costs of mental ill health, the public mental health field is increasingly recognizing the need for a comprehensive approach to mental health. It is noted that, although treatment for mental disorders can be very effective, this is only once mental ill health has already emerged. A public health policy that only comprises cure and maintenance would have clear disadvantages. In addition to the consequences of only starting to take action when there has already been long-lasting suffering of individuals and families, evidence shows that there is a large proportion of under-treated cases (Kazdin 1993) and high rates of relapse after treatment (Muñoz 1998).

A policy framework for promotion and prevention in mental health

This chapter builds on existing evidence and recent reviews (WHO 2004b, 2004c; Jané-Llopis *et al.* 2005) and presents the policy response for action in mental health promotion and mental disorder prevention (Jané-Llopis and Anderson 2005). The next section outlines examples of policies and programmes for mental health promotion across the lifespan. The following section presents a policy response to reduce the risk of some mental health problems: depression, anxiety, conduct disorders, substance use disorders and associated suicide. While there is strong evidence for the reduction of risk factors and the increase of protective factors related to mental disorders, there is to date less evidence available for the actual prevention of mental disorders. Several reasons for this have been described elsewhere (WHO 2004c), but one of the frequent explanations is the need for large numbers of people that need to be involved in efficacy studies to ensure sufficient power to prove reductions in onset of mental disorders, especially when populations are not at increased risk. However, there are a few studies that have shown actual prevention of new cases of major depression, especially in children and adolescents (Clarke *et al.* 1995, 2001). Box 8.2 summarizes preventive and promotion approaches from which some interventions have proven to be efficacious. Examples of such efficacious interventions are described across the different sections in this chapter, outlining a policy framework that could guide decision-making and implementation. However, it is important to note that not all interventions can be or are effective, and that it is crucial to base implementation on the knowledge of available efficacious interventions.

Mental health promotion policies across the lifespan

The implementation of policies specially designed to promote mental health in the whole population and to tackle mental health problems can lead to substantial gains in mental health and improve the social and economic development of society (WHO 2004c). This section reviews the options for designing a mental health policy composed of effective strategies across the lifespan to improve mental health and to reduce the risks of mental disorders.

Box 8.2   Some efficacious approaches for prevention and promotion in mental health

	Childhood/ adolescence	Adulthood	Older groups
Mental health policy and programmes	General school skill-building programmes, like life skills and problem-solving	Parenting visits for depressed mothers	Early screening interventions in primary care
	Changing school environment	Parenting group interventions for difficult children	Prescriptions of antidepressants to prevent suicide
	Holistic school interventions combining skill-building and changes in the environment	Mental health support and early treatment for those at risk	
	Cognitive-behavioural programmes for children at risk of depression	Stress management techniques	
	Stress management techniques	Cognitive-behavioural models for depression	
		Brief interventions for alcohol in primary health care	
		Prescription of antidepressants to prevent suicide	
Public health and public policy	Home visiting, healthy development	Pregnancy free of addictive substances	Physical activity
	Parenting interventions	Parenting interventions	Patient education
		Workplace task and technical improvement interventions	
		Workplace improvement role clarity and social relationships	
		Combined interventions addressing the organization and employees	

		Skills training for the unemployed	
	Taxation of alcohol and tobacco Comprehensive and media community interventions for alcohol Reduction of means to commit suicide Policies to reduce economic insecurity Social policies to promote social support and inclusion and prevent social exclusion Access to preschool education Housing improvement		

Infants and toddlers

During the first months and years of life there is more development in mental, social and physical functioning than at any other time across the lifespan (Unicef 2001). A healthy start in life greatly enhances a child's later functioning in school, with peers, in later intimate relationships and with broader connections with society. Interventions at the early start of life, including home-based parenting and preschool interventions, mostly focus on enhancing the resilience and competence of parents and families through educational strategies (WHO 2004c). Such interventions have proved successful in improving both parents' and children's physical and mental health, and children's competence, mental well-being and functioning in society, with an impact across generations (WHO 2004c; Brown and Sturgeon 2006).

Pregnancy free of addictive substances

The use of the addictive substances, alcohol, tobacco and illicit drugs during pregnancy can cause harm to the foetus and child (Tuthill *et al.* 1999). In particular, tobacco doubles the risk of low birth weight (Institute of Medicine 2001). Strategies that work include educational programmes to help pregnant women to quit smoking and increase the birth weight of infants with both immediate and long-term mental health gain (Institute of Medicine 2001). For instance, Windsor *et al.* (1993) evaluated a 15-minute behavioural intervention for pregnant smokers, showing a 6 per cent increase in smoking cessation. Among those who quit, their babies were 200 grams heavier at birth while cutting down on smoking increased birth weight by half this amount.

Home visits to first-time mothers

First-time pregnant women, especially those who are single, adolescent or from impoverished backgrounds, are at increased risk of mental health problems and more likely to fail in providing a healthy start to life for their children (WHO 2004c). Often associated, pre-term delivery and low birth weight increase the risk of cognitive and behavioural problems and mental disorders in childhood and adult life (Elgen *et al.* 2002).

Home-visiting interventions during pregnancy and early infancy, addressing maternal substance use, coping with stress, parental caregiving, and links to support systems and health services can lead to health, social and economic gain (Olds 1989, 1997, 2002; Olds *et al.* 1998). For example, the outcomes of several randomized trials in the Prenatal/Early Infancy Project, a nurse-led home-visiting programme, have shown increased birth weights for newborns by up to 400 grams, improvement in mental health outcomes in both mothers and children, less use of health services, reductions in child maltreatment, improvements in children's educational achievements and long-term reductions in child and adolescent problem behaviours (Olds 1989, 1997, 2002; Olds *et al.* 1998). It has been suggested that home-visiting interventions can be cost-effective, especially when long-term outcomes are taken into account (Olds 2002; Brown and Sturgeon 2006).

Parenting interventions

Positive, proactive parenting involving praise, encouragement, and affection can increase children's self-esteem, their social and academic competence, and protection against later disruptive behaviour and substance use disorders (Brown and Sturgeon 2006). Conversely, negative parenting is a major contributing factor to the development of physical and psychiatric disorders (Stewart-Brown *et al.* 2005).

Parental early interventions that promote basic reading skills can lead to improved literacy and cognitive, emotional and language growth, facilitating the transition to school. Group-based parent training programmes for families at risk can improve the behaviour of children between the ages of 3 and 10 years (Coren and Barlow 1999). It has also been suggested that these interventions are more cost-effective and successful in the long term than methods that involve working with parents on an individual basis (Barlow 1999). Parenting programmes can also be effective in promoting the short-term psychosocial health of mothers (Barlow *et al.* 2001). For example, depression, anxiety/stress, self-esteem and relationship problems all registered significant improvement in a meta-analysis combining the results of 17 parenting programmes, as compared to those in the control groups (Barlow and Coren 2004).

Children and adolescents

School has a significant influence on the behaviour and development of all children. Poor school performance and poor academic achievement increase the risk of social and mental problems, antisocial behaviour, delinquency, substance use disorders, teenage pregnancy, conduct problems and involvement in crime. Conversely, school achievement is related to positive social and emotional development, increased employment and earnings, and access to health, social, and community resources (Weare 2000). Achievement and adult support promotes mental health and can counteract a range of adversities such as poverty, living in high-crime neighbourhoods, parental substance use disorders and family conflict. Schools provide an efficient means of promoting the health, academic and emotional development of young people. There is no other setting where such a large proportion of children and adolescents can be reached systematically (Domitrovich *et al.* 2006).

Three types of mental health promotion programmes in the school setting have shown to be efficacious in enhancing the resilience of children and adolescents.

General skill-building programmes

General cognitive, problem-solving and social skill-building programmes in primary and middle school can significantly improve cognition, emotional knowledge and problem-solving skills, and reduce internalizing and externalizing problems, with 50 per cent reductions in depressive symptoms (Greenberg *et al.* 2001).

Changing school environments

Programmes that restructure school and classroom environments to promote positive behaviour and rule compliance through reinforcement can lead to sustained reductions in aggressive behaviour (Felner *et al.* 1993).

Combining both approaches: multi-component programmes

Prevention and promotion programmes that focus simultaneously on different levels, such as changing the school environment as well as improving students' individual skills and involving parents are more effective than those that intervene solely on one level (WHO 2004b; Domitrovich *et al.* 2006). Such programmes should adopt a school-wide approach and be implemented for more than one year (Weare 2000).

Working life

Stress factors such as noise, work overload, time pressure, repetitive tasks, interpersonal conflict and job insecurity can cause mental health problems and increase the risk of anxiety, depression and stress-related problems (Price and Kompier 2006). Effective strategies to improve mental health in the workplace and to prevent the risk of mental disorders include: task and technical interventions (e.g. job enrichment, ergonomic improvements, reduction of noise, lowering workloads); improving role clarity and social relationships (e.g. communication, conflict resolution); and interventions addressing multiple changes directed both at work and employees (Price and Kompier 2006). Notwithstanding the existence of (inter)national legislation with respect to the psychosocial work environment that emphasizes risk assessment and risk management, these strategies still remain underused (Schaufeli and Kompier 2001) and most programmes aim to reduce the cognitive appraisal of stress factors and their subsequent effects (Murphy 1996), rather than the reduction or elimination of the stress factors themselves. Similarly, organizational downsizing, involuntary job loss and long-term unemployment produce both stress and adverse health and mental health problems including depression, substance abuse and marital conflict (Price *et al.* 2002). Many of these problems associated with unemployment increase health and human service costs to society (Vinokur *et al.* 1991).

A number of intervention programmes have been developed and evaluated to help unemployed workers to re-enter the labour market. Such programmes combine basic instruction on job search skills, with enhancing motivation, skills in coping with setbacks and social support among job seekers (Price *et al.* 1992). For example, the Winning New Jobs programme (see Box 8.3) has been tested and replicated in large-scale randomized trials both in the United States and Finland, showing positive effects on rates of re-employment, the quality and pay of jobs obtained, increases in job search self-efficacy and mastery, and reductions in depression and distress (Price *et al.* 1992; Price and Vinokur 1995; Vuori *et al.* 2002; Vuori and Silvonen 2005).

Retirement and older age

Over the next 30 years, the proportion of people aged over 80, as a share of those aged over 65, will increase in Europe as a whole from 22 to 30 per cent (WHO 2002a). This rapid increase in the ageing population implies a shift in the demographic structures of society, bringing associated problems such as an increased risk of some mental illness (e.g. dementia), age-related chronic diseases and decreases in the quality of life (Levkoff *et al.* 1995). In addition to loss of health and functional and cognitive abilities, elder populations are more likely to experience individual losses both within their social network (e.g. bereavement, diminished social contacts) as well as within their personal positioning in life (e.g. facing retirement, loss of income), placing them at risk of suffering mental health problems (Reynolds *et al.* 2001).

The mental health of older populations has been successfully improved through interventions to increase physical activity (Deuster 1996; Mather *et al.* 2002), for example through practising tai chi (Chen *et al.* 2001; Li *et al.* 2001). A Cochrane review of patient education programmes that included an instruction component for people with arthritis identified 24 randomized controlled trials indicating short-term improvements in disability and the psychological status of patients, including depression (Riemsma *et al.* 2002). Early screening, interventions in primary care (Burns *et al.* 2000; Shapiro and Taylor 2002) have also proven to be successful in improving the mental health of older people who are at risk. The risk of dementia is likely to be reduced by preventing craniocerebral traumas, and lowering raised blood pressure and cholesterol levels (Cooper 2002), although there is still a need for more research in this area.

Box 8.3 Promoting re-employment and mental health

The Winning New Jobs Programme: promoting re-employment and mental health

The Winning New Jobs Programme was developed in the United States to assist unemployed workers to effectively seek re-employment and cope with the multiple challenges of unemployment and job-searching (Caplan *et al.* 1989; Price *et al.* 1992; Price and Vinokur 1995). The half-day workshops held over one week focus on identifying effective job-search strategies, improving participant job-search skills, increasing self-esteem, confidence and the motivation of participants to persist in job-search activities. Two trainers deliver the programme to groups of 12 to 20 people.

The programme has been evaluated in replicated randomized trials involving thousands of unemployed workers in the United States. Results indicated increased quality of re-employment, increased self-esteem and decreased psychological distress and depressive symptoms, over two years, particularly among those with a higher risk for depression (Price *et al.* 1992). In addition, the programme has been shown to inoculate workers against the adverse effects of subsequent job loss because they gain an enhanced sense of mastery over the challenges of seeking employment (Price 2003).

Cost-effectiveness analyses have shown a threefold return on the investment after two and a half years, and more than a tenfold return after five years (Vinokur *et al.* 1991).

The programme has been adopted in Finland as The Työhön Job Search Programme, to meet cultural differences in unemployment, duration of social and economic security and labour policies on the use of labour market programmes. A randomized controlled trial of its implementation, including more than 1000 unemployed job seekers, showed, after six months, increases in quality of re-employment, which was strongest for those at risk of becoming long-term unemployed, and reductions in levels of distress, which was strongest for those who were at high risk for depression. Decreases in depressive symptoms and increases in self-esteem were found two years after the programme implementation. Those in the intervention groups also indicated benefits regarding higher engagement in the labour market, either by being employed or participating in vocational training (Vuori *et al.* 2002; Vuori and Silvonen 2005).

Preventing the risk of mental disorders

Depression and anxiety

Depression is one of the most prevalent psychiatric disorders (WHO 2003), and in Europe, unipolar depression alone is the third leading cause of disability, accounting for 6.1 per cent of disability adjusted life years (DALYs) in 2002

(Üstun *et al.* 2004). Children who have suffered child abuse during infancy and childhood, those who have suffered parental loss or parental divorce, and those who have a mentally ill parent are up to 50 per cent more likely to suffer from school problems such as underachievement and mental health problems such as depression and anxiety (Beardslee *et al.* 1998; WHO 2004c).

Effective strategies such as school-based prevention programmes for children at risk that have used cognitive-behavioural models (Clarke *et al.* 1995), life skills problem-solving (Greenberg *et al.* 2001) and stress management techniques (Hains and Ellman 1994) have been shown to reduce depressive and anxiety symptoms by more than half, as indicated in a systematic review (Gillham *et al.* 2000) and a meta-analysis of programmes aiming to prevent depression (Jané-Llopis *et al.* 2003). Only a small number of randomized trials have proven to be efficacious in reducing the onset of anxiety (Dadds *et al.* 1997, 1999) and depressive disorders (Clarke *et al.* 1995, 2001) (see Box 8.4) in children and adolescents, showing overall reductions of over two-thirds.

Box 8.4   Depression prevention for adolescents at risk

The Coping with Stress Course is a group-based prevention programme attempting to prevent unipolar depressive episodes in high-school adolescents with an elevated risk of depressive disorder. The programme (Clarke *et al.* 1990), during its 15 sessions, focuses on training adolescents to identify and challenge irrational or highly negative thoughts, and teaching coping mechanisms to strengthen coping techniques. A total of 150 adolescents considered at risk for future depression were enrolled in an evaluation study and randomized to either a cognitive group prevention intervention or a 'usual care' control condition (Clarke *et al.* 1995). After 12 months, the total incidence rate of affective disorders for the intervention group was 14.5 per cent versus 25.7 per cent for those in the control condition; indicating a 43.5 per cent reduction in new cases of depressive disorder (Clarke *et al.* 1995).

The same intervention has recently been implemented and evaluated with 13- to 18-year-old offspring of depressed parents (Clarke *et al.* 2001). Youth/parent dyads (demoralized group) were included in the study on the basis of whether the youth had sub-diagnostic depressive symptoms or had a past episode of major depression. Demoralized youth were randomized to usual care or usual care plus a 15-session group prevention programme using cognitive therapy methods, where they were taught to identify negative thinking patterns and to generate more realistic and positive counter-thoughts. Significant prevention effects were found for self-reported depressive symptoms. Survival analysis of total incident major depressive episodes indicated a significant advantage for the experimental condition (9.3 per cent cumulative major depression incidence) compared to the usual care control condition (28.8 per cent) at the median of 14-month follow-up (Clarke *et al.* 2001).

Other interventions that have led to reductions in depressive symptoms in adults and older populations (Jané-Llopis *et al.* 2003) include cognitive behavioural models (Allart-van Dam *et al.* 2003), home-based interventions with families at risk (Aronen and Kurkela 1996), stress management policies in the workplace (Heaney *et al.* 1995a, 1995b), detection and management interventions in primary health care (Gilbody 2004), and the support of community networks and physical activities in older age (Jané-Llopis *et al.* 2006).

Conduct disorders, bullying, aggression and violence

Conduct disorders and developmental learning disorders are associated with educational failure, accidents, injuries, physical illness, unemployment and poor work performance, criminal activity, adult problems in intimate relationships, substance use disorders, anxiety disorders and depression (Yoshikawa 1994). The social and economic costs of conduct disorders, and of aggressive and violent behaviour, are enormous, including the costs of treatment, the criminal justice system, social services, academic failure, and the emotional and economic costs for individuals and families (Eddy 2006).

Effective programmes to improve the behaviour of children at risk of behavioural problems and later aggression are those that combine strategies of classroom behaviour management, social skills enhancement and parent involvement (Reid and Eddy 1997). Such programmes can cut disruptive behaviour and aggression, including bullying, theft, and vandalism by half (Olweus 1991). Similarly, programmes targeting children of parents with substance use disorders can reduce problem behaviour (Eddy 2006).

Addictive substances

Addictive substances (tobacco, alcohol and illicit drugs) can cause intoxication and injuries, a very wide range of harm and dependence (see Chapter 11). Together they cause over a fifth (tobacco 12 per cent, alcohol 8 per cent and illicit drugs 2 per cent) of the total burden of ill health and premature death in Europe (WHO 2002b). Such substances cause harm not only to users but also to those surrounding users and are a major cause of socioeconomic inequities in health. They cause an enormous economic burden to society and economic productivity. Some 10 to 15 per cent of the total health care budget arises from treating the harm done by substance use (WHO 2001). Substance use disorders are a classified mental disorder as well as being co-morbid with a wide range of mental and behavioural disorders including depression and suicide (WHO 1992).

Successful and cost-effective options to reduce substance use disorders are environmental measures that influence the price, availability and marketing of substances (Anderson 1999; WHO 2004a). Taxation is the most effective policy option, with increases in the price of tobacco and alcohol reducing both use and harm (Anderson *et al.* 2006). For alcohol, direct health and social outcomes of taxation policies include the reduction of the incidence and prevalence of alcohol-related liver disease, traffic accidents and other intentional and unintentional injuries, suicide, family violence and the associated negative mental health impacts of the consequences attributed to alcohol consumption. In the European Union (EU), it is estimated that with the tax on alcohol set to the current level plus a 25 per cent increase, 656,000 incidents a year of disability and premature death would be averted at a total administrative cost of €159 million each year (Anderson and Baumberg 2006, adopted from Chisholm *et al.* 2004). An increase in the cost of alcohol would lead to a reduction in the harm from neuropsychiatric disorders, reduce alcohol-related costs and increase government revenue per year from tax (Babor *et al.* 2003).

Increases in government revenue would also allow for the hypothecation or earmarking of such revenue to be used for additional mental health promotion policy measures. Advertising bans and restrictions on the availability of substances are also effective (Anderson *et al.* 2006). Other policy measures include media and comprehensive community interventions. Restrictions on smoking in public places and private workplaces reduce both smoking prevalence and average daily cigarette consumption among smokers (Fichtenberg and Glantz 2002). An econometric analysis found that workplace smoking bans reduced smoking prevalence by 4–6 per cent and reduced average daily cigarette consumption among smokers by 10 per cent (Evans *et al.* 1999). The introduction of public smoking bans in one jurisdiction of California led to a 40 per cent reduction in hospital admissions for myocardial infarction (Sargent *et al.* 2004). School-based interventions, although popular, unfortunately have limited effectiveness (Babor *et al.* 2003). In contrast, interventions based in primary health care are effective in reducing tobacco and alcohol-related disorders, being among the most cost-effective of all health care interventions (Anderson *et al.* 2006).

Suicide prevention

The most important risk factors for suicide are psychiatric disorders (mostly depression, alcohol dependence and schizophrenia), post or recent social stressors (e.g. childhood adversities, sexual or physical abuse, unemployment, social isolation, serious economic problems), suicide in the family or among friends or peers, low access to psychological help and access to means for committing suicide (Wasserman 2001).

Among youngsters, suicide education in school settings has produced mixed results, and has mostly failed to demonstrate an impact on suicide behaviours (Wasserman 2001). While some studies have shown changes in attitudes and reported attempts (Hosman *et al.* 2006b), others have suggested that school education may increase the number of students who consider suicide as a possible solution to their problems (Shaffer *et al.* 1990). These mixed results have led to the conclusion that school programmes should be developed according to the science-base and should not be left to enthusiastic amateur initiatives (Wasserman and Narboni 2001). One effective strategy for adolescent suicide prevention implemented in the United States encompasses a multi-component, school-based approach which includes a suicide prevention school policy, teacher training and consultation, education for parents, stress management and life skills curriculum for students, and the establishment of a crisis team in each school (Zenere and Lazarus 1997). A recent systematic review of the evidence for suicide prevention suggests that in the general school population, suicide prevention programmes based on behavioural change and coping strategies tended to be efficacious (WHO 2004d). Skill training and social support methods have shown reductions in risk factors and increases in protective factors for adolescents at high risk (WHO 2004d).

Some of the most effective strategies to prevent suicides in the adult population include the prescription of antidepressant drugs to patients suffering from depression (WHO 2004d) and the reduction of access to the means to commit suicide (Mann *et al.* 2005; Hosman *et al.* 2006b). The latter has shown the clearest and most dramatic results and includes strategies such as detoxification of domestic gas and car exhausts, safety measures on high buildings and bridges, limiting quantities of over-the-counter medicines and prescription quantities of particularly toxic drugs and limiting access to pesticides (Gunnell and Frankel 1994; Wasserman 2001). The WHO has proposed the reduction of access to means of suicide as an essential strategic component of its 'human-ecological' model for suicide prevention (WHO 1998).

Public policies and their potential impact on mental health

Adjustments in legislation, policy implementation and resource allocation across many sectors can result in substantial gains in the mental health of European citizens. This section reviews the consequences that sound and integrated public policies can have for improved mental health and for the reduced risk of mental disorders.

Reduce economic insecurity

Economic insecurity impairs mental health because the main determining factors for poor mental health include income, education and employment (Morris *et al.* 2000; The Netherlands Ministry of Health, Welfare and Sport 2001). Absolute income levels determine the poor mental health associated with poverty (Patel 2005) while relative income differences, irrespective of social class, are related to a gradient in mental ill health that stretches across all levels of the social hierarchy. Economic insecurity affects mental health at all ages, with lower socioeconomic groups having a greater incidence of premature and low birth-weight babies, depression and substance use disorders in adults (Barker 1998; van de Mheen *et al.* 1998; Bradshaw 2000; Patel and Kleinman 2003). The longer people live in stressful economic and social circumstances, the greater the mental strain they suffer, and the less likely they are to enjoy a mentally healthy old age. Income distribution is important not only for mental health but also for social cohesion. Societies with high levels of income inequality also tend to have higher levels of violent crime and lower social cohesion (Hsieh and Pugh 1993), which also leads to an increased risk of mental health problems (see next section).

The life course contains a series of critical transitions: emotional and material changes in early childhood, the move from primary to secondary education, starting work, leaving home and starting a family, changing jobs and facing possible redundancy, and eventually, retirement. Each of these changes can affect mental health by pushing people onto a more or less advantaged path. Because people who have been disadvantaged in the past are at the greatest risk in each subsequent transition, welfare policies need to provide not only safety nets but also springboards to offset earlier disadvantage (Bartley *et al.* 1997). Policies attempting to target families' well-being such as attempting to alleviate economic hardship, or provide access to child care, can lead to overall mental and physical health improvements in children and future adults (WHO 2004b, 2004c).

Improve social cohesion through social policies and social support

Social networks and support improve mental health, increase social cohesion and lead to safer communities (House *et al.* 1988). Social cohesion – defined as the quality of social relationships and the existence of trust, mutual obligations and respect in communities or in the wider society – helps to protect people and their mental health. Conversely, lack of social cohesion impairs mental health (Kawachi and Berkman 2003).

Social support and belonging to a social network of communication and mutual obligation give value and esteem to people, provide emotional and practical resources (WHO 2004b) and can protect against mental disorders (WHO 2004c). On the other hand, people who receive less social and emotional support from others are more likely to experience less well-being, more depression, a greater risk of pregnancy complications and higher levels of disability from chronic diseases (Oxman *et al.* 1992); the breakdown of social relations also reduces trust and increases levels of violence (Raudenbush and Earls 1997).

Social exclusion can be both a cause and an outcome of mental disorders. The unemployed, many ethnic minority groups, disabled people, people who live in, or have left, institutions such as prisons, children's homes and psychiatric hospitals, refugees and homeless people are particularly at risk from social exclusion and associated mental health problems (WHO 2004c). Racism, discrimination and stigmatization also lead to social exclusion. Social exclusion increases the risk of divorce and separation, disability, illness, addiction and social isolation and vice versa, forming vicious circles that deepen the predicaments people face (Townsend and Gordon 2002).

Integrated government policies that promote social cohesion through the development and stimulation of social networks and empowerment, and through decreases in material inequalities, will also contribute to the promotion of mental health and reduce the premature death and disability that results from mental ill health (WHO 2004b; Patel 2005).

Expand access to education

Educational levels produce a gradient in mental ill health similar to that produced by income (WHO 2004b). Lack of education limits the ability of individuals to access economic entitlements. Better education increases cognitive-emotional and intellectual competencies and job prospects, and reduces social inequity and the risk of mental disorders, including depression (Kuh and Ben-Shlomo 1997). Children who are raised in limited learning environments or enter school with depressed symptoms are less likely to benefit from primary school, and this poor start can lead to slower achievement and a higher rate of school failure later in life (Hertzman and Wiens 1996).

Access to preschool education can help break the link with deprivation and poor mental health. For example, as described in Box 8.5, a randomized controlled trial of preschool active learning with children from impoverished backgrounds, combined with home visits, has been proven to lead to improved cognitive development, educational achievement and less conduct and criminal problems through to early adulthood – also proving to be highly cost-effective over time (Schweinhart and Weikart 1998).

Box 8.5 Long-term effects of preschool education for at-risk children

One of the most convincing controlled studies of the long-term benefits of preschool intervention for children living in poverty is the High/Scope Perry Preschool Project (Schweinhart and Weikart 1998; Schweinhart 2000). Targeting at risk 3- to 4-year-old African-American children from impoverished backgrounds, the programme combines half a day preschool intervention using a developmentally appropriate curriculum with weekly home visits. In the short term children in the intervention groups showed improved cognitive development, lower levels of learning disability, improved academic achievement, better social adjustment and increased high-school completion. When followed up through to age 27, young adults showed increased social competence, a 40 per cent reduction in lifetime arrests, a 40 per cent increase in literacy and employment rates, less welfare dependence and improved social responsibility (Schweinhart and Weikart 1998). The costs of US$1000 per child were returned by the benefit produced by the programme, which was estimated to be over US$7000–8000 per child (Barnett 1993), due to decreased schooling costs, increased taxes paid on higher earnings, reduced welfare costs, decreased justice system costs and decreased crime victim costs (Schweinhart and Weikart 1998).

Implement health-conducive labour policies

Labour policy can also influence mental health. Both the quantity and quality of work have strong influences on mental health-related factors, including income, social networks and self-esteem. Conversely, unemployment puts mental health at risk, both because of its psychological consequences and the financial problems it brings, increasing both depression and anxiety (Price and Kompier 2006). The risk is higher in regions where unemployment is widespread (Bethune 1997). Because very unsatisfactory or insecure jobs can be as harmful as unemployment, merely having a job will not always protect mental health: job quality is also important. Within employment, there is a clear association between grade of employment and mental ill health, including sickness absence rates (Burchell 1994).

Government management of the economy that reduces the highs and lows of the business cycle can improve job security and reduce unemployment. For those out of work, higher unemployment benefits are likely to have a protective effect on mental health. A variety of workplace policies are available to be applied during times of economic difficulty to reduce the risk of job loss and unemployment, including job sharing, job security policies, cutbacks on pay and reduced hours, among others (Bartley and Plewis 2002). To equip people for the work available, high standards of education and good retraining schemes are important.

Improve housing and promote healthy urban planning

The home is the physical environment in which people spend most of their time and it should be conducive to positive mental health (Shaw *et al.* 1999). Poor housing conditions are related to impaired mental health and pose a risk of developing mental health problems (Thomson and Petticrew 2005). Interventions to improve housing conditions also improve mental health and have a positive impact on broader social factors such as increased safety, crime reduction and social and community participation (Raudenbush and Earls 1997). Interventions to improve housing include those generated by health needs, by relocation or community regeneration, and those aiming to improve energy efficiency such as heating (Thomson *et al.* 2001). A systematic review of the health effects of housing improvement has shown health and mental health outcomes such as improvements in self-reported physical and mental health, broader social impacts in social outcomes such as perceptions of safety, crime reduction and increased social and community participation (Thomson *et al.* 2001).

Similarly, cities can also have direct implications for mental health. Urban shape, zoning strategies, reduced noise levels and public amenities can reduce stress, social dislocation and violence (WHO 1999). Socially underprivileged and disintegrated neighbourhoods contribute to people's sense of stress and frustration and inhibit the development of supportive networks. Within urban environments, transport policies that promote cycling, walking and the use of public transport provide physical activity, reduce fatal accidents, increase social contact and stimulate social interaction on the streets (McCarthy 1999; WHO 1999). Recreation areas, safe streets, and access to public transport and basic amenities and services are essential resources for a healthy and safe community and strong social networks, and should be maintained and improved (Social Exclusion Unit 2003).

Promoting efficient transport management through urban road pricing, integrated public transportation, vehicle priority schemes, traffic calming, traffic bans in designated areas and parking controls can reduce air pollution, congestion, noise and accidents (Fletcher and McMichael 1996; WHO 1999; Dora and Phillips 2000). Well-planned urban environments, which separate cyclists and pedestrians from car traffic, increase the safety of cycling and walking. Housing and neighbourhood design should look for solutions to counteract loneliness and strengthen social networks (Kawachi and Berkman 2003), encouraging daily physical activity and making provision for groups with special needs, such as disabled and older people.

Making it happen

An integrated approach to mental health promotion policy

Mental health and mental ill health can be a result of the combined actions of society. Though many of the key mental health burdens are due to risk factors such as substance use or child abuse, the major causes of mental ill health are poverty and socioeconomic deprivation. It is important to note that for the same level of income, societies with less income inequality tend to have more social cohesion, less violent crime and lower death rates from mental disorders (Marmot and Wilkinson 1999). It follows that enlightened economic policies, social support and good social relations can make an important contribution to mental health. Policy initiatives, both in and outside of the health sector, can result in significant improvement in community mental health, and this in turn calls for an integrated and intersectoral approach to mental health development.

During the WHO European Ministerial conference on Mental Health, held in Helsinki in January 2005, the governments of the European region of the WHO endorsed the WHO *Declaration* (WHO 2005a) and *Action Plan* (WHO 2005b) for mental health. The prevention and promotion components in the *Action Plan*, along with a current initiative by the European Commission with the Green Paper for mental health (EC 2005a) and the consultation process that has been launched across EU member states, set out a framework for the development of comprehensive national action plans that include prevention and promotion in mental health. These broad recommendations for seeking solutions are expanded and translated into specific actions in the publication *Mental Health Promotion and Mental Disorder Prevention: A Policy for Europe* (Jané-Llopis and Anderson 2005) which identifies evidence-based options for action in ten different areas.

However, in addition to using evidence to inform and guide the choice of what to implement, the way implementation is carried out is as important as the programmes and policies to be implemented. There are a number of principles that ensure high quality of implementation and these have to be included from the outset in policy-making and implementation. In addition, it is crucial that monitoring systems and evaluation of implementation are in place so that it is possible to disseminate effective practice and be aware of the impact of implemented action. Some of these determinants for effective and sustained implementation are outlined in Box 8.6, and the issues of building capacity and engaging stakeholders are expanded in the next sections.

Box 8.6 Main determinants for effective implementation and sustainability

---

Stimulate and support evidence-based decision-making for implementation

Expand the knowledge base for mental health, through developing and supporting information systems that develop, monitor and make knowledge available on risk and protective factors, the mental health status of the population, the availability of prevention, promotion and other relevant interventions for mental health, including the development of strategies which address gaps in evidence and new approaches to deal with societal challenges, and support sustained monitoring and reporting.

Ensure high quality implementation of programmes

Support building capacity, through supporting training of staff and the development of necessary skills, providing supervision and organizational support, ensuring adequate resources, infrastructures and management instruments for implementation, developing guidelines for high quality implementation and engaging relevant stakeholders, including those from other relevant sectors, by the creation of partnerships.

Support evaluation, generation and improvement of knowledge

Develop and use appropriate indicators for mental health, its determinants and the outcomes of preventive and promotion interventions, support process and outcome evaluation of all implemented interventions and the evaluation of their cost-effectiveness, assess the impact of policies on mental health, stimulate the revision and improvement of programmes and policies on the basis of the knowledge generated and ensure the information generated is disseminated and used accordingly.

Source: Jané-Llopis and Anderson (2005); Barry *et al.* (2005); Herrman and Jané-Llopis (2005)

Building capacity and supporting implementation

The development of effective policies for mental health and an integrated approach to action needs to be supported by their dissemination and adoption across countries and communities, their adaptation and tailoring to new sites and cultures, their effective implementation, the evaluation and monitoring of their implementation and outcomes, and the sustainability of effective practices at the local and national levels (WHO 2004c).

To meet these requirements, national policies should be based on building partnerships between relevant stakeholders, promoting capacity-building and training to develop expertise, and developing resources and infrastructures that facilitate policy-making, programme development and implementation, and the provision of preventive services (WHO 2004e; Jané-Llopis and Anderson 2005).

A case example of engaging stakeholders

The mobilization of stakeholders can be developed at country and European levels. An example of an initiative to support development for mental health promotion is the IMHPA Network, the European network for mental health promotion and mental disorder prevention (www.imhpa.net). Co-financed by the European Commission, the network has the participation of 29 European countries and several European organizations and related networks. To support dissemination and implementation, and to stimulate partnership and action nationally, the IMHPA network's country focal points are building country expert groups or coalitions that involve mental health actors at different professional levels. The purpose of such country groups is to exchange information on mental health promotion and prevention of mental disorders, to build cooperation and to stimulate the development of the field. One of the initiatives undertaken by these coalitions is an exercise to map capacity in mental health promotion and mental disorder prevention at the country or regional level. Country expert groups have gathered information systematically on the available infrastructures, policies and resources for prevention and promotion in mental health (www.imhpa.net/infrastructures-database). Information includes, for example, availability of policies for mental health, training programmes for professionals, identification of key stakeholders and evaluation initiatives across countries. All the information has been collected in the publication *Mental Health Promotion and Mental Disorder Prevention Across European Member States: A Collection of Country Stories* (EC 2005b). The information depicted in the report helps increase awareness of what is available, can support the coordination of initiatives, and can be used to overcome the barriers to successful development and implementation of mental health promotion (Jané-Llopis 2005).

Conclusions

Mental health promotion and mental disorder prevention have been proven to lead to better health and to social and economic development (WHO 2004b, 2004c). An integrated policy framework that includes tackling prevention and promotion in mental health, inside and outside the health sector, can be efficient in decreasing mental health burdens and in improving the mental health of all.

When developing and implementing a mental health policy it is crucial to pay attention to the levels of evidence for effectiveness, the cultural appropriateness and acceptability of practices across implementation areas, the financial, personnel, technical and infrastructural requirements needed, along with the estimation of overall benefits and potential for large-scale and efficient application. The barriers to implementing effective programmes, especially in countries with low levels of resources, call for the collective efforts of all organizations, sectors and professionals with responsibility for mental health (WHO 2002c) to work together and support development at the country and European levels.

References

Allart-van Dam, E., Hosman, C., Hoogduin, C. and Schaap, C. (2003) Short term and mediating results of the Coping with Depression course as indicated prevention: a randomized controlled trial, *Behaviour Therapy*, 34: 381–96.

Anderson, P. (1999) *Tobacco, Alcohol and Illicit Drugs: The Evidence of Health Promotion Effectiveness*. A report for the European Commission by the International Union for Health Promotion and Education. Paris: International Union for Health Promotion and Education.

Anderson, P. and Baumberg, B. (2006) *Alcohol in Europe*. Report for the European Commission. London: Institute of Alcohol Studies.

Anderson, P., Biglan, A. and Holder, H. (2006) Preventing the harm done by substances, in C. Hosman, E. Jané-Llopis and S. Saxena (eds) *Prevention of Mental Disorders: Effective Strategies and Policy Options*. Oxford: Oxford University Press, in press.

Aronen, E.T. and Kurkela, S.A. (1996) Long-term effects of an early home-based intervention, *Journal of the American Academy of Child and Adolescent Psychiatry*, 35(12): 1665–72.

Babor, T.F., Caetano, R., Casswell, S., Edwards, G., Giesbrecht, N., Graham, K., Grube, J.W., Gruenewald, P.J., Hill, L., Holder, H.D., Homel, R., Österberg, E., Rehm, J., Room, R. and Rossow, I. (2003) *Alcohol: No Ordinary Commodity. Research and Public Policy*. Oxford: Oxford University Press.

Barker, D.J.P. (1998) *Mothers, Babies and Disease in Later Life*. Edinburgh: Churchill Livingstone.

Barlow, J. (1999) *Systematic Review of the Effectiveness of Parent Training Programmes in Improving Behaviour Problems in Children Aged 3–10 Years*. Oxford: Health Services Research Unit, University of Oxford.

Barlow, J. and Coren, E. (2004) Parent training programmes for improving maternal psychosocial health (Cochrane Review), in *The Cochrane Library*, Issue 3. Chichester: Wiley.

Barlow, J., Coren, E. and Stewart-Brown, S. (2001) *Systematic Review of the Effectiveness of Parenting Programmes in Improving Maternal Psychosocial Health*. Oxford: Health Services Research Unit, University of Oxford.

Barnett, W.S. (1993) Benefit-cost analysis of preschool education: findings from a 25-year follow-up, *American Journal of Orthopsychiatry*, 63(4): 500–8.

Barry, M., Domitrovich, C. and Lara, M.A. (2005) The implementation of mental health promotion programmes, *Promotion and Education*, Supplement, 2: 30–6.

Bartley, M. and Plewis, I. (2002) Accumulated labour market disadvantage and limiting long-term illness, *International Journal of Epidemiology*, 3(2): 336–41.

Bartley, M., Blane, D. and Montgomery, S. (1997) Socioeconomic determinants of health: Health and the life course: why safety nets matter, *British Medical Journal*, 314: 1194–6.

Beardslee, W.R., Versage, E.M. and Gladstone, T.R.G. (1998) Children of affectively ill parents: a review of the past 10 years, *Journal of the American Academy of Child and Adolescent Psychiatry*, 37(11): 1134–41.

Bethune, A. (1997) Unemployment and mortality, in F. Drever and M. Whitehead (eds) *Health Inequalities*. London: HMSO.

Bradshaw, J. (2000) Child poverty in comparative perspective, in D. Gordon and P. Townsend (eds) *Breadline Europe: The Measurement of Poverty*. Bristol: The Policy Press.

Brown, H. and Sturgeon, S. (2006) Healthy start of life and reducing early risks, in C. Hosman, E. Jané-Llopis and S. Saxena (eds) *Prevention of Mental Disorders: Effective Strategies and Policy Options*. Oxford: Oxford University Press.

Burchell, B. (1994) The effects of labour market position, job insecurity, and unemployment on psychological health, in D. Gallie, C. Marsh and C. Vogler (eds) *Social Change and the Experience of Unemployment*. Oxford: Oxford University Press.

Burns, R., Nichols, L.O., Martindale-Adams, J. and Graney, M.J. (2000) Interdisciplinary geriatric primary care evaluation and management: two-year outcomes, *Journal of the American Geriatrics Society*, 48(1): 8–13.

Caplan, R.D., Vinokur, A.D., Price, R.H. and van Ryn, M. (1989) Job seeking, reemployment, and mental health: a randomized field experiment in coping with job loss, *Journal of Applied Psychology*, 74(5): 759–69.

Chen, K.M., Snyder, M. and Krichbaum, K. (2001) Tai chi and well-being of Taiwanese community-dwelling elders, *Clinical Gerontologist*, 24(3–4): 137–56.

Chisholm, D., Rehm, J., Van Ommeren, M. and Monteiro, M. (2004) Reducing the global burden of hazardous alcohol use: a comparative cost-effectiveness analysis, *Journal of Studies in Alcohol*, 65(6): 782–93.

Clarke, G.N., Lewinsohn, P.M. and Hops, P. (1990) *Instructor's Manual for the Adolescent Coping with Depression Course*. Eugene: Castalia Press.

Clarke, G.N., Hawkins, W., Murphy, M., Sheeber, L., Lewinsohn, P.M. and Seeley, J.R. (1995) Targeted prevention of unipolar depressive disorder in an at-risk sample of high-school adolescents: a randomized trial of a group cognitive intervention, *Journal of the American Academy of Child and Adolescent Psychiatry*, 34(3): 312–21.

Clarke, G.N., Hornbrook, M., Lynch, F., Polen, M., Gale, J., Beardslee, W., O'Connor, E. and Seeley, J. (2001) A randomized trail of a group cognitive intervention for preventing depression in adolescent offspring of depressed parents, *Archives of General Psychiatry*, 58(12): 1127–34.

Cooper, B. (2002) Thinking preventively about dementia, *International Journal of Geriatric Psychiatry*, 17(10): 895–906.

Coren, E. and Barlow, J. (1999) Individual and parenting-based programmes for improving psychosocial outcomes for teenage parents and their children (Cochrane Review), in *The Cochrane Library*, Issue 1. Chichester: Wiley.

Dadds, M.R., Spence, S.H., Holland, D.E., Barrett, P.M. and Laurens, K.R. (1997) Prevention and early intervention for anxiety disorders: a controlled trial, *Journal of Consulting and Clinical Psychology*, 65(4): 627–35.

Dadds, M.R., Holland, D.E., Laurens, K.R., Mullins, M., Barrett, P.M. and Spence, S.H. (1999) Early intervention and prevention of anxiety disorders in children: results at 2-year follow-up, *Journal of Consulting and Clinical Psychology*, 67(1): 145–50.

Detels, R., McEwan, J., Beaglehole, R. and Tanaka, H. (2002) *Oxford Textbook of Public Health*, 4th edn. Oxford: Oxford University Press.

Deuster, P. (1996) Exercise in the prevention and treatment of chronic disorders, *Women's Health Issues*, 6(6): 320–31.

Domitrovich, C., Weare, K., Greenberg, M., Elias, M. and Weissberg, R. (2006) Schools as a context for the prevention of mental health disorders and promotion of mental health, in C. Hosman, E. Jané-Llopis and S. Saxena (eds) *Prevention of Mental Disorders: Effective Strategies and Policy Options*. Oxford: Oxford University Press, in press.

Dora, C. and Phillips, M. (eds) (2000) *Transport, Environment and Health*. Copenhagen: WHO Regional Office for Europe.

EC (2005a) *Improving the Mental Health of the Population: Towards a Strategy on Mental Health for the European Union*. Luxembourg: European Communities.

EC (2005b) *Mental Health Promotion and Mental Disorder Prevention across European Member States: A Collection of Country Stories*. Luxembourg: European Communities.

Eddy, M. (2006) The prevention of conduct disorders, violence and aggression, in C. Hosman, E. Jané-Llopis and S. Saxena (eds) *Prevention of Mental Disorders: Effective Strategies and Policy Options*. Oxford: Oxford University Press, in press.

Elgen, I., Sommerfelt, K. and Markestad, T. (2002) Population based, controlled study of behavioural problems and psychiatric disorders in low birthweight children at 11 years of age, *Archives of Disease in Childhood: Fetal and Neonatal Edition*, 87(2): 128–32.

Evans, W.N., Farrelly, M.C. and Montgomery, E. (1999) Do workplace smoking bans reduce smoking? *American Economic Review*, 89(4): 728–47.

Felner, R.D., Brand, S., Adan, A.M. and Mulhall, P.F. (1993) Restructuring the ecology of the school as an approach to prevention during school transitions: longitudinal follow-ups and extensions of the School Transitional Environment Project (STEP), *Prevention in Human Services*, 10: 103–36.

Fichtenberg, C. and Glantz, S. (2002) Effect of smoke-free workplaces on smoking behaviour: a systematic review, *British Medical Journal*, 325: 188–94.

Fletcher, T. and McMichael, A.J. (eds) (1996) *Health at the Crossroads: Transport Policy and Urban Health*. New York: Wiley.

Gilbody, S. (2004) *What is the Evidence on Effectiveness of Capacity Building of Primary Health Care Professionals in the Detection, Management and Outcome of Depression?* Copenhagen: WHO Regional Office for Europe's Health Evidence Network (HEN), World Health Organization.

Gillham, J.E., Shatte, A.J. and Freres, D.R. (2000) Preventing depression: a review of cognitive-behavioural and family interventions, *Applied and Preventive Psychology*, 9: 63–88.

Greenberg, M.T., Domitrovich, C. and Bumbarger, B. (2001) The prevention of mental disorders in school-aged children: current state of the field, *Prevention and Treatment*, 4.

Gunnell, D. and Frankel, S. (1994) Prevention of suicide: aspirations and evidence, *British Medical Journal*, 308: 1227–33.

Hains, A.A. and Ellman, S.W. (1994) Stress inoculation training as a preventive intervention for high school youths, *Journal of Cognitive Psychotherapy*, 8(3): 219–32.

Heaney, C.A., Price, R.H. and Rafferty, J. (1995a) The Caregiver Support Program: an intervention to increase employee coping resources and enhance mental health, in L.R. Murphy, J.J. Hurrell, S.L. Sauter and G.P. Keita (eds) *Job Stress Interventions*. Washington, DC: American Psychological Association.

Heaney, C.A., Price, R.H. and Rafferty, J. (1995b) Increasing coping resources at work: a field experiment to increase social support, improve work team functioning, and enhance employee mental health, *Journal of Organizational Behavior*, 16: 335–52.

Herrman, H. and Jané-Llopis, E. (2005) Mental health promotion in public health, *Promotion and Education*, Supplement, 2: 42–7.

Herrman, H., Moodie, R. and Saxena, S. (eds) (2005) *Promoting Mental Health: Concepts, Evidence, Practice*. Geneva: World Health Organization.

Hertzman, C. and Wiens, M. (1996) Child development and long-term outcomes: a population health perspective and summary of successful interventions, *Social Science and Medicine*, 43(7): 1083–95.

Hosman, C. and Jané-Llopis, E. (1999) Political challenges 2: mental health, in *The Evidence of Health Promotion Effectiveness: Shaping Public Health in a New Europe*. Brussels: ECSC-EC-EAEC.

Hosman, C., Jané-Llopis, E. and Saxena, S. (eds) (2006a) *Prevention of Mental Disorders: Effective Strategies and Policy Options*. Oxford: Oxford University Press, in press.

Hosman, C., Wasserman, D. and Bertolotte, J. (2006b) Prevention of suicide, in C. Hosman, E. Jané-Llopis and S. Saxena (eds) *Prevention of Mental Disorders: Effective Strategies and Policy Options*. Oxford: Oxford University Press, in press.

House, J.S., Landis, K.R. and Umberson, D. (1988) Social relationships and health, *Science*, 241: 540–5.

Hsieh, C.C. and Pugh, M.D. (1993) Poverty, income inequality, and violent crime: a meta-analysis of recent aggregate data studies, *Criminal Justice Review*, 18(22): 182–202.

Institute of Medicine (2001) *Clearing the Smoke*. Washington, DC: National Academy Press.

Jané-Llopis, E. (2005) From evidence to practice: mental health promotion effectiveness, *Promotion and Education*, Supplement, 1: 21–7.

Jané-Llopis, E. and Anderson, P. (2005) *Mental Health Promotion and Mental Disorder Prevention: A Policy for Europe*. Nijmegen: Radboud University Nijmegen.

Jané-Llopis, E., Hosman, C., Jenkins, R. and Anderson, P. (2003) Predictors of efficacy in depression prevention: meta-analysis, *British Journal of Psychiatry*, 183: 384–97.

Jané-Llopis, E., Barry, M., Hosman, C. and Patel, V. (eds) (2005) Evidence of mental health promotion effectiveness, *Promotion and Education*, Supplement, 2.

Jané-Llopis, E., Muñoz, R. and Patel, V. (2006) Prevention of depression, in C. Hosman, E. Jané-Llopis and S. Saxena (eds) *Prevention of Mental Disorders: Effective Strategies and Policy Options*. Oxford: Oxford University Press, in press.

Kawachi, I. and Berkman, L. (eds) (2003) *Neighborhoods and Health*. Oxford: Oxford University Press.

Kazdin, A. (1993) Adolescent mental health: prevention and treatment programs, *American Psychologist*, 48(2): 127–41.

Kuh, D. and Ben-Shlomo, Y. (1997) *A Life Course Approach to Chronic Disease Epidemiology*. Oxford: Oxford University Press.

Levkoff, S., MacArthur, I. and Bucknall, J. (1995) Elderly mental health in the developing world, *Social Science and Medicine*, 41(7): 983–1003.

Li, F., Duncan, T.E., Duncan, S.C., McAuley, E., Chaumeton, N.R. and Harmer, P. (2001) Enhancing the psychological well-being of elderly individuals through tai chi exercise: a latent growth curve analysis, *Structural Equation Modelling*, 8(1): 53–83.

Mann, J., Apter, A., Bertolote, J., Beautrais, A. *et al.* (2005) Suicide prevention strategies: a systematic review, *Journal of the American Medical Association*, 294(16): 2064–74.

Mather, A.S., Rodriguez, C., Guthrie, M.F., McHarg, A.M., Reid, I.C. and McMurdo, M.E.T. (2002) Effects of exercise on depressive symptoms in older adults with poorly responsive depressive disorder: randomized controlled trial, *British Journal of Psychiatry*, 180(5): 411–15.

McCarthy, M. (1999) Transport and health, in M.G. Marmot and R. Wilkinson (eds) *The Social Determinants of Health*. Oxford: Oxford University Press.

Morris, J.N., Donkin, A.J.M., Wonderling, D., Wilkinson, P. and Dowler, E.A. (2000) A minimum income for healthy living, *Journal of Epidemiology and Community Health*, 54(12): 885–9.

Mrazek, P. and Haggerty, R. (eds) (1994) *Reducing Risks for Mental Disorders: Frontiers for Preventive Intervention Research*. Washington, DC: National Academy Press.

Muñoz, R.F. (1998) Preventing major depression by promoting emotion regulation: a conceptual framework and some practical tools, *The International Journal of Mental Health Promotion*, 1(1): 23–33.

Murphy, L.R. (1996) Stress management in work settings: a critical review of the health effects, *American Journal of Health Promotion*, 11(2): 112–35.

Murray, C. and Lopez, A. (1996) *The Global Burden of Disease*. Harvard: Harvard University Press.

Netherlands Ministry of Health, Welfare and Sport Programme Committee on Socio-economic Inequalities in Health (SEGV-II) (2001) *Reducing Socioeconomic Inequalities in Health*. The Hague: Ministry of Health, Welfare and Sport.

Olds, D. (1989) The Prenatal/Early Infancy Project: a strategy for responding to the needs of high-risk mothers and their children, *Prevention in Human Services*, 7: 59–87.

Olds, D. (1997) The Prenatal/Early Infancy Project: fifteen years later, in G.W. Albee and T.P. Gullotta (eds), *Primary Prevention Works*. Thousand Oaks, CA: Sage.

Olds, D.L., Henderson, C.R., Cole, R., Eckenrode, J., Kitzman, H., Luckey, D., Pettitt, L., Sidora, K., Morris, P. and Powers, J. (1998) Long-term effects of nurse home visitation on children's criminal and antisocial behaviour: 15-year follow-up of a randomized controlled trial, *Journal of the American Medical Association*, 280(8): 1238–44.

Olds, D.L. (2002) Prenatal and infancy home visiting by nurses: from randomized trials to community replication, *Prevention Science*, 3(3): 153–72.

Olweus, D. (1991) Bully/victim problems among schoolchildren: basic facts and effects of a school based intervention program, in D. Pepler and K. Rubin (eds) *The Development and Treatment of Childhood Aggression*. Hillsdale, NJ: Lawrence Erlbaum.

Oxman, T.E., Berkman, L.F., Kasl, S., Freeman, D.H. Jr. and Barrett, J. (1992) Social support and depressive symptoms in the elderly, *American Journal of Epidemiology*, 135(4): 356–68.

Patel, V. (2005) Poverty, gender and mental health promotion in a global society, *Promotion and Education*, Supplement 2. www.iuhpe.org.

Patel., V. and Kleinman, A. (2003) Poverty and common mental disorders in developing countries, *Bulletin of the World Health Organization*, 81(8): 609–15.

Price, R. and Kompier, M. (2006) Work stress and unemployment: risks, mechanisms, and prevention, in C. Hosman, E. Jané-Llopis and S. Saxena (eds) *Prevention of Mental Disorders: Effective Strategies and Policy Options*. Oxford: Oxford University Press, in press.

Price, R.H. (2003) Understanding and improving the mental health of populations, in J.S. House, R.L. Kahn, F.T. Juster, H. Schuman and E. Singer (eds) *Telescope on Society: Survey Research and Social Science at the University of Michigan and Beyond*. Ann Arbor, MI: The University of Michigan Press.

Price, R.H. and Vinokur, A.D. (1995) Supporting career transitions in a time of organizational downsizing: the Michigan JOBS Program, in M. London (ed.) *Employees, Careers, and Job Creation: Developing Growth-oriented Human Resource Strategies and Programs*. San Francisco, CA: Jossey-Bass.

Price, R., Van Ryn, M. and Vinokur, A. (1992) Impact of a preventive job search intervention on the likelihood of depression among the unemployed, *Journal of Health and Social Behaviour*, 33(June): 158–67.

Price, R.H., Choi, J.N. and Vinokur, A. (2002) Links in the chain of adversity following job loss: how economic hardship and loss of personal control lead to depression, impaired functioning and poor health, *Journal of Occupational Health Psychology*, 7(4): 302–12.

Raudenbush, S.W. and Earls, F. (1997) Neighborhoods and violent crime: a multilevel study of collective efficacy, *Science*, 277: 918–24.

Reid, J.B. and Eddy, J.M. (1997) The prevention of antisocial behavior: some considerations in the search for effective interventions, in D.M. Stoff, J. Breiling and J.D. Maser (eds) *Handbook of Antisocial Behavior*. New York: Wiley.

Reynolds, C.F., Alexopoulos, G.S., Katz, I.R. and Lebowitz, B.D. (2001) Chronic depression in the elderly: approaches for prevention, *Drugs & Aging*, 18(7): 507–14.

Riemsma, R.P., Kirwan, J.R., Taal, E. and Rasker, J.J. (2002) Patient education for adults with rheumatoid arthritis (Cochrane Review), in *The Cochrane Library*, Issue 4. Oxford: Update Software.

Sargent, R.P., Shepard, R.M. and Glantz, S.A. (2004) Reduced incidence of admissions for myocardial infarction associated with public smoking ban: before and after study, *British Medical Journal*, 328: 977–83.

Schaufeli, W. and Kompier, M. (2001) Managing job stress in the Netherlands, *International Journal of Stress Management*, 8(1): 15–34.

Schweinhart, L.J. (2000) The High/Scope Perry preschool study: a case study in random assignment, *Evaluation and Research in Education*, 14(3&4): 136–47.

Schweinhart, L.J. and Weikart, D.P. (1998) High/Scope Perry preschool program effects at age twenty-seven, in J. Crane (ed.) *Social Programs that Work*. New York: Russell Sage Foundation.

Shaffer, D., Garland, A., Gould, M., Fisher, P. and Trautman, P. (1990) Preventing teenage suicide: a critical review, in S. Chess and M.E. Hertzig (eds) *Annual Progress in Child Psychiatry and Child Development*. New York: Brunner/Mazel.

Shapiro, A. and Taylor, M. (2002) Effects of a community-based early intervention program on the subjective well-being, institutionalization, and mortality of low-income elders, *The Gerontologist*, 42(3): 334–41.

Shaw, M., Dorling, D. and Brimblecombe, N. (1999) Life chances in Britain by housing wealth and for the homeless and vulnerably housed, *Environment and Planning*, 31(12): 2239–48.

Social Exclusion Unit (2003) *Making the Connections: Transport and Social Exclusion*. London: Office of the Deputy Prime Minister.

Stewart-Brown, S.L., Fletcher, L. and Wadsworth, M.E.J. (2005) Parent-child relationships and health problems in adulthood in three UK national birth cohort studies, *European Journal of Public Health*, 15(6): 640–6.

Thomson, H. and Petticrew, M. (2005) *Is Housing Improvement a Potential Health Improvement Strategy?* Copenhagen: WHO Regional Office for Europe's Health Evidence Network (HEN).

Thomson, H., Petticrew, M. and Morrison, D. (2001) Housing interventions and health – a systematic review, *British Medical Journal*, 323: 187–90.

Townsend, P. and Gordon, D. (2002) *World Poverty: New Policies to Defeat an Old Enemy*. Bristol: The Policy Press.

Tuthill, D.P., Stewart, J.H., Coles, E.C., Andrews, J. and Cartlidge, P.H. (1999) Maternal cigarette smoking and pregnancy outcome, *Paediatrics and Perinatal Epidemiology*, 13(3): 245–53.

Unicef (2001) *State of the World's Children 2001: Early Childhood*. New York: Unicef.

Üstun, T.B., Ayuso-Mateos, J.L., Chatterji, S., Mathers, C. and Murray, C.J.L. (2004) Global burden of depressive disorders in the year 2000, *British Journal of Psychiatry*, 184: 386–92.

van de Mheen H., Stronks K., Looman C.W. and Mackenbach, J.P. (1998) Role of childhood health in the explanation of socioeconomic inequalities in early adult health, *Journal of Epidemiology and Community Health*, 52(1): 15–19.

Vinokur, A., van Ryn, M., Gramlich, E. and Price, R. (1991) Long-term follow-up and benefit-cost analysis of the jobs program: a preventive intervention for the unemployed, *Journal of Applied Psychology*, 76(2): 213–19.

Vuori, J. and Silvonen, J. (2005) The benefits of a preventive job search program on re-employment and mental health at two-year follow-up, *Journal of Occupational and Organizational Psychology*, 78(1): 43–52.

Vuori, J., Silvonen, J., Vinokur, A. and Price, R. (2002) The Tyohon Job Search Program in Finland: benefits for the unemployed with risk of depression or discouragement, *Journal of Occupational Health Psychology*, 7(1): 5–19.

Wasserman, D. (ed.) (2001) *Suicide, an Unnecessary Death*. London: Martin Dunitz.

Wasserman, D. and Narboni, V. (2001) Examples of suicide prevention : programmes in schools, in D. Wasserman (ed.) *Suicide, An Unnecessary death*. London: Martin Dunitz.

Weare, K. (2000) *Promoting Mental, Emotional and Social Health: A Whole School Approach*. London: Routledge.

Windsor, R.A., Lowe, J.B., Perkins, L.L., Smith-Yoder, D., Artz, L., Crawford, M., Amburgy, K. and Boyd, N.R. (1993) Health education for pregnant smokers: its behavioral impact and cost benefit, *American Journal of Public Health*, 83(2): 201–6.

World Health Organization (1992) *The ICD-10 Classification of Mental and Behavioural Disorders: Clinical Descriptions and Diagnostic Guidelines*. Geneva: World Health Organization.

World Health Organization (1998) *Primary Prevention of Mental, Neurological and Psychosocial Disorders*. Geneva: World Health Organization.

World Health Organization (1999) *Health for All in the 21st century*. Copenhagen: WHO Regional Office for Europe.

World Health Organization (2001) *The World Health Report 2001: Mental Health, New Understanding, New Hope*. Geneva: World Health Organization.

World Health Organization (2002a) *Healthy Aging*. Copenhagen: WHO Regional Office for Europe.

World Health Organization (2002b) *The World Health Report 2002: Reducing Risks, Promoting Healthy Life*. Geneva: World Health Organization.

World Health Organization (2002c) *Prevention and Promotion in Mental Health*. Geneva: World Health Organization.

World Health Organization (2003) *The World Health Report 2003: Shaping the Future*. Geneva: World Health Organization.

World Health Organization (2004a) *CHOICE Global Programme On Evidence for Health Policy: Improving Health System Performance*, www3.who.int/whosis.

World Health Organization (2004b) *Promoting Mental Health: Concepts, Emerging Evidence, Practice*. A report from the World Health Organization, Department of Mental Health and Substance Abuse in collaboration with the Victorian Health Promotion Foundation and the University of Melbourne. Geneva: WHO.

World Health Organization (2004c) *Prevention of Mental Disorders: Effective Interventions and Policy Options*. A report of the World Health Organization Department of Mental Health and Substance Abuse in collaboration with the Prevention Research Centre of the Universities of Nijmegen and Maastricht. Geneva: WHO.

World Health Organization (2004d) *For Which Strategies of Suicide Prevention is there Evidence of Effectiveness?* Copenhagen: WHO Regional Office for Europe's Health Evidence Network (HEN).

World Health Organization (2004e) *Mental Health Promotion and Mental Disorder Prevention*, briefing sheet for the WHO European Ministerial Conference on Mental Health. Copenhagen: WHO Regional Office for Europe.

World Health Organization (2005a) *Mental Health Declaration for Europe: Facing Challenges, Building Solutions*. Copenhagen: WHO Regional Office for Europe.

World Health Organization (2005b) *Mental Health Action Plan for Europe: Facing Challenges, Building Solutions*. Copenhagen: WHO Regional Office for Europe.

Yoshikawa, H. (1994) Prevention as cumulative protection: effects of early family support and education on chronic delinquency and its risks, *Psychological Bulletin*, 115(1): 28–54.

Zenere, F.J. and Lazarus, P.J. (1997) The decline of youth suicidal behaviour in an urban, multicultural public school system following the introduction of a suicide prevention and intervention program, *Suicide and Life-Threatening Behaviour*, 27(4): 387–402.

chapter nine

Common mental health problems in primary care: policy goals and the evidence base

Simon Gilbody and Peter Bower

Mental health problems, such as anxiety and depression, are especially common in primary care settings and are responsible for substantial morbidity, impairment and lost productivity. Most of these problems can be appropriately and effectively managed in primary care settings, either by primary care workers or in collaboration with specialist secondary care services. However, care is often less than satisfactory, due to a mixture of three (often interrelated) factors: (1) inappropriate recognition and management of common mental health problems by clinicians; (2) a low priority being given to mental health problems by decision-makers at all levels; and (3) inadequate resources being made available for common mental health problems.

The World Health Organization (WHO) (WHO 2001a) suggests that all mental health policies should be anchored by the four guiding principles of access, equity, effectiveness and efficiency. In this chapter we examine the potential impact of mental health policies directed at improving the *organization and delivery* of primary mental health care from this perspective. Primary care mental health policies can be linked to high quality clinical and economic evidence, and the potential to improve the quality of care is substantial. Policies need to be tailored within individual health care settings, with due consideration of the total resources available.

Mental health policy and primary care

The WHO Atlas survey of mental health resources worldwide defined mental health policies as 'a specifically written document of the government or Ministry of Health containing the goals for improving the mental health situation of the country, the *priorities* among those goals and the main *directions* for attaining them'.[1] Policies provide a common vision and plan for all programmes and services related to mental health, and avoid inefficiency and fragmentation. The Atlas survey found that 67 per cent of European countries had a mental health policy (WHO 2001a).

One key policy recommended by the WHO *World Health Report 2001* concerned the importance of providing treatment for mental health problems in primary care (WHO 2001b). *Primary health care* was defined by the Alma Ata declaration as 'essential health care based on practical, scientifically sound and socially acceptable methods and technology made universally accessible to individuals and families in the community through their full participation and at a cost that the community and country can afford to maintain at every stage of their development in the spirit of self-reliance and self-determination'. Descriptions of the core content of primary care vary (Starfield 1992; Fry and Horder 1994), but key aspects include:

- first contact care, with direct patient access;
- care characterized by patient-centredness, family orientation, and continuity;
- a role in the coordination of care; and
- a 'gatekeeping' function in relation to access to specialist care.

The structure of health care systems in Europe varies widely, and the degree to which particular systems can be characterized as 'primary care-led' varies (Boerma *et al.* 1993; Fry and Horder 1994; Saltman *et al.* 2006). There is some evidence that the degree of primary care focus in a health care system (especially the gatekeeping role) is a key driver of the cost-effectiveness and efficiency of health care provision (Starfield 1992).

Mental health care in primary care is defined as 'the provision of basic preventive and curative mental health care at the first point of contact of entry into the health care system'. Usually this means that care is provided by a non-specialist primary care clinician, such as a general practitioner (GP) or nurse, who can refer complex cases to a more specialized mental health professional (Boerma and Verhaak 1999; WHO 2001a). The Atlas survey found that 96 per cent of European countries identified mental health activity in primary care, and 62 per cent reported training facilities, although implementation was highly variable among countries (WHO 2001a). In particular, a number of countries in central and eastern Europe still have the overwhelming majority of resources for mental health tied up in long-stay institutions, with little role for primary care practitioners. For instance, in Lithuania more than 70 per cent of state expenditure for mental health services was allocated to such institutions in 2003 (Murauskiene 2003).

Mental health disorders in primary care

A distinction is often made between 'severe and long-term mental health disorders' (most often associated with schizophrenia), and 'common mental health disorders' (most often associated with anxiety and depression). Although primary care has an important role to play in the management of more severe disorders, recent policy in the United Kingdom has highlighted the role of specialist services (such as community mental health teams – CMHTs) in their management. 'Common' disorders are viewed as being more appropriately within the remit of primary care, partly by default, as specialist services have refocused their energies, and partly by design, as primary care is seen as being able to provide appropriate, patient-sensitive care to this population.

'Common' disorders can be described using the standard diagnostic classifications (WHO 1992; Ustun *et al.* 1995), but a more useful typology for present purposes has been presented (Goldberg and Gournay 1997) which defines three key categories of disorders in terms of the availability of relevant pharmacological and non-pharmacological treatments, and the roles of the primary care team. The categories are:

1 Well-defined disorders which are also associated with disability, for which there are effective pharmacological and psychological treatments. Even when these disorders remit, they are likely to relapse once more. These include anxious depression, pure depression, generalized anxiety, panic disorder and obsessive-compulsive disorder. These disorders can usually be managed entirely within primary care.
2 Disorders where drugs have a more limited role, but where psychological therapies are available, including somatized presentations of distress, panic disorders with agoraphobia and eating disorders. These disorders are rarely treated within primary care, and only a small proportion of cases are treated by specialist services.
3 Disorders which resolve spontaneously, including bereavement and adjustment disorder. In these cases, supportive help, rather than a specific mental health skill, is required.

Primary care services for common mental disorders

Generally, primary care services for mental health problems are viewed in terms of a 'pathways to care' model (Goldberg and Huxley 1980, 1992). The pathway has five levels and four filters (see Figure 9.1). Of all those individuals in the community, a high proportion consult their doctor in any one year while a lesser number suffer an episode of psychological illness during the same time span. These patients pass the first filter ('the decision to consult'). Of those reaching primary care services, a proportion is recognized by the primary care clinician as suffering from psychiatric disturbance and thus pass the second filter ('ability to detect a disorder'). Passing the third and fourth filters involves referral to specialist psychiatric services or admission as inpatients. Although there may be exceptions to this referral process, and variations depending on the local

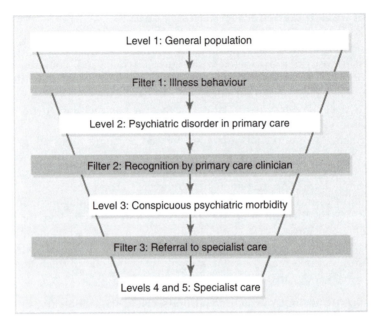

Figure 9.1 Pathways to care for common mental health problems

Source: Bower and Gilbody (2005)

structure of services (Gater *et al.* 1991), it provides an adequate general model for the bulk of psychiatric morbidity in any primary care-led service.

This model highlights the fact that effective mental health provision depends on accurate recognition and management of disorders in primary care, but significant problems have been identified. Stigma within society and poor knowledge about the nature of psychiatric disorders often prevents people from consulting a doctor about psychiatric problems in the first instance (Goldberg and Huxley 1980). For those that do consult, a wealth of evidence has indicated that levels of recognition of disorders are low (Andersen and Harthorn 1989; Ormel *et al.* 1990; Paykel and Priest 1992; Tiemens *et al.* 1996), and furthermore there is wide variation in recognition rates between primary care clinicians (Marks *et al.* 1979). Patients who are recognized often do not receive quality of care in line with current guidelines, either in relation to pharmacological treatments or the provision of evidence-based psychological therapies (Schulberg and McClelland 1987; Katon *et al.* 1992; Katon *et al.* 1997; Schulberg *et al.* 1998). Finally, provision of specialist services (such as psychological therapists working on-site in practices) often varies widely (Sibbald *et al.* 1993; Corney 1996).

Policy goals in primary mental health care

As noted above, mental health policies are characterized by two main elements: a statement of goals (and priorities among goals) and a statement of ways of achieving those goals. The WHO suggests that all mental health policies are anchored by four guiding principles:

1 *Access*: service provision should meet the need for services in the community. In addition, the right to obtain treatment should depend on the need for services, not ability to pay or geographic location. As outlined in Goldberg's 'pathways to care' model, there are problems in access to care in primary care, related to the fact that people do not consult as a consequence of stigma or inadequate knowledge, and a significant proportion of disorders presenting in this setting are not recognized by the gatekeeping primary care clinician. Patients failing to pass the first 'filter to care' are unable to access effective care from health services.

2 *Equity*: mental health care resources should be distributed fairly across the population at large, so that patients with similar problems receive similar services (horizontal equity) and patients with more severe problems receive more care than those with minor problems (vertical equity). There are two main sources of inequity in current services, which relate to the wide variation in the ability of individual practitioners to recognize disorders, and inequity in the provision of specialist services within practices. In addition, the inherent under-investment in mental health services and stigma that is associated with mental health problems means that allocation of resources is inequitable compared to other disease groups.

3 *Effectiveness*: mental health services should do what they are intended to do: improve health. Health may be defined in terms of health status, or broader definitions may involve wider function and quality of life, and not just the absence of disease (WHO 1948). Patient satisfaction with services is an additional, if somewhat more controversial, measure of effectiveness. Current management of mental health problems can involve the provision of ineffective treatments or those of unknown effectiveness (such as some forms of psychological therapy), or the ineffective delivery of effective treatments (such as inappropriate use of medication).

4 *Efficiency*: given that resources for any health care system are limited, they should be distributed in such a way as to maximize health gains to society. Clearly, the problems with access, equity and effectiveness identified above limit the degree to which current services can be efficient.

The relationships between these different goals are complex, and satisfying multiple criteria requires a population approach to planning care, rather than a focus on the particular patient which characterizes the philosophy of primary health care (Sibbald 1996; Katon *et al.* 1997).

Models to improve mental health care in primary care settings

Broadly, there are four main models available to improve mental health care in primary care (Bower and Gilbody 2005), which are described below. Additional consideration should be given to the promotion of mental well-being and the reduction of stigma associated with mental health problems is also important. Mental health promotion is considered in Chapter 8 and is not considered in any detail here. The impact of campaigns to reduce stigma (such as the Defeat Depression Campaign in the United Kingdom – Paykel and Priest 1992) have generally not been evaluated in any rigorous way. One exception is the Nuremberg Alliance Against Depression Project, which has been rolled out nationally in Germany, and which will be subjected to evaluation (Hegerl *et al.* 2003). This programme has now been extended to a number of cities across the EU (see www.eaad.net).

Complex models of the relationships between primary care and specialist services have been described (Pincus 1987), but for our present purposes the key dimension along which they differ relates to the amount of responsibility taken by the primary care clinician in managing common mental health problems, compared to the role of specialist mental health staff:

1 *Training primary care staff*: this is defined as the provision of essential knowledge and skills in the identification, prevention and care of mental disorders to primary health care personnel (WHO 2001a). Care includes both pharmacology and psychological therapy (King *et al.* 2002). Referral to specialist care is expected to be required in only a small proportion of cases. Methods of improving the skills of primary care staff include large-scale public relations campaigns (Priest 1991), dissemination of evidence-based guidelines (Cornwall and Scott 2000), simple practice-based education (Thompson *et al.* 2000), or more complex teaching strategies (Gask 1998).

2 *Consultation-liaison*: this is a variant of the training model. Rather than the provision of one-off training interventions, in this model specialists enter into an ongoing educational relationship with the primary care team, in order to support them in caring for specific patients who are currently undergoing care (Gask *et al.* 1997; Bower and Gask 2002). Referral to specialist care is again only expected to be required in a small proportion of cases, and only occurs after discussion between the primary care team and the specialist.

3 *Collaborative care*: this complex model has elements of both the educational and consultation-liaison model (Bower and Gask 2002), but in addition requires fundamental changes in the system of care. The full range of interventions in this model varies, but generally includes practitioner education and the provision of guidelines, screening, patient education, case management and consultation (Von Korff and Goldberg 2001). The implementation of such systems may require changes in practice routines and developments in information technology (Wagner *et al.* 1996). Most importantly, collaborative care is based on changes in the roles of primary care providers and specialists such as psychiatrists (Katon *et al.* 2001), as well as changes in the workforce, which can involve retraining existing staff or the introduction of new mental health worker roles to undertake tasks such as 'case management' (Bower *et al.* 2001).

4 *Replacement/referral*: although primary care clinicians always have overall clinical responsibility for their patients, in this model the management of the presenting problem is passed onto a mental health professional for the duration of the treatment (Bower 2002). This is most frequently related to the provision of psychological therapies in primary care, such as cognitive-

behavioural therapy (Scott and Freeman 1992), problem-solving (Corney and Briscoe 1977), counselling (Ward *et al.* 2000) and interpersonal therapy (Schulberg *et al.* 1996).

It should be noted that these models are not designed to capture the complexity of actual service provision, but to provide broad categories which are of use in prioritizing different methods of achieving mental health policy goals.

How do these methods assist in the achievement of policy goals?

Access

Key goals of mental health policies (such as those in the United Kingdom and other EU countries) relate to improvements in access and effectiveness. There are two key criteria which determine the effect of each model on access.

The first relates to the *impact of the model on the confidence and skills on the primary care clinician*. As noted above, the models differ in the degree to which responsibility for care remains with the primary care clinician, or is passed to the specialist. In primary care-led services, the primary care clinician acts as a gatekeeper to mental health care, and thus interventions which leave responsibility in the hands of primary care clinicians and target interventions towards that group theoretically have the greatest impact on access, because changes in the skills and confidence of primary care clinicians in mental health issues can potentially impact on *all* patients with mental health problems in the community. In contrast, interventions which require significant specialist involvement to achieve their effects can only impact on the small number of patients to which specialist assistance can be provided. Therefore, training of the primary care team has the greatest potential impact on access, followed by consultation-liaison and collaborative care models. Replacement models have potentially little or no impact.

Efficiency

The second criteria relates to the *efficiency of specialist interventions* within the model. Within all primary care-led mental health care systems, the numbers of specialist staff are insufficient to meet the demand for mental health care, and thus specialist resources must be allocated efficiently. Thus, treatments (such as medication from the primary care clinician) which may not need specialist input at all are the most efficient because limitations in the availability of specialists have no impact on access to this form of care. The consultation-liaison approaches spread specialist resources efficiently, as most specialist time is spent in training a large number of primary care clinicians, and only a small proportion in direct patient contact. Collaborative care and replacement models are least efficient because both require significant specialist time for all patients (for case management and the delivery of therapy). Efficiency issues in these models relate to the amount of specialist time required per patient, and the seniority (and cost) of the specialist involved.

It should be noted that these impacts are theoretical, as there is very little empirical work on levels of access to mental health care, compared to the amount of research on effectiveness (see below).

Effectiveness

Effectiveness has traditionally been conceptualized as clinical effectiveness; that is, changes in health status, such as reductions in depression symptoms. However, as noted earlier and in line with WHO definitions of health, there is increasing interest in wider outcomes such as social function and quality of life and issues of efficiency mean that issues of cost are also increasingly important. Compared with issues of access, the effectiveness of treatments has received much greater scientific evaluation.

The next section summarizes the evidence for each of the models described above, based on a number of systematic overviews or reviews completed by the authors of organizational and educational interventions to improve the management of common mental health problems in primary care (Bower and Sibbald 2000a, 2000b; Bower 2002; Bower *et al.* 2003a, 2003b; Gilbody *et al.* 2003; Bower and Gilbody 2005). Systematic reviews represent the highest form of evidence relating to clinical and cost-effectiveness data, and these reviews have been conducted under the auspices of the Cochrane Collaboration and the United Kingdom NHS Centre for Reviews and Dissemination. The methodological details of this important approach to synthesizing clinical and cost-effectiveness data are elaborated in Box 9.1. Most of the data relates to the management of depression, but the broad principles are likely to apply to all common mental health disorders. The data focuses on randomized controlled trials (RCTs), given the advantages associated with this design, but other designs of relevance are considered where applicable (Gilbody *et al.* 2003). For example, reviews of educational and organizational interventions look beyond the conventional RCT, and consider evidence from non-randomized and observational designs (Black 1996; Gilbody and Whitty 2002).

Box 9.1 A systematic review of the clinical and cost-effectiveness of strategies to improve the management of depression in primary care conducted by the Cochrane Effective Practice and Organization of Care (EPOC) group

Context

Depression is common in primary care settings, yet is often missed or suboptimally managed. A number of organizational and educational strategies to improve the management of depression have been proposed. The clinical and cost-effectiveness of these strategies have not yet been subject to systematic review.

Objective

To systematically evaluate the effectiveness of guidelines, organizational, and educational interventions to improve the recognition and management of depression in primary care settings.

Data sources

Electronic medical and psychological databases from inception to March 2003. (MEDLINE, PsycLIT, EMBASE, CINAHL, Cochrane Controlled Trials Register, NHS Economic Evaluations Database, Cochrane Depression Anxiety and Neurosis Group register, Cochrane Effective Professional and Organizational Change group specialist register.) Correspondence with authors and searches of reference lists.

Study selection

We selected 36 studies including: 29 randomized controlled trials (RCTs) and non-randomized controlled clinical trials (CCTs); 5 controlled before and after (CBA) studies; and 2 interrupted time series (ITS) studies. Outcomes relating to recognition, management and outcome of depression were sought.

Data extraction

Methodological details and outcomes were extracted and checked by two reviewers. Summary risk ratios were, where possible, calculated from original data and attempts were made to correct for unit of analysis error.

Data synthesis

A narrative synthesis was conducted. Twenty-one positive studies were found. Strategies effective in improving patient outcome were generally complex interventions that incorporated clinician education, an enhanced role of nurses (nurse case management) and a greater degree of integration between primary and secondary care (consultation-liaison). Telephone medication counselling delivered by practice nurses or trained counsellors was also effective. Simple guideline implementation and educational strategies were generally ineffective.

Conclusion

There is substantial potential to improve the recognition and management of depression in primary care. Commonly used guidelines and educational strategies are likely to be ineffective. The implementation of the findings from this research will require substantial investment in primary care services and a major shift in the organization and delivery of care.

Evidence concerning the effectiveness of the models

Training

Although this model is theoretically one of the most attractive, and has been the subject of large-scale interventions in both Europe and the United States, the evidence is generally unconvincing that training alone can improve the effectiveness of primary care for depression. Simple passive dissemination of guidelines is ineffective, as are the sort of short-term, pragmatic training courses that can be delivered within current educational systems (certainly in the United Kingdom) (Kendrick 2000). Although there is evidence that more intensive and complex training packages can influence primary care clinician behaviour (Gask *et al.* 1987, 1995), it may not always impact on patient outcome when delivered alone (King *et al.* 2002). The training model may be limited by the paradox that feasible training is not effective, while effective training may be unfeasible. An additional problem is that, although the training model has the greatest theoretical impact on access, training courses which rely on voluntary attendance may only attract those clinicians with an interest in mental health problems, who may be least likely to benefit. Therefore, advantages in access may be unrealized, and inequities may occur.

Consultation-liaison

The current evidence concerning consultation-liaison is sparse, and the studies that do exist do not provide evidence of effectiveness. Given the theoretical possibility that this model could be highly efficient, the lack of empirical evidence is surprising. One of the problems may relate to the fact that the evaluation of this model has important methodological considerations which makes evaluation problematic (Gask *et al.* 1987). One reason for the lack of effectiveness may be that the presumed causal mechanisms underlying consultation-liaison are themselves ineffective in changing professional behaviour (Bower and Gask 2002).

Collaborative care

Although the exact nature of the interventions varies from study to study, there is a large amount of high quality evidence for the general approach of collaborative care (Gilbody *et al.* 2003). Several issues remain. The key 'mechanisms of change' in these interventions are unclear, and it may be the case that the effectiveness of this approach derives in part from the large number of components (e.g. patient and clinician education; enhanced physician support; compliance monitoring; structured patient follow-up; audit and feedback). Importantly, almost all the studies emanate from the United States, and it is not clear whether they will generalize to different populations or European health care settings; for instance, collaborative care interventions in the United Kingdom have not been as uniformly successful (Wilkinson *et al.* 1993; Mann *et al.* 1998; Peveler *et al.* 1999), although it should be noted that they are generally much less intensive in terms of the number of interventions involved. Qualitative research might therefore be used to examine factors inherent in the adaptation of these models of health care to different health care systems and local contexts. Most of the interventions are dependent on willingness to use antidepressants, which is problematic given the negative attitudes towards medication in Europe (Priest *et al.* 1996). Finally, where economic evidence has been presented, most of the studies indicate that collaborative care is both more effective, and more costly (Gilbody *et al.* 2003).

Replacement

There is good evidence that psychological therapies in primary care are clinically effective. Information on cost-effectiveness is poor (Byford and Bower 2002; Barrett *et al.* 2005), although the high cost associated with specialist therapists' time is likely to be a key factor (Bower *et al.* 2003a, 2003b). However, there is significant interest in the potential for less therapist-intensive minimal interventions (such as written or computerized self-help), which may both increase access and reduce costs (Bower *et al.* 2001; Kaltenthaler *et al.* 2002). One significant disadvantage associated with the use of this model relates to the possibility that the lack of involvement of primary care staff may lead to them becoming deskilled. Certainly, there is little evidence that the presence of a psychological therapist in a practice leads to widespread increases in diagnosis or treatment (Bower and Sibbald 2002).

Deciding priorities according to available resources

Key issues in implementing evidence-based policies within primary care are likely to relate to the total resources available for mental health, both in absolute terms and in relation to the total health care budget. In deciding priorities for mental health policy and practice, the WHO gives guidance in relation to resources by dividing systems into low, medium and high resource countries. Each of these scenarios will now be examined to establish which priorities within mental health and primary care might follow from the evidence base which has already been presented.

Low resource countries

This scenario refers to low income countries where mental health resources are completely absent or very limited. Such countries have no mental health policy programmes or if they exist they are outdated and not implemented effectively. Governmental finances available to mental health are tiny, often less than 0.1 per cent of the total health budget. There are no mental health services in primary or community care, and essential psychotropic drugs are seldom available. While this scenario applies mostly to low income countries, in many high income countries essential mental health services remain beyond the reach of rural populations, indigenous groups and others. Even within these scenarios, it is clear that the integration of mental health services and awareness within primary care, rather than the establishment of a high-cost specialist service, has the greatest impact in terms of increasing access and promoting the equitable and efficient delivery of mental health care. From within the interventions outlined above, it is the low-cost interventions which improve access to services which have the greatest potential to improve the health of the population. Educational strategies, together with funding for a limited list of essential drugs such as antidepressants and antipsychotics, delivered within primary care, are a feasible strategy, although the effectiveness of educational strategies, by themselves, has not been determined within low resource health care systems. Costly collaborative care strategies are not realistic, nor should they be a priority.

Medium resource countries

In countries in this scenario, some resources are available for mental health, such as centres for treatment in big cities or pilot programmes for community care. But these resources do not provide even essential mental health services to the total population. These countries are likely to have mental health policies, programmes and legislation, but they are often not fully implemented. The government budget for mental health is typically less than 5 per cent of the total health budget, a situation that is relevant to a number of countries undergoing economic transition in central and eastern Europe.

In these countries, unlike medium resource countries in other parts of the world, there is usually no shortage of psychiatrists; in fact, the opposite may be the case. However, the system is usually heavily institutionalized with little availability of community-based professionals such as social workers or community-based psychiatric nurses to serve the population. Primary care providers are largely untrained in mental health care. Within these scenarios, the development of a comprehensive primary care-led mental health service and a rebalancing of institutional compared with community-based care is more of a priority than the development of a fully functioning and comprehensive specialist mental health service. Education and training of primary care professionals and the devolution of the management of common mental health problems to primary care workers such as nurses should become a priority, and these strategies can be well supported from some low intensity collaborative care and educational strategies. There are, however, many barriers to the greater development and investment in the provision of mental health services within the primary care sector, not least perverse incentives in the way in which mental health systems may be funded that may not easily allow resources to be transferred away from institutional based care (see Chapter 4).

High resource countries

This scenario relates mostly to industrialized countries in the EU with a relatively high level of resources for mental health. Mental health policies, programmes and legislation are implemented reasonably effectively. The proportion of the total health budget allocated to mental health is above 5 per cent or more, and most primary care providers are trained in mental health care. Efforts are made to identify and treat major mental disorders in primary care, though effectiveness and coverage may be inadequate. Specialized care facilities are more comprehensive, but most may still be located in psychiatric hospitals. Psychotropic drugs are readily available and community-based services generally available.

Even within these countries, as has been seen, there remains substantial opportunity to improve the quality of mental health care within primary care settings and the key strategies should lie in the integration of primary and secondary care services, and in the efficient management of resources by providing specialist input within primary care settings and changing the organization and delivery of care. Collaborative care remains the most effective and efficient strategy in this scenario.

Key issues for the future development of primary care mental health services

A number of issues relating to the future development of primary care mental health services follow on from the evidence already presented. These can be linked to a series of recommendations made by the WHO in deciding future priorities.

Developing the workforce

Many health care systems, including those from medium and high resource countries, are seeking to increase and change the emphasis of the primary care workforce. For example, in the United Kingdom, 1000 graduate mental health workers are to be recruited and trained (Bower 2002). Much needs to be decided about their core function, the level of skills that they will require and how best to organize their training. Evidence-based interventions from within the models of collaborative care, such as case management for depression, are likely to be both effective and efficient (Von Korff and Goldberg 2001). These are interventions that can be readily adopted by non-mental health nurses working in primary care, staff with a counselling or social care background and graduate psychologists, who can be offered a postgraduate training programme of up to one year. Simple training programmes have been shown to produce autonomous practitioners capable of dealing with the range of problems that occur in primary care. A substantial issue for the future is likely to be the retention and further training of these professional groups in order that they remain within primary care, rather than seeking more specialist challenges in secondary care settings.

Developing information technology

Many primary care systems operate in an 'information free' environment and it is difficult to know what treatments are offered to whom, and if the quality of care is improving. The WHO recommends that primary care information systems be developed or enhanced to take on board the needs of mental health care. Such systems provide the potential for better integration of care and can form a component of case identification and monitoring of treatment and follow-up visits – all key components of collaborative care models. Examples include case registers of those with depression in order to monitor relapse prevention and to flag up the presence of depression as a presenting problem within the primary care consultation. Other innovations include: (computerized) decision aids on the optimum management of depression; specific computerized algorithms to ensure evidence-based prescribing and referral, and that follow-up is offered at the appropriate time; and links to pharmacy refill records in order to check when patients do not order their medication on time.

Raising the profile of mental health and reducing stigma

Mental health suffers from a low profile within the general medical profession and within the wider population. Strategies aimed at improving awareness and reducing stigma at each of these levels are needed. As mentioned above, the evidence to support interventions that target awareness and stigma is scarce – largely because this field is not well researched. The Nuremberg Depression Alliance provides an example of a coherent and multi-faceted strategy that is being evaluated alongside its implementation. Financial levers might also be needed to raise the profile and quality of care for mental health problems. A new employment contract for United Kingdom primary care physicians provides financial incentives for the improved recognition and management of depression and might form a model for other health care systems. Many of the performance targets that are set in order to provide better quality care for depression are those that are outlined in this chapter – including case management and structured follow-up. However, concerns have been raised that enhanced care for depression is just one of a number of performance indicators that are sought in primary care, and that others (such as immunization and physical screening programmes) are technically easier to comply with. Therefore, depression may be not seen as a priority in comparison with other performance targets.

Research into policy and practice – making it happen

A cohesive series of priorities have emerged recently from the WHO (2005), which provide an agenda for action for improving mental health and reflect the primary care focus outlined in this chapter. Decision-makers are likely to look for concrete examples of the implementation of policy initiatives that are underpinned by research evidence and a theoretical framework. Fortunately, examples do exist.

From low and middle income countries, examples include the adaptation of a collaborative care model within the Chilean health care system (Araya *et al.* 2003), and problem-focused, psychosocial interventions among those with depression and HIV in Uganda (Bolton *et al.* 2003).

In the Chilean example, a multi-component intervention was led by a non-medical health worker and included group psychoeducation about depression, systematic monitoring of symptoms and a structured drug programme for those with more severe or persistent depression. After six months, 70 per cent of the collaborative care group had recovered. This study, and others in the developing world, has shown that small investments in the treatment of depression can have a huge impact, especially in socially deprived populations. Importantly, in adapting this model for a low income health care setting, a specific aim was to ensure cross-cultural adaptability and acceptance. Due consideration was made of cultural factors such as the local acceptability of specific interventions; health system factors such as the availability of human resources to implement interventions; and the cost and availability of medications. The structured approach facilitated an increased role for non-medical staff and patients. One of the outcomes of the programme was greater patient involvement, and in some places women's groups started by the programme were still functioning after two years. The outcomes would be considered to be appropriate for many inner-city areas in high income countries (McKenzie *et al.* 2004).

From higher income countries, the primary care focus has been reflected in the development of evidence-based guidelines. For example, in the United Kingdom recent guidelines on the management of depression have made strong policy recommendations on the use of collaborative care models in primary care (NICE 2004). A key issue in the implementation of this model of care is the integration of primary and secondary care, and the question of who will coordinate and deliver this care. A reconfiguration of existing roles and the expansion of the primary care workforce are required. A specific role has emerged for new graduate mental health workers, and national training programmes have emerged which seek to produce workers who can implement these packages of care within one year of postgraduate training (versus the several years required to train specialist nurses, clinical psychologists and psychiatrists). Clear 'how to do it' guides have been published to act as a template for local services, which can be used by commissioners of health care services to ensure that primary care shows fidelity to evidence-based models (NIMHE 2004).

Cost-effectiveness

Decision-makers at every level increasingly require evidence of both clinical effectiveness and cost-effectiveness. There are a number of cost-effectiveness studies on the organizational enhancements of primary care for common mental health problems (Gilbody *et al.* 2003). Short-term cost-effectiveness studies of collaborative care have tended to show improved outcome, but with increased health care costs (Schoenbaum *et al.* 2001). This has implications for allocative efficiency as providing such care to a population will require either more resources to be provided overall, or for resources to be removed from other forms of mental health care.

Depression has its greatest impact on productive societal costs (see Chapter 1), and it is this area where the economic benefits of effective interventions might be most readily realized. Unfortunately, economic evaluations of models of care, such as collaborative care, have tended to focus on short-term health care costs alone. The longer-term and wider economic impact from a societal perspective have not been adequately studied. However, the economic benefits, in terms of relapse prevention and reduced health care utilization might become apparent over the longer term. There is now emerging evidence from longer-term cost-effectiveness studies that collaborative care may have a longer-term cost offset effect and might be a more technically efficient method of delivering care (Wells *et al.* 2004).

Economic evaluations have also included cost per quality adjusted life year (QALY) assessments and the incremental health gains have been shown to be achieved at a cost that is the same as, or less than, other interventions (such as breast screening), which are funded. Interestingly, the work of Schoenbaum *et al.* (2001) and longer-term follow-up (Wells *et al.* 2004) have shown that costs per QALY estimates of cognitive-behavioural interventions delivered in primary care are similar to those achieved through medication management programmes. The caveat to this research is that such cost utility analyses have been conducted within US managed care settings and it is difficult to know to what extent these costs and health care gains can be directly extrapolated to the lower funded and more socialized health care systems in Europe. However, primary care organizational programmes remain a strong candidate in improving health at a population level and the overall funding of these programmes will be a question of allocative efficiency and health gain within finite resources.

Future policy and research

In addition to the extensive research presented in this chapter, a more solid evidential base is likely to emerge in coming years to help guide decision-makers and to help make a case for a more equitable provision of primary care focused health care, where mental health competes more readily with other conditions and specialties. These priorities were reflected in the Declaration of the WHO European Ministerial Conference on Mental Health in Helsinki (WHO 2005) where 12 key aims were outlined. Primary care was seen as being central to the successful transformation of mental health services and care, where the declaration highlights the need to: 'build up the capacity and ability of general practitioners and primary care services, networking with specialized medical and non-medical care, to offer effective access, identification and treatments to people with mental health problems' (p. 3). The Declaration had a final explicit aim to: 'initiate research and support evaluation and dissemination of [these] actions'. An evaluation programme is therefore needed to more fully explore the application and implementation of primary care programmes at a micro and macro level throughout each of the health care systems represented in the EU.

References

Andersen, S. and Harthorn, B. (1989) The recognition, diagnosis and treatment of mental disorders by primary care physicians, *Medical Care*, 27(9): 869–86.

Araya, R., Rojas, G., Fritsch, R., Gaete, J., Rojas, M., Simon, S. and Peters, T.J. (2003) Treating depression in primary care in low income women in Santiago, Chile: a randomised controlled trial, *Lancet*, 361: 995–1010.

Barrett, B., Byford, S. and Knapp, M. (2005) Evidence of cost-effective treatments for depression: a systematic review, *Journal of Affective Disorders*, 84(1): 1–13.

Black, N. (1996) Why we need observational studies to evaluate the effectiveness of health care, *British Medical Journal*, 312: 1215–18.

Boerma, W., de Jong, F. and Mulder, P. (1993) *Health Care and General Practice Across Europe*. Utrecht: NIVEL, Netherlands Institute of Primary Health Care.

Boerma, W. and Verhaak, P. (1999) The general practitioner as the first contacted health professional by patients with psychosocial problems: a European study, *Psychological Medicine*, 29(3): 689–96.

Bolton, P., Bass, J., Neugebauer, R., Verdeli, H., Clougherty, K.F., Wickramartne, P., Speelman, L., Ndogoni, L. and Weissman, M. (2003) Group interpersonal psycho-therapy for depression in rural Uganda, *Journal of the American Medical Association*, 289(23): 3117–24.

Bower, P. (2002) Primary care mental health workers: models of working and evidence of effectiveness, *British Journal of General Practice*, 52(484): 926–33.

Bower, P. and Gask, L. (2002) The changing nature of consultation-liaison in primary care: bridging the gap between research and practice, *General Hospital Psychiatry*, 24(2): 63–70.

Bower, P. and Gilbody, S. (2005) Managing common mental health disorders in primary care: conceptual models and evidence base, *British Medical Journal*, 330, 839–42.

Bower, P. and Sibbald, B. (2000a) Systematic review of the effect of on-site mental health professionals on the clinical behaviour of general practitioners, *British Medical Journal*, 320: 614–17.

Bower, P. and Sibbald, B. (2000b) Do consultation-liaison services change the behaviour of primary care providers? A review, *General Hospital Psychiatry*, 22(2): 84–96.

Bower, P. and Sibbald, B. (2002) On site mental health workers in primary care: effects on professional practice (Cochrane Review), *The Cochrane Library*, Issue 2. Oxford: Update Software.

Bower, P., Richards, D. and Lovell, K. (2001) The clinical and cost-effectiveness of self-help treatments for anxiety and depressive disorders in primary care: a systematic review. *British Journal of General Practice*, 51(471): 838–45.

Bower, P., Byford, S., Barber. J, Beecham, J., Simpson, S., Friedli, K., Corney, R., King, M. and Harvey, I. (2003a) Meta-analysis of data on costs from trials of counselling in primary care: using individual patient data to overcome sample size limitations in economic analyses, *British Medical Journal*, 326: 1247.

Bower, P., Rowland, N. and Hardy, R. (2003b) The clinical effectiveness of counselling in primary care: a systematic review and meta-analysis, *Psychological Medicine*, 33(2): 203–15.

Byford, S. and Bower, P. (2002) Cost-effectiveness of cognitive-behaviour therapy for depression: current evidence and future research priorities, *Expert Review of Pharmaco-economics and Outcomes Research*, 2: 457–66.

Corney, R. (1996) Links between mental health professionals and general practices in England and Wales: the impact of GP fundholding, *British Journal of General Practice*, 46(405): 221–4.

Corney, R. and Briscoe, M. (1977) Social workers and their clients: a comparison between primary health care and local authority settings, *Journal of the Royal College of General Practitioners*, 27(405): 295–301.

Cornwall, P. and Scott, J. (2000) Which clinical practice guidelines for depression? An overview for busy practitioners, *British Journal of General Practice*, 50(178): 908–11.

Donaldson, C., Currie, G. and Mitton, C. (2002) Cost effectiveness analysis in health care: contraindications, *British Medical Journal*, 325: 891–4.

Fry, J. and Horder, J. (1994) *Primary Health Care in an International Context*. Abingdon: Wace Burgess.

Gask, L. (1998) Small group interactive techniques utilizing videofeedback, *International Journal of Psychiatry and Medicine*, 28(1): 97–113.

Gask, L., McGrath, G., Goldberg, D.P. and Millar, T. (1987) Improving the psychiatric skills of established general practitioners: evaluation of group teaching, *Medical Education*, 21(4): 362–8.

Gask, L., Williams, L. and Harrison, J. (1995) Teaching cognitive-behavioural skills for the management of depression to general practice trainees: a pilot study of training, *Primary Care Psychiatry*, 1: 201–5.

Gask, L., Sibbald, B. and Creed, F. (1997) Evaluating models of working at the interface between mental health services and primary care, *British Journal of Psychiatry*, 170: 6–11.

Gater, R., De Almeida e Sousa, B., Barrientos, G., Caraveo, J. *et al.* (1991) The pathways to psychiatric care: a cross-cultural study, *Psychological Medicine*, 21(3): 761–4.

Gilbody, S. and Whitty, P. (2002) Improving the delivery and organization of mental health services: beyond the conventional randomized controlled trial, *British Journal of Psychiatry*, 180: 13–18.

Gilbody, S., Whitty, P., Grimshaw, J. and Thomas, R. (2003) Educational and organizational interventions to improve the management of depression in primary care: a systematic review, *Journal of the American Medical Association*, 289(23): 3145–51.

Goldberg, D. and Gournay, K. (1997) *The General Practitioner, the Psychiatrist and the Burden of Mental Health Care*. Maudsley: Maudsley Hospital, Institute of Psychiatry.

Goldberg, D. and Huxley, P. (1980) *Mental Illness in the Community: The Pathway to Psychiatric Care*. London: Tavistock.

Goldberg, D. and Huxley, P. (1992) *Common Mental Disorders: A Biosocial Model*. London: Routledge.

Hegerl, U., Althaus, D. and Stefanek, J. (2003) Public attitudes towards treatment of depression: effects of an information campaign, *Pharmacopsychiatry*, 36(6): 288–91.

Kaltenthaler, E., Shackley, P., Stevens, P., Beverley, C., Parry, G. and Chilcott, J. (2002) A systematic review and economic evaluation of computerized cognitive behaviour therapy for depression and anxiety, *Health Technology Assessment*, 6(22): 1–89.

Katon, W., Von Korff, M., Lin, E., Bush, T. and Ormel, J. (1992) Adequacy and duration of antidepressant treatment in primary care, *Medical Care*, 30(1): 67–76.

Katon, W., Von Korff, M., Lin, E., Unutzer, J., Simon, G., Walker, E., Ludman, E. and Bush, T. (1997) Population-based care of depression: effective disease management strategies to decrease prevalence, *General Hospital Psychiatry*, 19(3): 169–78.

Katon, W., Von Korff, M., Lin, E. and Simon, G. (2001) Rethinking practitioner roles in chronic illness: the specialist, primary care physician and the practice nurse, *General Hospital Psychiatry*, 23(3): 138–44.

Kendrick, T. (2000) Why can't GPs follow guidelines on depression? *British Medical Journal*, 320: 200–1.

King, M., Davidson, O., Taylor, F., Haines, A., Sharp, D. and Turner, R. (2002) Effectiveness of teaching general practitioners skills in brief cognitive behaviour therapy to treat patients with depression: randomized controlled trial, *British Medical Journal*, 324: 947–52.

Mann, A., Blizard, R., Murray, J., Smith, J.A., Botega, N., MacDonald, E. and Wilkinson, G. (1998) An evaluation of practice nurses working with general practitioners to treat people with depression, *British Journal of General Practice*, 48(426): 875–9.

Marks, J., Goldberg, D. and Hillier, V. (1979) Determinants of the ability of general practitioners to detect psychiatric illness, *Psychological Medicine*, 9(2): 337–53.

McKenzie, K., Patel, V. and Araya, R. (2004) Learning from low income countries: mental health, *British Medical Journal*, 329: 1138–40.

Murauskiene, L. (2003) *Economic Assessment*. Vilnius: Community Mental Health Services.

National Institute for Clinical Excellence (NICE) (2004) *Depression: Core Interventions in the Management of Depression in Primary and Secondary Care*. London: HMSO.

National Institute for Mental Health in England (NIMHE) (2004) *Enhanced Services Specification for Depression Under the New GP Contract*. Manchester: NIMHE North West.

Ormel, J., Van Den Brink, W., Koeter, M., Geil, R., Van Der Meer, K., Van De Willige, G. and Wilmink, F.W. (1990) Recognition, management and outcome of psychological disorders in primary care: a naturalistic follow up study, *Psychological Medicine*, 20(4): 909–23.

Paykel, E. and Priest, R. (1992) Recognition and management of depression in general practice: consensus statement, *British Medical Journal*, 305: 1198–202.

Peveler, R., George, C., Kinmonth, A., Campbell, M. and Thompson, C. (1999) Effect of antidepressant drug counselling and information leaflets on adherence to drug treatment in primary care: randomized controlled trial, *British Medical Journal*, 319: 612–15.

Pincus, H. (1987) Patient-oriented models for linking primary care and mental health care, *General Hospital and Psychiatry*, 9(2): 95–101.

Priest, R. (1991) A new initiative on depression, *British Journal of General Practice*, 41(353): 487.

Priest, R., Vize, C., Roberts, A., Roberts, M. and Tylee, A. (1996) Lay people's attitudes to treatment of depression: results of opinion poll for Defeat Depression Campaign just before its launch, *British Medical Journal*, 313: 858–9.

Saltman, R., Rico, A. and Boerma, W. (eds) (2006) *Primary Care in the Driver's Seat?* Buckingham: Open University Press.

Schoenbaum, M., Unutzer, J., Sherbourne, C., Duan, N., Rubenstein, L.V., Miranda, J., Meredith, L.S., Carney, M.F. and Wells, K. (2001) Cost-effectiveness of practice-initiated quality improvement for depression: results of a randomized controlled trial, *Journal of the American Medical Association*, 286(11): 1325–30.

Schulberg, H. and McClelland, M. (1987) A conceptual model for educating primary care providers in the diagnosis and treatment of depression, *General Hospital and Psychiatry*, 9(1): 1–10.

Schulberg, H., Block, M., Madonia, M., Scott, C.P., Rodriguez, F., Inbar, S.D., Perel, J., Lave, J., Houch, P.R. and Coulehan, J.L. (1996) Treating major depression in primary care practice: eight month clinical outcomes, *Archives of General Psychiatry*, 53(10): 913–19.

Schulberg, H., Katon, W., Simon, G. and Rush, J. (1998) Treating major depression in primary care practice: an update of the Agency for Health Care Policy and Research practice guidelines, *Archives of General Psychiatry*, 55(12): 1121–7.

Scott, A. and Freeman, C. (1992) Edinburgh primary care depression study: treatment outcome, patient satisfaction, and cost after 16 weeks, *British Medical Journal*, 304: 883–7.

Sibbald, B. (1996) Skill mix and professional roles in primary care, in *What is the Future for a Primary Care-Led NHS?* Oxford: Radcliffe Medical Press.

Sibbald, B., Addington-Hall, J., Brenneman, D. and Freeling, P. (1993) Counsellors in English and Welsh general practices: their nature and distribution, *British Medical Journal*, 306: 29–33.

Starfield, B. (1992) *Primary Care: Concept, Evaluation and Policy.* New York: Oxford University Press.

Thompson, C., Kinmonth, A., Stevens, L., Peveler, R.C., Stevens, A., Ostler, K.J., Pickering, R.M., Baker, N.G., Henson, A., Preece, J., Cooper, D. and Campbell, M.J. (2000) Effects of a clinical practice guideline and practice-based education on detection and outcome of depression in primary care: Hampshire Depression Project randomized controlled trial, *Lancet*, 355(9199): 185–91.

Tiemens, B., Ormel, J. and Simon, G. (1996) Occurrence, recognition and outcome of psychological disorders in primary care, *American Journal of Psychiatry*, 153(5): 636–44.

Ustun, T., Goldberg, D., Cooper, J., Simon, G. and Sartorius, N. (1995) New classification for mental disorders with management guidelines for use in primary care: ICD-10 PHC chapter five, *British Journal of General Practice*, 45(393): 211–15.

Von Korff, M. and Goldberg, D. (2001) Improving outcomes in depression, *British Medical Journal*, 323: 948–9.

Wagner, E., Austin, B. and Von Korff, M. (1996) Organizing care for patients with chronic illness, *Milbank Quarterly*, 74: 511–43.

Ward, E., King, M., Lloyd, M., Bower, P., Sibbald, B., Farrelly, S., Gabbay, M., Tarrier, N. and Addington-Hall, J. (2000) Randomized controlled trial of non-directive counselling, cognitive-behaviour therapy and usual GP care for patients with depression – I: clinical effectiveness, *British Medical Journal*, 321: 1383–8.

Wells, K., Sherbourne, C., Schoenbaum, M., Ettner, S., Duan, N., Miranda, J., Unutzer, J. and Rubenstein, L. (2004) Five-year impact of quality improvement for depression: results of a group-level randomized controlled trial, *Archives of General Psychiatry*, 61(4): 378–86.

Wilkinson, G., Allen, P., Marshall, E., Walker, J., Browne, W., and Mann, A. (1993) The role of the practice nurse in the management of depression in general practice: treatment adherence to antidepressant medication, *Psychological Medicine*, 23(1): 229–37.

World Health Organization (1948) *Constitution.* Geneva: WHO.

World Health Organization (1992) *The ICD-10 Classification of Mental and Behavioural Disorders – Clinical Descriptions and Diagnostic Guidelines.* Geneva: WHO.

World Health Organization (2001a) *Atlas – Mental Health Resources in the World 2001.* Geneva: WHO.

World Health Organization (2001b) *The World Health Report 2001: Mental Health, New Understanding, New Hope.* Geneva: WHO.

World Health Organization (2005) European Ministerial Conference on Mental Health: *Mental Health Action Plan for Europe: Facing Challenges, Building Solutions.* Copenhagen: WHO.

chapter ten

Reforms in community care: the balance between hospital and community-based mental health care

*Francesco Amaddeo, Thomas Becker,
Angelo Fioritti, Lorenzo Burti and
Michele Tansella*

Mental health services in many countries are currently subjected to change and are being reviewed and redesigned. These changes reflect, in part, the growing evidence of what constitutes cost-effective care, and also an acknowledgement of the failures of the system of care that was based on old-fashioned and remote institutions. Asylums do not offer the quality of care that is expected today, both by patients and their families. There is also an increasing worldwide focus on chronically disabling conditions, including mental disorders, rather than infectious and communicable diseases. This is reflected in the attention given not only to mortality but also to a wider concept of morbidity that goes beyond symptoms to attach importance to disability, quality of life and the impact of responsibilities on caregivers (Thornicroft and Tansella 2004).

A broad consensus to move towards deinstitutionalization has taken place across most of western Europe for more than 20 years. This change is now underway in central and eastern Europe. Despite this, the rate of change has varied markedly, and support service models vary substantially. For instance, a survey of European psychiatrists reported community mental health services existed in fewer than half of the localities in Spain, Portugal, Greece and Ireland, and only as pilot schemes in eastern Europe (Goldberg 1997).

In the last two decades of the twentieth century there has been debate between those in favour of the provision of mental health treatment and care within hospitals and those who prefer treatment and care in community settings, where the two are seen as mutually exclusive. This false dichotomy should be replaced by a new agenda, in which balanced care includes both modern community-based and modern hospital-based care (Thornicroft and Tansella 2004).

Without investment in community-based structures during a period of transition from institutional to community-based care, the burden of care may be shifted from the formal sector to informal care provided by families. Moreover, it should be noted that in some cases the motivation for hospital closures may be to reduce financial costs rather than to change care delivery settings.

Changes in policies in European countries

The philosophy of psychiatric reforms in European countries has implicitly or explicitly been based upon some key principles of community psychiatry and incorporated actions along the following axes: i) the deinstitutionalization process and closure of old mental hospitals; ii) the development of alternative community services and programmes; iii) integration with other health services; and iv) integration with social and community services (Becker and Vázquez-Barquero 2001). Wide differences are present within the member states of the European Union (EU), with different levels of implementation of the principles of community psychiatry.

Table 10.1 summarizes some indicators derived from the *Atlas* of the World Health Organization's (WHO) *World Health Report* 2001 (WHO 2001a) on the 25 EU member states. The total number of psychiatric beds available in each country ranges from 1.7 per 10,000 population in Italy to 25 per 10,000 in Belgium (see Figure 10.1). The mean number of beds in the world is 4.4 per 10,000 population. Thirteen countries have more than 10 beds per 10,000 population: Belgium, the Czech Republic, Denmark, Estonia, France, Ireland, Latvia, Lithuania, Luxembourg, Malta, the Netherlands, Finland and Slovenia. Only five countries (Austria, Cyprus, Spain, Italy and the United Kingdom) have less than 6 beds per 10,000 population. Excluding Italy and Finland, all the other countries still have psychiatric beds in mental hospitals.

Moreover, although the majority of EU countries have a national mental health programme (absent in Austria, Spain, Slovakia, Slovenia and Sweden), regional and local variations are present in most countries (Becker and Vázquez-Barquero 2001).

Many countries, which have already chosen to switch to a community-based mental health system (e.g. the United Kingdom) or have incorporated substantial community services in a hospital-based system (e.g. the Netherlands, Portugal, some Länder in Germany), have a high number of psychiatric beds. The WHO *Atlas* 2001 (WHO 2001a) provides an overview of the development of mental health services worldwide and a description of the shift from hospital-based to community-based mental health care is available for some EU countries. In each of the EU-25 member states community facilities are available to psychiatric patients at different levels.

In Austria, there are some mental health plans at the level of the provinces. Since 1997, there has been a national hospital plan, which places a certain

Table 10.1 Mental health care in the 25 EU member states

	Total psychiatric beds	Psychiatric beds in mental hospitals	Psychiatric beds in general hospitals	Psychiatric beds in other settings	Number of psychiatrists	Number of social workers	National mental health programme	Latest mental health legislation	Total health budget for mental health care (%)
	Per 10,000 population				*Per 100,000 population*				
Austria	5.2	4.7	0.5	–	10	103	No	1997	–
Belgium	25.0	16.4	2.4	6.6	18	–	Yes	2000	6.0
Cyprus	5.2	4.7	0.6	0.0	5	25	Yes	1997	7.0
Czech Republic	11.3	9.7	1.4	0.2	12	–	Yes	1966	3.0
Denmark	15.1	4.0	3.6	7.5	16	7	Yes	1998	–
Estonia	10.2	8.0	2.1	0.0	13	0	Yes	1997	–
Finland	11.6	0.0	10.4	1.2	16	165	Yes	1990	5.0
France	12.1	7.3	2.3	2.2	20	–	Yes	1990	–
Germany	7.6	4.8	–	–	7	–	Yes	1999	–
Greece	8.7	4.3	0.3	4.1	6	56	Yes	1999	–
Hungary	9.6	2.3	7.2	0.1	9	1	Yes	1997	8.0
Ireland	11.5	10.0	1.6	0.8	5	37	Yes	1991	7.7
Italy	1.7	0.0	0.8	0.9	9	3	Yes	1998	–
Latvia	15.5	15.1	0.4	–	10	0.6	Yes	1997	5.0
Lithuania	11.8	10.8	0.7	0.3	13	–	Yes	1995	7.0
Luxembourg	10.1	7.5	3.0	0.0	12	35	Yes	2000	13.4
Malta	18.9	18.8	0.1	0.0	5	2	No	1981	9.0
Netherlands	18.7	15.4	1.0	2.3	9	176	Yes	1994	7.0
Poland	7.5	5.9	1.0	0.6	6	1	Yes	1994	–
Portugal	7.7	2.1	1.2	4.4	5	7	Yes	2000	–
Slovakia	9.0	6.0	3.0	0.0	10	–	No	1994	2.0
Slovenia	11.9	6.8	1.1	4.0	8	–	No	1999	–
Spain	4.4	3.7	0.6	0.1	4	–	No	1986	–
Sweden	6.7	–	–	3.2	20	–	No	2000	11.0
United Kingdom	5.8	–	–	–	11	58	Yes	1983	10.0

Source: WHO (2001a)

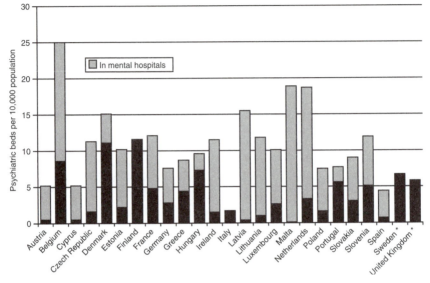

Figure 10.1 Total psychiatric beds and psychiatric beds in mental hospitals per 10,000 population in the 25 EU member states

* Data on psychiatric beds in mental hospitals not available.

degree of obligation on individual provinces to fulfil stipulated requirements. These include a few pages on psychiatry, with a subsection on community services. This plan is continuously adapted (latest version January 2001) and contains suggestions for the establishment of psychiatric units in general hospitals. However, up to now, only a few such units exist, with some others in the planning stage.

Greece developed a ten-year national plan for mental health that was submitted for financial assistance to the EU in 1997 (*Psychoargos*), part of which has already been approved and is now in progress. The main points of this plan are: the continuation of deinstitutionalization and destigmatization; sectorization of psychiatric services throughout the country; continuation of the development of primary health care units and psychiatric units in general hospitals; continuation and intensification of the development of rehabilitation facilities; establishment and development of patient cooperatives in order to promote the social, economic and occupational reintegration into society of patients with severe psychiatric problems; and establishment of detailed guarantees and procedures for the protection of patients' rights. During the period 2000–6, there has been a special emphasis on the areas of child psychiatry, psychogeriatrics and the reform of psychiatric hospitals (WHO 2001b). Plans are also underway in Ireland to further develop community-based services and to organize services for the disturbed mentally ill.

In Italy, the 1978 reform law inaugurated fundamental changes in the mental health care system (prohibiting admissions to state mental hospitals, stipulating community-based services, allowing hospitalization only in small general hospital units) and the year 1998 marked the end of the state mental hospital system (Burti 2001). The most recent legislation, known as the 'Target Project 1998–2000' provides for the establishment of local 'Departments for Mental Health' at health-district level (about 100,000 population). The main points covered by the project are: mental health promotion during a person's whole life; early detection of mental health problems; prevention of relapses and their psychological and social consequences; attention to the life of patients' families; and prevention of suicide and self-harm behaviour.

The Dutch government has developed a policy (the National Mental Health Plan) to create a mental health care sector with the following characteristics: demand-driven care that is tailored to the care needs of the individual client and his or her specific social or cultural characteristics, generated through consult-ation with the client, easily accessible and consisting of both medical and psy-chiatric treatment and social assistance; effectively organized provision of care in accordance with a clear profile from 'light and general care to heavy and specialized care'; disorders that can be treated in the short term and by general means are dealt with in the locally-organized, first echelon of mental health care by general practitioners (GPs), health care psychologists and social workers; disorders that are beyond the capacities of the first echelon are referred to the regionally-organized specialist mental health care centres, which are preferably located in or near the general hospital. These regional centres offer a complete range of facilities (prevention, diagnosis, crisis care, outpatient and short-term inpatient treatment, resocialization and sheltered accommodation); super-specialist help is provided at the supraregional or national level in university hospitals and in a number of designated mental health care institutions.

In the United Kingdom, despite relatively low expenditure, substantial pro-gress has been made in deinstitutionalization and the development of com-prehensive community-based services. The closure of large asylums has largely been achieved (Johnson *et al.* 2001).

Recently, an international multi-centre study (EPSILON study) compared provision of services in five European regions (Becker *et al.* 2002). Using the European Service Mapping Schedule (ESMS), differences in mental health ser-vices across the five centres were identified. The study found that there was some heterogeneity in outpatient and community services across the sites with a focus on community mental health teams in London (United Kingdom) and Verona (Italy) and in outpatient care in Santander (Spain). Amsterdam (the Netherlands) took an intermediate position. However, in spite of substantial inter-site differences in service provision all the centres shared some elements of community mental health care.

WHO recommendations on mental health policies

Principles of deinstitutionalization and the public health approach

The WHO has embraced, developed and disseminated the principle of deinsti-tutionalization and the public health approach since the 1970s when a long-term programme of the WHO Regional Office for Europe was approved. The

WHO Regional Office had monitored changes in the psychiatric services delivery systems in different European countries every ten years, adjusting its recommendations on service provision accordingly. For example, in 1953, when 3 beds per 1000 population was the rule in most western European countries, 1 psychiatric bed per 1000 was recommended. This figure went down to 0.5–1.0 per 1000 in the 1972 report, when the survey reported a growing provision of new types of community-based facilities. The WHO later stressed that the different geographic characteristics of areas, available resources, including staff, service organization and style of intervention made it problematic to derive a single global ratio as an index of adequate service provision. In the meantime, extramural facilities had evolved from simple dispensaries to more complex facilities for the treatment and rehabilitation of mental health patients, including those with severe conditions, in the community. Often, these community facilities represented the pivot of the system. Mental hospitals were decreasing in number and size, while general hospital psychiatric beds were opened instead, but in most countries the latter represented only 10 per cent or less of all the available psychiatric beds in the mid-1970s. In the 1982 survey, large mental hospitals, those with 2000 or more beds, had disappeared, while those with more than 1000 had fallen by 50 per cent. Italy, with a reduction from 55 to 20 large hospitals, and the United Kingdom, with a reduction from 65 to 23, contributed most to these results. However, the numerous intermediate-size mental hospitals had decreased only slightly. Unfortunately, again, the number of psychiatric beds in general hospitals remained relatively small. Variations during the period 1982–92 were even more striking with respect to the hospital categories mentioned above.

A WHO document containing recommendations for the immediate future (WHO 2001c) strongly emphasizes the importance of developing community care under the umbrella of public health principles. The need for a shift away from institutional to community care is taken for granted, as is the decentralization of health services and the need to integrate mental health into general health services. The evidence is that stand-alone mental hospitals are not the preferred service option and present a number of barriers to effective treatment and care: they are associated with a number of human rights violations; living conditions are often sub-standard; and stigmatization and isolation of people with mental disorders is sustained (WHO 2001c). It is noteworthy that WHO definitely endorses community mental health in times when mistrust and prejudice affect public opinion and the media, while prudent support or even overt criticism is found within national governments and the international literature (Leff 2001; Geller 2002).

Mental health policies

A basic WHO recommendation concerns the establishment, in all countries, of explicit mental health policies endorsed at the highest level of government so that they have maximum influence in giving higher priority to mental health. Guiding principles should include: community participation in mental health services; deinstitutionalization and community care; and accessibility and integration through primary health care. An important aspect of policy is legislation. Such legislation should be consistent with the *UN Principles for the Protection of Persons with Mental Illness and the Improvement of Mental Health Care* (United Nations 1991). Money should follow services and shifting of funds should occur from institutions to community care according to local planning based on specific needs and negotiation with local authorities, instead of sticking to global norms. Financial disincentives to discourage care in psychiatric institutions should be used as well as incentives to promote care through general hospitals and in the community. The real needs of the population should guide the establishment of services, with a public health approach in mind. In fact, in many developing countries, services are missing or nominal, while in many industrialized countries there may be a large range of mental health services but they do not always meet population needs. As to the training of health care professionals, a need to retreat from disease-based medical models to include psychosocial theories and practices is stressed: a recommendation that is at odds with the universal upheaval of biological orientations in psychiatry.

Another WHO document, reporting on the latest developments in mental health globally (WHO 2001b), stresses community-based mental health; continuity of care; a wide range of accessible services to respond to the different needs of the population; partnership with families; and integration into primary care. A broad range of ingredients of care is suggested to meet both medical and social needs, including medication, psychotherapy, psychosocial rehabilitation, vocational rehabilitation, employment and housing. The importance of legislation to form the basis of mental health policy and to guarantee the human rights of patients is stressed once more. Unfortunately, numbers are not encouraging: of 160 countries worldwide reporting to the WHO, nearly a quarter have no legislation on mental health (WHO 2001d) and a fifth of existing legislation is rather old. In Europe, only 4 per cent of countries are without legislation, yet 37 per cent have no mental health policy.

Ten statements (see Box 10.1) condense the WHO's overall recommendations. Such recommendations identify specific actions in accordance with scenarios defined by the level of resources available in every country. For instance,

---

Box 10.1 WHO recommendations on mental health policy

- Provide treatment in primary care
- Make psychotropic drugs available
- Provide care in the community
- Educate the public
- Involve communities, families and consumers
- Establish national policies, programmes and legislation
- Develop human resources
- Link with other sectors
- Monitor community mental health
- Support more research

Source: WHO (2001b)

'provide care in the community' implies moving people out of prison, down-sizing mental hospitals and improving care within them in countries with low levels of resources. In countries with greater resources the same recommendation implies completing the closure of remaining custodial mental hospitals and assuring 100 per cent coverage of community care.

However, reports from European areas indicate that psychiatric hospitals still provide inpatient care, including acute hospitalization, in most countries (Becker and Vázquez-Barquero 2001) and the range of acute inpatient beds per 100,000 population varies between 17 in Italy (where the process of closing all mental hospitals has been accomplished) and 165 in France. Thus, it is clear that the process of psychiatric reform in Europe is still far from complying with the WHO recommendations. In addition – as Becker and Vázquez-Barquero observe – Europe is not equivalent to the EU; in eastern Europe physical and mental health conditions have worsened considerably in the last decade. The decrease in life expectancy by ten years in some eastern European countries dramatically epitomizes the severity of the problem.

Involvement of carers and users in planning, evaluation and managing services

While evidence demonstrates the benefits of involving families to improve patient outcomes in a number of mental health conditions (WHO 2001b; Chamberlin 2005; Thornicroft and Tansella 2005), and the WHO stresses the need for partnership with patients and families, carers' and users' organizations continue to complain about their far from satisfactory levels of involvement and lack of recognition by the psychiatric establishment. This is unfortunate and unjust as between 40 and 80 per cent of the chronically mentally ill now live with their families and, consequently, relatives carry the greatest part of the burden of care. Relatives are partners and their role should be fully acknowledged. Family organizations have been in existence for decades, but only more recently have they been successful in influencing health authorities in policy-making decisions and been consulted over the functioning of mental health services. A European network of family organizations, the European Federation of Associations of Families of Mentally Ill People (EUFAMI) was founded in 1992 and has been actively coordinating efforts ever since. The needs most often emphasized by families include: livelihood/subsistence; crisis management; case management/community social interventions; work services for the mentally ill; rehabilitation services; inpatient care; and innovative pharmacological treatments (Brand 2001a, 2001b).

Users of mental health services have been recognized as partners only recently because of the long-lasting prejudice that they were unable to have an accountable say, let alone be considered responsible for their own destiny, and as such were not consulted by professionals and administrators. Nonetheless, since the 1990s, in some European countries users have had an influence on their personal treatment plans, have councils in mental hospitals and their representatives participate in psychiatric services advisory boards at local and regional levels (Schene and Faber 2001).

In 1991, ENUSP (www.enusp.org), the European Network of (ex-) users and survivors of psychiatry was founded. Selecting a name for the organization among all the descriptions commonly used by different groups[1] was an important issue. Finally, the term (ex-) users and survivors of psychiatry was chosen (Hölling 2001). Every two years ENUSP delegates from 40 different countries meet in congress. The movement supports the concept of user/survivor-controlled services, advocating that for every psychiatric bed there should be one bed in an anti- or non-psychiatric 'runaway house'. The prototype of this kind of facility is, in fact, Runaway House in Berlin, a crisis centre operated by the clients themselves. The house has been in existence since the mid-1990s and has accommodated more than 300 people.

Comprehensiveness of health and social care

Besides improving patients' competencies and increasing the resources available in the care settings offered to service users, rehabilitation has to secure patients' rights to self-determination and help them to resume meaningful social roles. Having a job is central in the process of recovery. A movement stemming from the worker cooperatives (known as 'the social enterprise') has been successful in Italy in offering (ex-) users jobs and opportunities to become actively involved in companies as associates (Warner 1994).

Psychiatric consumer groups are also effective in meeting users' practical needs with regard to work, accommodation and social life while promoting members' emancipation and empowerment. There are examples of joint programmes where users collaborate with mental health services and/or non-profit organizations to run such programmes. In Verona, a programme has now been in operation for almost ten years, with encouraging results. It is attended by about 400 users per year, offering 150 vocational rehabilitation interventions, 350 interventions for job placements and support at work, housing for 60 users and about 40 regular activities per week (Burti *et al.* 2005).

The economic impact of shifting care from institutions to the community

A consequence of shifting care from institutions to the community is the rising indirect costs sustained by caregivers – mainly families, voluntary or self-help organizations – and society as a whole. Very few countries have available data on the percentage of their total health budget spent on mental health (see Table 10.1). Despite the international diversity of health care systems, most developed nations spend approximately 10 per cent of their total health care expenditures on the treatment of mental disorders (Souetre 1994). Among EU countries, it seems that the amount of money allocated to mental health is generally close to that of other developed countries; it ranges from 13.4 per cent in Luxembourg to 2 per cent in Slovakia.

From an economic point of view, the planning of mental health services' reform should consider several points: i) human rights; ii) the public impact of mental disorders (severity, burden due to illness); and iii) social cohesion. It is demonstrated that, for example, in Italy 70 per cent of the total burden for schizophrenia is due to indirect costs (Tarricone *et al.* 2000) while Murray and Lopez (1997) estimate that neuropsychiatric conditions account for 10.5 per cent of the worldwide burden (in Disability Adjusted Life Years – DALYs) of illnesses, and exceed the contributions of cardiovascular conditions (9.7 per cent) and malignant neoplasm (5.1 per cent).

The economic impact of shifting from hospital to community-based care was analysed by Knapp *et al.* (1994). This study used a randomized controlled trial to compare the comprehensive costs of a programme (Daily Living Programme – DLP) that offered problem-oriented, home-based care for people aged 17–64 with severe mental illness against standard inpatient care. The DLP was significantly less costly than standard treatment in both the short and medium term. A further randomized study conducted by Merson *et al.* (1996) found that the total cost of treatment for the community group (GBP £56,000) was much lower than for the hospital group (GBP £130,000), although the median patient cost was 50 per cent higher in the community group (GBP £938 versus GBP £610), with a greater proportion of the community service expenditure (10 per cent versus 2 per cent) due to failed contacts. Taken together with clinical outcomes, which showed no advantages for the hospital-based service over the community-based service, this study suggests that this form of community psychiatric service is a cost-efficient alternative to hospital-based care for this group of patients.

As a recent review of the literature has demonstrated, acute day hospitals are a means of providing intensive psychiatric care without the high overheads and restriction on liberty that are associated with inpatient care. Moreover, assertive community treatment, when used to divert patients from hospital, can achieve a 55 per cent reduction in admissions compared with 23 per cent achieved by day hospitals. From an economic point of view, community care produces savings of up to 65 per cent (Marshall *et al.* 2001). Psychiatric reforms, begun in all European countries, also enabled financial weaknesses within health systems to become apparent and consequently economic studies examining health production processes and resource distribution were required in order to avoid previous management problems experienced by both hospital managers and policy decision-makers. In particular, it has become essential to implement new financing systems that should help to respond to patients' needs while taking into account the quality of services, patient satisfaction and outcomes.

For the WHO, there are three principles to be followed. Firstly, people should be protected from catastrophic financial risk, which means minimizing out-of-pocket payments and, in particular, requiring such payments only for small expenses on affordable goods or services. All forms of prepayment, whether this be via general taxation, mandatory social insurance or voluntary private insurance, are preferable in this respect, because they pool risks and allow the use of services to be at least partly separated from direct payments by patients. Mental problems are often chronic; therefore what matters is not only the cost of a specific treatment or service but the likelihood of it being repeated over long intervals. That is, what an individual or a household can afford once, in a crisis, may be unaffordable in the long term.

Secondly, the healthy should subsidize the sick. Any prepayment mechanism will do this in general – as out-of-pocket payment will not – but whether or not subsidies flow in the right direction for mental health depends on whether prepayment covers the specific needs of the mentally ill. A financing system could be adequate in this respect for many services but still not transfer resources from the healthy to the sick where mental or behavioural problems are concerned, simply because such problems are not covered. The effect of a particular financing arrangement on mental health therefore depends on the choice of interventions to be funded.

Finally, a good financing system will also mean that the well-off subsidize the poor, at least to some extent. This is the hardest characteristic to ensure as it depends on the coverage and progressivity of the tax system and on who is covered by social or private insurance. For example, insurance allows for the well-off to subsidize the worse-off only if both groups are included in the scheme rather than insurance coverage being limited to the well-off. Moreover, cross subsidies only work if contributions or premiums are at least partly income-related and subject to risk-pooling, rather than uniform or related to individual risk profiles. As always, the magnitude and direction of subsidies also depends on what services are covered.

Legal frameworks for mental health care

Cross-national comparison of legal provisions can be very helpful in outlining models and trends and in supporting the drafting of new legislation (Saraceno 2002). A recent comparison of legal texts relating to mental health in all EU countries (Fioritti 2002) allows us to produce an outline of the different models regulating this complex issue in Europe. This study updates previous research (Ferrari *et al.* 1986) conducted 19 years earlier, and serves to highlight historical trends. Mental health legislation became a focus in most countries during the 1990s. When Ferrari *et al.* conducted their study in 1986, the Italian (1978) and British (1984) Mental Health Acts represented the most recent legislation in this area; today they are the oldest. All other countries modified their legislation during the 1990s, and some changed it more than once (e.g. the Netherlands). The amendments may reflect the impact of major changes in public attitudes and treatment methods in mental health care, which have promoted greater debate and a remodelling of the legal frameworks for care. At the time of writing, reform proposals are again before Parliament in both Italy and the United Kingdom. Therefore, one thing does appear to be clear: if in the 1970s the average duration of a mental health law was 30 years, it is now 15.

A second trend highlights that the distinction between the functions of a general/federal law (encompassing provisions on general principles, patients' rights and procedures for involuntary care), and a local/regional law (regarding the organization of services, standards for mental health care personnel and care itself) has become clearer. This is natural given the radical differences that can exist within large nations where standards for staff may depend on local needs and the availability of resources, and in the light of the broader political trend towards devolution.

Current legislation has completely abolished most terms that formed the basis of national legislation only 20 years ago. Words such as 'lunatic' or 'insane' in English or *'alienè'* in French have been amended and terms such as 'citizen', 'user' or 'patient' have taken their place. The words 'asylum' or 'mental hospital' also have been replaced by terms such as 'mental health departments'. These changes, which may seem obvious, can be seen to be a result of the transformations that have occurred independently within the mental health profession and its institutions. They may also influence the direction of policy in countries which have not yet embarked on mental health reform.

Current legislation emphasizes the protection of patients' rights rather than protecting society from disturbing or criminal behaviour on the part of the mentally ill. Dangerousness is no longer the unique grounds for compulsory treatment (dangerousness criterion); most legislation contains provisions which allow for the treatment of patients for their own benefit ('treatability' criterion) and on the basis of the clinical judgement of one or more physicians ('need for care' criterion). Some legislation (e.g. in the United Kingdom) has different procedures for different situations – and one criterion prevails over the others depending on the circumstances. Moreover, the direct involvement of judicial authorities in compulsory admission procedures is now much less commonplace, and usually occurs only in the case of appeals. Instead, mental health administrative authorities (e.g. in Italy, France, Greece, Ireland and the United Kingdom) are responsible for most activities regarding case assessment, decision-making and implementing the procedures for obligatory treatment. This reflects significant changes in public attitudes and in mental health philosophies over the last few decades.

There is now a far greater level of variety in the locations where care can be delivered (voluntarily or involuntarily) and in the procedures for commitment, including emergency commitment, inpatient commitment, outpatient-mandated care, and medium and long-term commitment. This differentiation reflects the search for a more modulated response to patient care, in terms of balancing protection and coercion, and in the light of the primary goal of protecting patients' rights.

The role of the medical profession in compulsory treatment is split around two major models: the medical model and the legal model. The medical model emphasizes that although it is coercive, compulsory treatment is treatment nevertheless, that only skilled clinicians know what is in their patients' best interests, and that making such decisions is part of their professional activity. A broad criterion ('need for treatment') is usually preferred, and doctors can either admit patients directly or after their decision has been formally validated by an administrative authority. Controls for preventing abuses are implemented through, for example, the involvement of judicial authorities.

The legal model emphasizes that compulsory treatment is always a restriction of personal freedom and therefore should be determined only through the decision of a legal authority, preferably judicial. Physicians can recommend treatment but their proposal should be thoroughly examined by a non-clinical authority, which should ensure that formal criteria to justify compulsory treatment are met, procedures are properly followed and that no other alternatives exist. This is the case in the United Kingdom where an approved social worker must personally verify all aspects of a compulsory treatment proposal and make a decision on the behalf of the local government authority. A behavioural criterion (e.g. dangerousness, self-neglect) is often preferred and the role of the medical profession is limited to the input phase.

Finally, a few countries have introduced into their mental health laws some provisions which mandate future trends and developments, such as: implementing clinical governance and quality management; involving users and carers in the planning and evaluation of services; adapting procedures to emerging clinical profiles (personality disorders, learning disabilities, drug abuse); increasing health promotion; and preventing stigma. Mental health legislation must be viewed as a process: it reflects changes, it promotes changes. As a result, it is destined to be at the core of the debate on mental health systems. However, to produce benefits mental health legislation must also include provisions that require and monitor its implementation and evaluation.

Cross-national comparisons may be helpful to outline historical and cultural trends and to provide a framework for drafting a nation's mental health laws (Dressing and Salize 2004; Salize and Dressing 2004). European countries have been shown to attach great importance to legislative activities during the last two decades, which has been crucial in acknowledging consolidated changes and promoting new approaches.

Further directions for change

Countries that have, to some degree, already adopted a community-based system of care are likely to develop their mental health policies in a number of key areas. The first is in the implementation of clinical governance and quality management in mental health care. Clinical governance represents an organization-wide strategy for improving quality and is a framework through which health organizations are accountable for continually improving the quality of their services, and safeguarding high standards by creating an environment in which excellence in clinical care will flourish (Department of Health 1998). This approach seeks to combine previous managerial and professional approaches to quality management, such as quality assurance and quality improvement (Buetow and Roland 1999). A second future direction lies in the establishment of collaborative programmes between community mental health services and consumer organizations. In these programmes, consumer participation seems to improve the use of patients' resources and initiative in their own treatment and care (Corrigan *et al.* 2002). Thirdly, more and more patients, especially young patients, may have dual diagnoses, present multiple needs and be subject to high risks of their conditions becoming chronic. The prevention of this kind of new chronicity requires the additional integration of clinical and social actions: that is, mental health services providing psychiatric treatment to these clients have to work in tandem with social agencies to meet their personal, social and financial needs and expectations.

Last but not least, health promotion and the prevention of stigma must become a priority in mental health plans. A wide range of strategies are now available to improve mental health and prevent mental disorders. These strategies can also contribute to a reduction in other problems such as youth delinquency, child abuse, dropping out of school and work days lost to illness. Stigma plays a negative role in the recovery process and the effectiveness of psychosocial rehabilitation. The stigma attached to mental illnesses creates social isolation, an inability to work, alcohol or drug abuse, homelessness, or excessive institutionalization, which decreases a person's chance of recovery and their quality of life (WHO 2001b).

Note

1 Names in use include consumers, users, survivors of psychiatry, psychiatric survivors, clients, victims of psychiatry, ex-users, ex-patients, ex-inmates, lunatics . . .

References

Becker, T. and Vázquez-Barquero, J.L. (2001) The European perspective of psychiatric reform, *Acta Psychiatrica Scandinavica*, 104 (Suppl. 410): 8–14.

Becker, T., Hülsmann, S., Knudsen, H.C., Martiny, K., Amaddeo, F., Herran, A., Knapp, M., Schene, A.H., Tansella, M., Thornicroft, G., Vázquez-Barquero, J.L., EPSILON Study Group (2002) Provision of services for people with schizophrenia in five European regions, *Social Psychiatry and Psychiatric Epidemiology*, 37(10): 465–74.

Brand, U. (2001a) Mental health care in Germany: carers' perspectives, *Acta Psychiatrica Scandinavica*, 104 (Suppl. 410): 35–40.

Brand, U. (2001b) European perspectives: a carer's view, *Acta Psychiatrica Scandinavica*, 104 (Suppl. 410): 96–101.

Buetow, S.A. and Roland, M.O. (1999) Clinical governance: bridging gap between managerial and clinical approaches to quality of care, *Quality in Health Care*, 8(3): 184–90.

Burti, L. (2001) Italian psychiatric reform 20 plus years after, *Acta Psychiatrica Scandinavica*, 104 (Suppl. 410): 41–6.

Burti, L., Amaddeo, F., Ambrosi, M., Bonetto, C., Cristofalo, D., Ruggeri, M. and Tansella, M. (2005) Does additional care provided by a consumer self-help group improve psychiatric outcome? A study in an Italian community-based psychiatric service, south Verona (submitted). Available from the authors.

Chamberlin, J. (2005) User/consumer involvement in mental health service delivery, *Epidemiologia e Psichiatria Sociale*, 14(1): 10–14.

Corrigan, P.W., Calabrese, J.D., Diwan, S.E., Keogh, C.B., Keck, L. and Mussey, C. (2002) Some recovery processes in mutual-help groups for persons with mental illness; I: qualitative analysis of program materials and testimonies, *Community Mental Health Journal*, 38(4): 287–301.

Department of Health (1998) *A First Class Service: Quality in the New NHS*. London: Department of Health.

Dressing, H. and Salize, H.J. (2004) Compulsory admission of mentally ill patients in European Union Member States, *Social Psychiatry and Psychiatric Epidemiology*, 39(10): 797–803.

Ferrari, G., Fioritti, A., Piazza, A. and Pileggi, F. (1986) Legge e salute mentale: rassegna delle legislazioni psichiatriche nel mondo, *Fòrmazione Psichiatrica*, VII(2): 29–54.

Fioritti, A. (2002) *Leggi e Salute Mentale: Panorama Europeo delle Legislazioni di Interesse Psichiatrico*. Torino: Centro Scientifico Editore.

Geller, J.L. (2002) Does 'in the community' mean anything any more? *Psychiatric Services*, 53(10): 1201.

Goldberg, D. (1997) Community psychiatry in Europe, *Epidemiologia e Psichiatria Sociale*, 6 (Suppl. 1): 217–27.

Hölling, I. (2001) About the impossibility of a single (ex-) user and survivor of psychiatry position, *Acta Psychiatrica Scandinavica*, 104 (Suppl. 410): 102–6.

Johnson, S., Zinkler, M. and Priebe, S. (2001) Mental health service provision in England, *Acta Psychiatrica Scandinavica*, 104 (Suppl. 410): 47–55.

Knapp, M., Beecham, J., Koutsogeorgopoulou, V., Hallam, A., Fenyo, A., Marks, I.M., Connolly, J., Audini, B. and Muijen, M. (1994) Service use and costs of home-based versus hospital-based care for people with serious mental illness, *British Journal of Psychiatry*, 166: 120–2.

Leff, J. (2001) Why is care in the community perceived as a failure? *British Journal of Psychiatry*, 179: 381–3.

Marshall, M., Crowther, R., Almaraz-Serrano, A., Creed, F., Sledge, W., Kluiter, H., Roberts, C., Hill, E., Wiersma, D., Bond, G.R., Huxley, P. and Tyrer, P. (2001) Systematic reviews of the effectiveness of day care for people with severe mental disorders; 1) Acute day hospital versus admission; 2) Vocational rehabilitation; 3) Day hospital versus outpatient care, *Health Technology Assessment*, 5(21): 1–75.

Merson, S., Tyrer, P., Carlen, D. and Johnson, T. (1996) The cost of treatment of psychiatric emergencies: a comparison of hospital and community services, *Psychological Medicine*, 26 (4): 727–34.

Murray, C.J.L. and Lopez, A.D. (1997) Regional patterns of disability-free life expectancy and disability-adjusted life-expectancy: Global Burden of Disease Study, *The Lancet*, 349: 1347–52.

Salize, H.J. and Dressing, H. (2004) Epidemiology of involuntary placement of mentally ill people across the European Union, *British Journal of Psychiatry*, 184: 163–8.

Saraceno, B. (2002) *Prefazione*, in A. Fioritti (ed.) *Leggi e Salute Mentale. Panorama Europeo delle Legislazioni di Interesse Psichiatrico*. Torino: Centro Scientifico Editore.

Schene, A. and Faber, A.M.E. (2001) Mental health care in the Netherlands, *Acta Psychiatrica Scandinavica*, 104 (Suppl. 410): 74–81.

Souetre, F. (1994) Economic evaluation in mental disorders: community versus institutional care, *Pharmachoeconomics*, 6(4): 330–6.

Tarricone, R., Gerzeli, S., Montanelli, R., Frattura, L., Percudani, M. and Racagni, G. (2000) Direct and indirect costs of schizophrenia in community psychiatric services in Italy. The GISIES study, *Health Policy*, 51: 1–18.

Thornicroft, G. and Tansella, M. (2004) Components of a modern mental health service: a pragmatic balance of community and hospital care – overview of systematic evidence, *British Journal of Psychiatry*, 185: 283–90.

Thornicroft, G. and Tansella, M. (2005) Growing recognition of the importance of service user involvement in mental health planning and evaluation, *Epidemiologia e Psichiatria Sociale*, 14 (1): 1–3.

United Nations (1991) *The Protection of Persons with Mental Illness and the Improvement of Mental Health Care*. UN General Assembly resolution A/RES/46.119 (available at:http://www.un.org/ga/documents/gadocs.htm).

Warner, R. (1994) *Recovery from Schizophrenia*, 2nd edn. London: Routledge.

World Health Organization (2001a) *Atlas: Country profiles*. Geneva: World Health Organization.

World Health Organization (2001b) *The World Health Report 2001, Mental Health: New Understanding, New Hope*. Geneva: World Health Organization.

World Health Organization (2001c) *Mental Health Policy Project: Policy and Service Guidance Package, Executive Summary*. Geneva: World Health Organization.

World Health Organization (2001d) *Mental Health Resources in the World: Initial Results of Project Atlas*. Geneva: World Health Organization.

chapter eleven

Addiction and alcohol use disorders

Peter Anderson

Of the 2 billion people who consume alcoholic beverages worldwide, over 76 million are diagnosed with alcohol use disorders at any one time (World Health Organization 2004a). Globally, alcohol causes 3.2 per cent of deaths (1.8 million) and 4 per cent of ill health and premature death (58.3 million years) (World Health Organization 2002a); it is the leading risk factor for disease burden in low mortality, low income countries, and the third largest risk factor in high income countries. Apart from being a drug of dependence and aside from the 60 or so different types of disease and injury it causes, alcohol is responsible for widespread social, mental and emotional harms, including crime and family violence, leading to enormous costs to society (Babor *et al.* 2003). Alcohol not only harms the user, but those surrounding the user, including the unborn child, children, family members and the sufferers of crime, violence and drink driving accidents. This can be termed environmental alcohol damage or 'passive drinking'.

The use of alcohol brings with it a number of benefits, a point emphasized by the beverage alcohol industry (Peele and Grant 1999). The notion that light consumption of alcohol is good in various ways for health is possibly as old as the history of alcohol itself (Thom 2001) and is embedded in folk wisdom on the subject. Alcohol has been medically recommended for pain and stress relief and for a variety of minor ailments. The perceived health benefits have received much support with the findings that small amounts of alcohol consumption can reduce the risk of coronary heart disease.

That alcohol improves the drinker's mood in the short term is perhaps the main reason why most people drink. There is, indeed, a large amount of experimental evidence that the acute effects of alcohol include increased enjoyment, euphoria, happiness and the general expression of positive moods – feelings that are experienced more strongly in group situations than when drinking alone (Pliner and Cappell 1974), and very much influenced by expectancies

(Brown *et al.* 1980). Alcohol is an anxiolytic drug that reduces anxiety and the physiological response to stress, as well as possibly self-awareness (Baum-Baicker 1987).

Alcohol plays a role in everyday social life, marking such events as births, weddings and deaths, as well as marking the transition from work to play and easing social intercourse. Throughout history and in many different cultures, alcohol is a principal means by which many groups of friends enhance the enjoyment of each other's company and generally have fun. So entrenched are these beliefs about alcohol that people become observably more sociable when they merely think that they have consumed alcohol but actually have not (Darkes and Goldman 1993).

Alcohol is drunk primarily for its intoxicating effects, even by those who are light or moderate consumers of wine. Many drinkers, and in particular younger men, deliberately and self-consciously use alcohol to pursue intoxication, i.e. to get drunk. The benefits of moderate drinking occur in spite of, not because of, the basic nature of the substance (Heather 2001).

The harm from alcohol arises from it being a toxic substance (harmful use), an intoxicating substance and a dependence-producing substance. Alcohol is a toxic substance in terms of its direct and indirect effects on a wide range of body organs and systems. The prevalence of hazardous and harmful alcohol use in western European populations (aged 15+ years) is estimated to be 14.1 per cent for men and 11.1 per cent for women, with an annual incidence of 1.7 per cent and 1.2 per cent respectively, a mean duration of 10.2 years and an annual case fatality of 0.36 per cent (Rehm *et al.* 2004).

Alcohol intoxication can be defined as a more or less short-term state of functional impairment in psychological and psychomotor performance induced by the presence of alcohol in the body. The impairments that can be produced by alcohol are mostly dose-related, often complex and involve multiple body functions. The prevalence of serious intoxication occasions is very widespread, with, across European countries, some 10–30 per cent of drinking occasions including consumption of at least six drinks (Rehn *et al.* 2001).

Alcohol dependence is a recognized disorder within the ICD classification of mental and behavioural disorders (World Health Organization 1992). The prevalence of alcohol dependence ranges from 3 to 5 per cent in European countries (World Health Organization 2002b). No matter how drinking is measured, the risk of alcohol dependence begins at low levels of drinking and increases linearly with both the volume of alcohol consumption and a pattern of drinking larger amounts on occasion (Caetano and Cunradi 2002).

This chapter will discuss alcohol in the European Union (EU) of 25 countries. It will consider alcohol's contribution to individual and societal harm, and outline the policy options that can be put in place to reduce such harm. Existing alcohol policy in Europe will be described and the EU's approaches will be discussed in terms of opportunities and threats to alcohol policy. Most of what is written in this chapter applies to the other non-EU western European countries, as well as the accession countries Bulgaria and Romania (Anderson and Baumberg 2006). With over 80 per cent of the population being lifetime abstainers, and with a per capita consumption level of 1.45 litres of alcohol, Turkey faces a different position (although the consumption per drinker is as high in Turkey as in the rest of

Europe) (Anderson and Baumberg 2006). Going further east to the countries of the former Soviet Union, different problems emerge. Alcohol consumption has been increasing, and patterns of drinking remain particularly harmful, particularly in terms of injuries and cardiovascular diseases (McKee and Sholnikov 2001; McKee *et al.* 2001; Rehm *et al.* 2004). Coupled with this, there remains the difficulty of policy implementation (World Health Organization 2004a).

Alcohol in Europe

Alcohol consumption

Europe has the highest proportion of drinkers worldwide and has the highest levels of alcohol consumption per population (Rehm *et al.* 2003). There has been a harmonization of drinking levels between the 25 EU countries between the years 1970 and 2001. This is clearly illustrated in Figure 11.1, which shows the changes in alcohol consumption for the four countries with the highest consumption in 1970, and the four countries with the lowest consumption in 1970. Furthermore, there is no evidence that the addition of the ten new countries has increased the overall consumption of the EU (see Figure 11.2). The harmonization of drinking levels has also been matched by a harmonization of drinking patterns and beverage choice (Norström 2001).

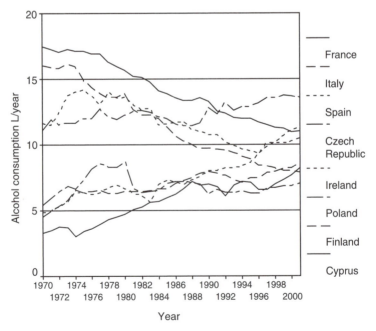

Figure 11.1 Alcohol consumption in the four countries with the highest consumption in 1970, and the four countries with the lowest consumption, EU 1970–2001

Source: World Health Organization (2004c)

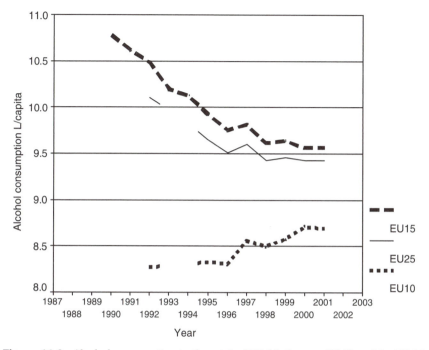

Figure 11.2   Alcohol consumption in the original EU-15, the new EU-10 and the EU-25, 1970–2001

Source: World Health Organization (2004c)

The use of alcohol is unevenly distributed throughout the population (Skog 1991); most of the alcohol in a society is drunk by a relatively small minority of drinkers. Lemmens (2001) estimated that the top tenth of drinkers in the Netherlands in the mid-1980s consumed more than a third of the total alcohol, and that the top 30 per cent of drinkers accounted for up to three-quarters of all consumption.

One of the biggest determinants of alcohol consumption is purchasing power (Norström 2001). Economic analyses find a strong relationship between pre- dicted economic growth and alcohol consumption in both western, and more particularly, eastern Europe (Anderson and Baumberg 2006).

Alcohol-related harm

As there has been a harmonization of drinking levels between the 25 EU coun- tries between the years 1970 and 2001, there has been a similar harmonization in death rates from chronic liver disease and cirrhosis, one of the best indicators of alcohol-related harm. Unlike the situation with drinking levels, there is some evidence that the addition of the ten new countries has increased the average death rate from chronic liver disease and cirrhosis (and probably, thus, other alcohol-related harms) (see Figure 11.3). Figure 11.3 excludes data from

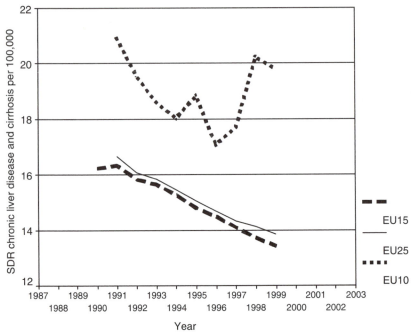

Figure 11.3 SDR chronic liver disease and cirrhosis in the original EU-15, the new EU-10 and the EU-25, 1970–2001 (excluding Hungary)

Source: World Health Organization (2004c)

Hungary, which has more than four times the average cirrhosis death rate of the EU, possibly due to aliphatic alcohol congeners arising from home-made spirits (Szucs *et al.* 2005); this might also suggests a higher rate of unrecorded alcohol consumption in the new member states, compared with the 15.

Alcohol and the burden of harm in individuals and societies

Alcohol and individuals

The relationship between alcohol consumption and individual harm is summarized in Table 11.1. For many conditions there is an increasing risk with increasing levels of alcohol consumption, with no evidence of a threshold effect. The slopes of the risks vary by gender and the geographical areas in which studies are performed. The absolute risk of death from alcohol-related cancers (mouth, oesophagus, pharynx, larynx and liver) increases from 13 per 100,000 at no alcohol consumption to 37 per 100,000 at four or more drinks (40+g) per day (Thun *et al.* 1997). The cumulative incidence of breast cancer by age 80 years increases from 8.8 per 100 women in non-drinkers to 13.3 per 100 women consuming an average of 60g each day (Collaborative Group on Hormonal Factors in Breast Cancer 2002). The absolute risk of death from liver cirrhosis

Table 11.1 Relative risks for stated conditions based on alcohol consumption

	Women			Men		
	Alcohol consumption, g/day					
	0–19.99	20–39.99	40+	0–39.99	40–59.99	60+
Conditions arising during the perinatal period						
Low birth weight (RR refers to drinking of mother)	1.00	1.40	1.40	1.00	1.40	1.40
Malignant neoplasms						
Mouth and oropharynx cancers	1.45	1.85	5.39	1.45	1.85	5.39
Oesophageal cancer	1.8	2.38	4.36	1.8	2.38	4.36
Liver cancer	1.45	3.03	3.60	1.45	3.03	3.60
Breast cancer	1.14	1.41	1.59	N/A	N/A	N/A
under 45 years of age	1.15	1.41	1.46	N/A	N/A	N/A
45 years and over	1.14	1.38	1.62	N/A	N/A	N/A
Other neoplasms	1.10	1.30	1.70	1.10	1.30	1.70
Diabetes mellitus	0.92	0.87	1.13	1.00	0.57	0.73
Neuropsychiatric conditions						
Unipolar major depression	Attributable fraction = 6%					
Epilepsy	1.34	7.22	7.52	1.23	7.52	6.83
Alcohol use disorders	Attributable fraction = 6%					
Cardiovascular (CVD) diseases						
Hypertensive disease	1.40	2.00	2.00	1.40	2.00	4.10
Coronary heart disease	0.82	0.83	1.12	0.82	0.83	1.00
Cerebrovascular disease						
Ischaemic stroke	0.52	0.64	1.06	0.94	1.33	1.65
Haemorrhagic stroke	0.59	0.65	7.98	1.27	2.19	2.38
Digestive diseases						
Cirrhosis of the liver	1.30	9.50	13.00	1.30	9.05	13.00

Source: Rehm *et al.* (2003)

increases from 5 per 100,000 at no alcohol consumption to 41 per 100,000 at four or more drinks (40+g) per day (Thun *et al.* 1997).

People with depression have an increased risk of alcohol dependence and vice versa. An American study found that 12 per cent of people with unipolar depression were dependent on alcohol (Regier *et al.* 1990). Conversely, 28 per cent of people dependent on alcohol had a major depressive disorder. Although depression may precede heavy alcohol consumption or alcohol use disorders, there is a substantial proportion of co-morbidity where the onset of alcohol use disorders precedes the onset of depressive disorders. Alcohol-dependent individuals demonstrate a two- to threefold increase in the risk of depressive disorders, and there is evidence for a continuum in the magnitude of co-morbidity as a function of the level of alcohol use problems (Kessler *et al.* 1996).

Alcohol, in low doses, reduces the risk of coronary heart disease but higher quality studies find less of a protective effect than lower quality studies. A review of 28 higher quality studies found that the risk of coronary heart disease decreased to 80 per cent of the level of non-drinkers at 20g (two drinks) of alcohol per day (Corrao *et al.* 2000). Most of the reduction in risk occurred by the level of one drink every second day. However, beyond two drinks a day, the risk of heart disease increases. The protective effect of alcohol is greater for non-fatal heart attacks than for fatal heart attacks, for men rather than for women and for people studied in Mediterranean countries than those in non-Mediterranean countries.

Whereas low doses of alcohol may protect against heart disease, high doses increase the risk, and high volume drinking occasions may precipitate myocardial ischemia or infarction and coronary death (Anderson 2003). The relationship between alcohol consumption and the risk of coronary heart disease is biologically plausible. Alcohol consumption raises levels of high density lipoprotein cholesterol (HDL) (Klatsky 1999). HDL removes fatty deposits in blood vessels and thus is associated with a lower risk of coronary heart disease deaths. Moderate alcohol intake favourably affects blood clotting profiles, in particular, through its effects on platelet aggregation (McKenzie and Eisenberg 1996) and fibrinolysis (Reeder *et al.* 1996; Gorinstein *et al.* 2003). Alcohol's impact on coagulation mechanisms is likely to be immediate and, since lipid modification in older age groups produces significant benefit, the impact mediated through the elevation of HDL cholesterol can probably be achieved by alcohol consumption in middle and older age. The biochemical changes that might reduce the risk of heart disease result equally from beer, wine or spirits; they do not particularly result from grape juice or wine from which the alcohol has been removed (Sierksma 2003).

Although the relationship between lower levels of alcohol consumption and reduced risk of coronary heart disease is found in many studies, some studies have not found the relationship. For example, a study of a group of employed Scottish men aged over 21 years found no elevated risk for coronary heart disease among abstainers, compared to light and moderate drinkers (Hart *et al.* 1999). Other studies of the general population where respondents might be expected to have reduced their drinking due to poor health have found no differences in death rates between light drinkers and abstainers (Fillmore *et al.* 1998a, 1998b; Leino *et al.* 1998).

Some studies in England and the United States found that light drinkers had generally healthier lifestyles in terms of diet, physical activity and not smoking than people who did not drink, all of which could have explained the apparent increased risk of heart disease in non-drinkers compared with light drinkers (Wannamethee and Shaper 1999; Barefoot et al. 2002). An Australian study found that non-drinkers had a range of characteristics known to be associated with anxiety, depression and other facets of ill health, such as low status occupations, poor education, current financial hardship, poor social support and recent stressful life events, as well as an increased risk of depression, all of which could explain an increased risk of heart disease among non-drinkers compared with light drinkers (Rodgers et al. 2000). Controlling for depression interacts with the protective effect of alcohol (Greenfield et al. 2002). One recent American study found that, whereas alcohol consumption reduced the risk of coronary heart disease in white men, it increased the risk in black men, suggesting that the cardio-protective effect could be explained by the consistent confounding of lifestyle characteristics of drinkers (Fuchs et al. 2004).

Alcohol can harm people other than the drinker, and can have negative consequences for communities as a whole (Babor et al. 2003). It increases the risk of social harms, drink-driving, injuries, suicide, violence, divorce, child abuse and decreased work productivity. A causal link between alcohol intoxication and violence is supported not only by epidemiological and experimental research but also by research indicating specific biological mechanisms that link alcohol to aggressive behaviour (Bushman 1997).

When examining the relationship between alcohol consumption and death, the shape of the relationship depends on the distribution of causes of death among the population studied and on the level and patterns of alcohol consumption within the population. At younger ages, deaths from accidents and violence (which are increased by alcohol consumption) predominate, while coronary heart disease deaths (which are reduced by alcohol consumption) are rare. The position is reversed at older ages.

In the United Kingdom it has been estimated that the level of alcohol consumption with the lowest risk of death for women is 0g per day aged under 35 years, 1g per day aged 35 to 64 years and 4g per day aged 65 years and over (White et al. 2002). For men, the levels are 0g per day aged under 35 years, 5g per day aged 35–64 years, and 9g per day aged 65 years and over. Above these levels, the risk of death increases with increasing alcohol consumption. For men aged 35 to 69 years at death, the risk of death increases from 1167 per 100,000 at 10g of alcohol per day to 1431 per 100,000 at 60 or more grams per day (Thun et al. 1997). For women, the risk increases from 666 per 100,000 at 10g of alcohol per day to 828 per 100,000 at 60 or more grams per day.

In Sweden, up to 30 per cent of the differential mortality for middle-aged men by socioeconomic group is explained by alcohol consumption (Hemström 2001).

Alcohol and societies

Just as there is a relationship between the level of alcohol consumption and harm at the individual level, there is also a link at the societal level. Between societies, the lower the level of per capita alcohol consumption, the lower the level of the proportion of heavy drinkers (see Figure 11.4) and the lower the level of death from chronic liver disease and cirrhosis (see Figure 11.5).

When alcohol consumption levels increase in any given society there tends to be an increase in the prevalence of heavy drinkers, defined in terms of a high annual alcohol intake. For example, in Finland, following liberalization of the

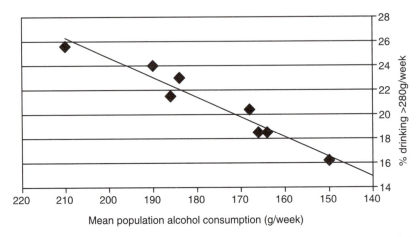

Figure 11.4   The proportion of heavy drinkers by alcohol consumption: eight English regions

Source: Academy of Medical Sciences (2004)

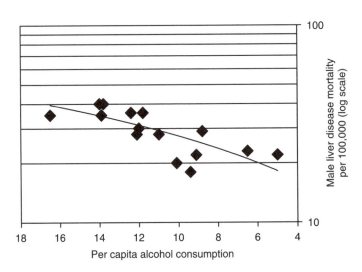

Figure 11.5   Death from liver disease by per capita alcohol consumption in 15 European countries

Source: Ramstedt (2001)

availability of alcohol, total alcohol consumption increased by 46 per cent from 1968 to 1969. The increase in consumption was influenced more by the addition of new heavy drinking occasions than by new drinkers (Mäkelä 1970), and the increase was greater in heavier consumption groups (Mäkelä 2002).

Within societies there is a direct relationship between levels of per capita consumption and alcohol-related harm. The European Comparative Alcohol Study reviewed the post-war experience of alcohol and mortality in EU countries (Norström 2001). Time series analysis demonstrated that there is a positive and significant relationship between changes in alcohol consumption and changes in both overall and alcohol related death for both men and women (see Table 11.2). The relationship applies to all types of alcohol-related harm, and is stronger in countries with lower overall alcohol consumption than in countries with higher overall alcohol consumption.

Due to the highly positively skewed distribution of alcohol consumption in populations, it is likely that the level of alcohol consumption with the lowest risk of death for a population will be considerably lower than that for an individual. How much lower this is will depend on the shape of the individual risk function and on how the distribution of alcohol consumption changes, as the overall consumption level of the population changes. In not too unrealistic circumstances (proportional changes in consumption), the minimum risk consumption level for the population could be less than that for an individual drinker by a factor of as much as five (Skog 1996). In countries with high rates of coronary heart disease, the per capita level associated with minimum risk for mortality may be in the order of about three litres of absolute alcohol. In countries with low rates of coronary heart disease, the level is likely to be

Table 11.2 Change in death rates (%) from a 1-litre increase in alcohol consumption per capita in low, medium and high consuming European countries for men (M) and women (F)

Country group (alcohol consumption)	Low		Medium		High	
	M	F	M	F	M	F
Cirrhosis	32*	17*	9*	5*	10*	11*
Alcohol dependence, psychosis and poisoning	35*	75*	18*	27*	3	1
Accidents	9*	10*	3*	3*	2*	2*
Suicide	9*	12*	0	3*	0	1
Homicide	18*	8	11*	7*	7*	2
IHD	−1	1	1	2*	1	0
Total mortality (M+F)	3*		1*		1*	

* $p<.05$.

Source: Norström (2001)

substantially lower. Thus, as all European countries already consume in excess of this level, reductions in alcohol consumption will also result in a net reduction in harm.

In 2002 it was estimated that alcohol was responsible for 7.5 per cent of the total burden of ill health and premature death in the EU, the third most important risk factor after tobacco and raised blood pressure (Anderson and Baumberg 2006, adapted from World Health Organization 2002b). Globally, injuries account for the largest portion of disease burden due to alcohol, with 40 per cent in total, with unintentional injuries by far outweighing intentional injuries (see Table 11.3) (Rehm *et al.* 2003). The second largest category is alcohol-attributable neuropsychiatric diseases and disorders with 38 per cent. Other alcohol-attributable, non-communicable diseases (diabetes and liver cirrhosis), malignant neoplasms and cardiovascular disease each contribute 7 to 8 per cent of the total. These are net figures, for which the alcohol-related beneficial effects on disease have already been subtracted. They do not include the social costs of alcohol which are probably of much greater importance.

The social costs of alcohol have been estimated in 15 European countries (see Table 11.4) (Anderson and Baumberg 2006). They range from some €50 per capita in Slovenia to €1200 per capita in Sweden.

Table 11.3 Global burden of disease (DALYs[1] in 1000s) attributable to alcohol by major disease categories for year 2000

Disease conditions	DALYs	%
Cancers: head and neck cancers, cancers of the gastrointestinal tract including liver cancer, female breast cancer	4,201	7.2
Neuropsychiatric conditions: alcohol dependence syndrome, depression, anxiety disorder, organic brain disease	21,904	37.7
Cardiovascular conditions: ischaemic heart disease, cerebrovascular disease	3,983	6.9
Gastrointestinal conditions: alcoholic liver cirrhosis, cholelithiasis, pancreatitis	4,555	7.8
Maternal and perinatal conditions: low birth weight, intrauterine growth retardation	123	0.2
Accidents and unintentional injuries: road and other transport injuries, falls, drowning and burning injuries, occupational and machine injuries, alcohol poisoning	15,767	27.2
Intentional and self-inflicted injuries: suicide and assaults	7,514	12.9
Alcohol-related disease burden all causes (DALYs)	58,047	100

[1] Disability Adjusted Life Years (DALYs), a methodology introduced in the global burden of disease, accounts for the disability and chronicity caused by disorders. The DALY is a measure of health gap, which combines information on disability and other non-fatal health outcomes and premature death. One DALY is one lost year of 'healthy life'.

Source: Rehm *et al.* (2003)

Table 11.4 Summary of studies looking at the social cost of alcohol

Country	Year of cost	Total cost per capita (PPS)[1]	Health[2]	Crime[3]	Mortality[4]	Absenteeism[4]
Belgium	1999	586	2.6%	–	0.5%	0.00%
Denmark						
Finland	1990	496–850	0.9–1.4%	**13–14%**	0.6–1.0%	**0.05–0.06%**
France	1997	261–310	2.4%			**0.04–0.05%**
Germany	1995	254	**2.3%**		0.4%	**0.08%**
Ireland	2003	556	4.4%	8%		0.78%
Italy	1994	134–153	1.7–1.9%		0.1–0.2%	0.17–0.18%
Netherlands	2000	192	0.3%	**14%**		**0.06%**
Norway	2001	429–472	0.7–1.3%	**2%**	0.1%	**0.10–0.11%**
Portugal	1995	73	0.5%	1%	0.1%	0.00%
UK (Scotland)	2001–2	296–360	1.4%	**14%**		**0.09%**
Slovak Republic	1994	292	4.9%	17%	0.5%	0.66%
Slovenia	2002	50	0.5%		0.3%	0.01%
Spain	1998	129	2.4%	3%		0.14%
Sweden	1998	1,194	5.5%	4%	1.0%	0.71%
UK (England & Wales)	2001	485–527	**2.8–3.3%**	**11%**	0.3%	**0.14–0.20%**

[1] Inflated to 2003 prices using the Consumer Price Index (base Euro); [2] as a % of total health expenditure; [3] as a % of total public order expenditure; [4] as a % of GDP.
* Figures in bold are higher quality studies

Source: Anderson and Baumberg (2006)

Policy options to reduce the harm done by alcohol

Over the last 25 years considerable progress has been made in the scientific understanding of the relationship between alcohol policies, alcohol consumption and alcohol-related harm (Bruun *et al.* 1975; Edwards *et al.* 1994; Babor *et al.* 2003). The evidence finds three types of policies that are effective in reducing alcohol's burden (see Table 11.5): 1) population-based policies such as those on taxation, advertising, regulation of the density of outlets, hours and days of sale, drinking locations and minimum drinking ages; 2) problem-directed policies aimed at specific alcohol-related problems such as drink-driving; and 3) interventions directed at individual drinkers, such as primary care based brief interventions for hazardous and harmful alcohol consumption.

In general, effectiveness is strong for the regulation of physical availability and the use of alcohol taxes (Babor *et al.* 2003). Given the broad reach of these

Table 11.5 Summary ratings of policy-relevant interventions and strategies

	Effectiveness[1]	Breadth of research support[2]	Cross-cultural testing[3]	Cost efficiency[4]	Target group[5] (TG) and comments
Pricing and taxing					
Taxes	+++	+++	+++	+++	TG = GP; effectiveness dependent on government oversight and control of alcohol production and distribution. High taxes can result in increased smuggling and illicit production
Regulating alcohol promotion					
Advertising bans	+	+	++	+++	TG = GP; strongly opposed by alcoholic beverage industry; can be circumvented by product placements on TV and in movies
Advertising content controls	?	0	0	++	TG = GP; often subject to industry self-regulation agreements, which are rarely enforced or monitored
Regulating physical availability					
Total ban on sales	+++	+++	++	+	TG = GP; substantial adverse side-effects from criminalized black market, expensive to suppress. Ineffective without enforcement
Minimum drinking age	+++	+++	+	++	TG = HR; reduces hazardous drinking, but does not eliminate drinking. Ineffective without enforcement
Rationing	++	++	++	+	TG = HD; particularly affects heavy drinkers; difficult to implement
Government retail outlets	+++	+++	++	+++	TG = GP; effective only if operated with public health and public order goals

Hours and days of sale	++	+++	++	+++	TG = GP; effective in certain circumstances. Ineffective without enforcement
Density of outlets	++	+	+	+++	TG = GP; much easier to implement before drinking establishments have become concentrated because of vested economic interests
Server liability	+++	+	+	+++	TG = HR; required legal definition of liability mostly limited to North America
Different availability by alcohol strength	++	++	+	+++	TG = GP; mostly tested for strengths of beer
Drinking-driving countermeasures					
Sobriety checks	+	+++	+++	++	TG = GP; effects of police campaigns typically short-term
Random breath testing (RBT)	+++	++	+	+	TG = GP; somewhat expensive to implement. Effectiveness depends on number of drivers directly affected
Lowered BAC levels	+++	+++	++	+++	TG = GP; diminishing returns at lower levels (e.g. .05% – .02%), but still significant
Administrative license suspension	+++	++	++	++	TG = HD
Graduated licensing	++	++	++	+++	TG = HR
Low BAC for youth ('zero tolerance')	+++	++	+	+++	TG = HR
Designated drivers and ride services	0	+	+	++	TG = HR; programmes are effective in getting drunk people not to drive but have not been shown to affect alcohol-related accidents
Treatment and early intervention					
Brief intervention	++	+++	+++	++	TG = HR; primary care practitioners lack training and time to conduct screening and brief interventions

Continue overleaf

Table 11.5 *Continued*

	Effectiveness[1]	Breadth of research support[2]	Cross-cultural testing[3]	Cost efficiency[4]	Target group[5] (TG) and comments
Alcohol problems treatment	+	+++	+++	0	TG = HD; population reach is low because most countries have limited treatment facilities
Mutual help/self-help attendance	+	+	++	+++	TG = HD; a feasible, cost-effective complement or alternative to formal treatment in many countries
Mandatory treatment of repeat drinking-drivers	+	++	+	++	TG = HD; punitive and coercive approaches tend to have time-limited effects, and sometimes distract attention from more effective interventions
Altering the drinking context					
Training servers to not serve persons to intoxication	+	+++	++	++	TG = HR; external signs of intoxication often difficult to recognize
Training bar staff and managers to prevent and better manage aggression	+	+	+	++	TG = HR
Voluntary codes of bar practice	0	+	+	+++	TG = HR; ineffective without enforcement
Enforcement of on-premise regulations	++	+	++	+	TG = HR; compliance depends on perceived likelihood of enforcement
Safer bar environment/containers	?	+	+	++	TG = HR; one controlled study questions whether tempered glassware is actually safer
Community mobilization	++	++	+	+	TG = GP; sustainability of changes has not been demonstrated
Education and persuasion					
Alcohol education in schools	0	+++	++	+	TG = HR; may increase knowledge and change attitudes but has no effect on drinking

College student education	0	+	+	+	TG = HR; may increase knowledge and change attitudes but has no effect on drinking
Public service messages	0	+++	++	++	TG = GP; refers to messages to the drinker about limiting drinking; messages to strengthen policy support untested
Warning labels	+	+	0	+++	TG = GP; effect on message awareness, none shown on behaviour
Promotion of alternatives	?	+	?	?	TG = GP; not enough research to draw conclusions about this strategy
Alcohol-free activities	0	++	++	++	TG = GP; evidence mostly from youth alternative programmes

[1] Evidence of effectiveness – This criterion refers the scientific evidence demonstrating whether a particular strategy is effective in reducing alcohol consumption, alcohol-related problems or their costs to society. To be considered in this compendium, at a minimum the strategy had to be carefully investigated in at least one well designed study which accounted for alternative and competing explanations. The following rating scale was used as a guide:

0   Evidence indicates a lack of effectiveness
+   Evidence for limited effectiveness
++   Evidence for moderate effectiveness
+++ Evidence of a high degree of effectiveness
?   No studies have been undertaken or there is insufficient evidence upon which to make a judgement

[2] Breadth of research support. The highest rating was influenced by the availability of integrative reviews and meta-analyses. Breadth of research support was evaluated independent of the rating of effectiveness (i.e. it is possible for a strategy to be rated low in effectiveness but to also have a high rating on the breadth of research supporting this evaluation). The following scale was used:

0   No studies of effectiveness have been undertaken
+   Only one well designed study of effectiveness completed
++   From two to four studies of effectiveness have been completed
+++ Five or more studies of effectiveness have been completed
?   There is insufficient evidence on which to make a judgement

[3] Tested across cultures. This criterion is concerned with the diversity of geography and culture in which each strategy has actually been applied and tested. It refers to the robustness of international or multinational testing of a strategy as well as the extent to which a strategy applies to multiple countries and cultures. The following scale was used:

0   The strategy has not been tested adequately
+   The strategy has been studied in only one country or appears to be unique to one country
++   The strategy has been studied in two to four countries or appears relevant to more than one country but perhaps is culturally bounded
+++ The strategy has been studied in five or more countries or appears to be relevant to a large number of countries
?   There is inadequate information on which to make a judgement

[4] Cost efficiency. This criterion seeks to estimate the relative monetary cost to the state to implement, operate and sustain this strategy, regardless of effectiveness. For instance, increasing alcohol excise duties does not cost much to the state but may be costly to alcohol consumers. In this criterion, the lowest possible cost is the highest standard. Therefore, the higher the rating, the lower the relative cost to implement and sustain this strategy. The following scale was used:

0   Very high cost to implement and sustain

Continue overleaf

+   Relatively high cost to implement and sustain
++   Moderate cost to implement and sustain
+++ Low cost to implement and sustain
?   There is no information about cost or cost is impossible to estimate
[5] Each strategy applies to one of the following three target groups (TG): 1) the general population (GP) of drinkers; 2) high risk (HR) drinkers or groups considered to be particularly vulnerable to the adverse effects of alcohol (e.g. adolescents); and 3) persons already manifesting harmful drinking (HD) and alcohol dependence.

Source: Babor *et al.* (2003)

strategies, and the relatively low expense of implementing them, the expected impact of these measures on public health is relatively high. Most of the drinking-driving countermeasures are highly effective, particularly random breath testing, lowered BAC levels, administrative licence suspension and 'zero tolerance' for young offenders.

There is limited research on the effects of altering the drinking context. From the studies published so far, it appears likely that strategies in this area will have some impact, often without being too costly. However, these strategies are primarily applicable to on-premise drinking in bars or restaurants, which somewhat limits their public health significance. One theme that recurs in this literature is the importance of enforcement. Passing a minimum drinking age law, for instance, will have rather little effect if it is not backed up with a credible threat to cancel the licences of outlets that repeatedly sell to the under-aged.

At the other extreme of policy options, the expected impact is low for education and for public service messages about drinking (Babor *et al.* 2003). Although the reach of educational programmes is thought to be excellent (because of the availability of captive audiences in schools), the population impact of these programmes is poor due to their lack of effectiveness. Similarly, while feasibility is good, cost-effectiveness and cost-benefit are poor.

The World Health Organization (WHO) has estimated the cost-effectiveness and impact of different policy options (Baltussen *et al.* 2004; Chisholm *et al.* 2004; Murray *et al.* 2004; World Health Organization 2004b). The data has been reworked for the EU countries, grouping them by the WHO classification based on infant and adult mortality rates. The impact of different policy options is summarized in Figure 11.6, and their cost-effectiveness in Figure 11.7 (Anderson and Baumberg 2006, adapted from Chisholm *et al.* 2004).

In all three groups of countries, taxation has the greatest impact in preventing years of ill health or premature death as measured by disability-adjusted life years (DALYs). Taxation is not only effective in reducing alcohol consumption but also reduces a wide range of harms, including liver cirrhosis, drink-driving accidents, violence and crime (Anderson and Baumberg 2006). It is estimated that raising the price of alcohol by 10 per cent through taxation would lead to a reduction in alcohol consumption of 2 per cent in southern Europe, 5 per cent in central Europe and 8 per cent in northern Europe. For the EU-15 countries, it is estimated that this would prevent over 9000 deaths each year (Anderson and Baumberg 2006).

When applied to 25 per cent of the at-risk population, brief interventions

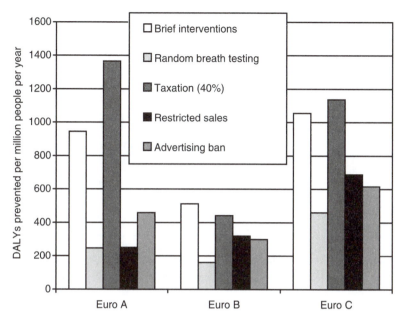

Figure 11.6 Impact of different policies in preventing DALYs per 1 million population per year

Euro A countries: Austria, Belgium, Czech Republic, Denmark, Finland, France, Germany, Greece, Ireland, Italy, Luxembourg, Malta, Netherlands, Portugal, Slovenia, Spain, Sweden, United Kingdom
Euro B countries: Cyprus, Poland, Slovakia
Euro C countries: Estonia, Hungary, Latvia, Lithuania

Source: Anderson and Baumberg (2006) adapted from Chisholm *et al.* (2004)

delivered by primary care physicians to help hazardous and harmful consumers of alcohol to reduce their consumption also have a large impact in reducing ill health and premature death.

When considering the cost-effectiveness of different policy options, taxation is found to be the most cost-effective in preventing ill health and premature death (see Figure 11.7). In all three country groupings, random breath testing is the least cost-effective. Surprisingly, there are no remarkable differences between the country groupings in terms of the impact of different policy options.

Alcohol policy in Europe

Just as there has been a harmonization in alcohol consumption and alcohol-related harm across Europe, there also has been a harmonization in alcohol policy (see Figure 11.8), particularly those policies that deal with marketing and social and environmental controls (see Figure 11.9). There is a relationship between a change in alcohol policy and a change in alcohol consumption in

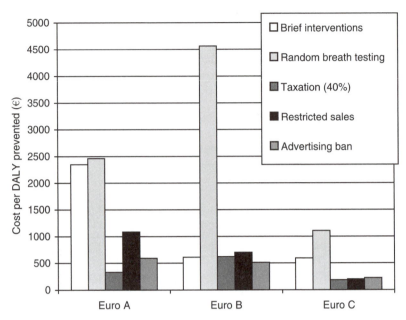

Figure 11.7 Cost-effectiveness of different policy options (€ per DALY prevented)

Source: Anderson and Baumberg (2006), adapted from Chisholm *et al.* (2004)

that strengthening alcohol policies is associated with reduced alcohol consumption (see Figure 11.10). Although European countries as a whole have been strengthening their alcohol policies, they lag behind the rest of the world in many regulatory areas, with the exception of measuring blood alcohol levels in drivers (see Figure 11.11).

In the EU, alcohol policy is influenced by the market's policies to encourage the free flow of goods, services, labour and capital across the national borders of the member states. Alcohol policy is determined by a balance of those articles which protect public health and those policies which relate to the free trade of products, taxation and agriculture.

Health protection

In the EC Treaty, articles which accord a protection of public health include Article 3, 'a contribution to the attainment of a high level of health protection'; Article 152, 'a high level of human health protection should be ensured in the definition and implementation of all Community policies and activities'; and Article 95, 'a high level of health protection in all legislative activities which have as their objective to establish and maintain the functioning of the internal market'.

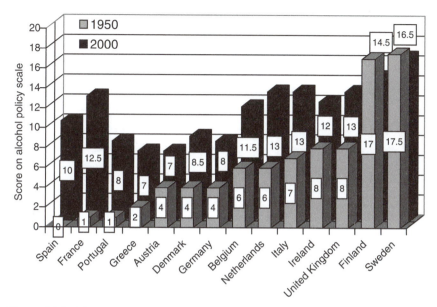

Figure 11.8 The strictness and comprehensiveness of alcohol control policies in 15 European countries, 1950 and 2000

Source: Österberg and Karlsson (2004)

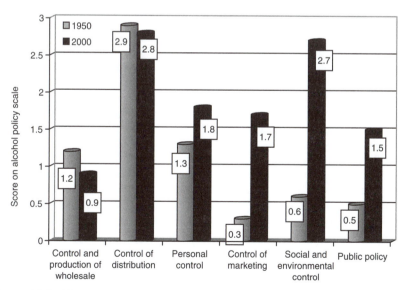

Figure 11.9 The strictness and comprehensiveness of alcohol control policies in the European Comparative Alcohol Study (ECAS) countries according to subgroups of alcohol control, 1950 and 2000

Source: Österberg and Karlsson (2004)

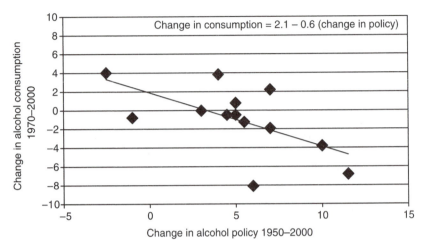

Figure 11.10   The relationship between change in alcohol policy 1950–2000 and the change in alcohol consumption (adjusted for changes in purchasing power) 1970–2000

Source: World Health Organization (2004c); Österberg and Karlsson (2004)

The European Court of Justice

Increasingly, the European Court of Justice has played an important role in shaping the approach to alcohol policy (Holder *et al.* 1998). In its case law, the Court has acknowledged that reducing the harm done by alcohol is a legitimate public health goal. In case C-189/95 (Franzen), the existence of the Swedish stated-owned alcohol monopoly was contested. In its conclusions, the Court stated that the purpose of Article 31 (ex 37) of the EC Treaty is to reconcile the possibility for member states to maintain certain monopolies of a commercial character as instruments for the pursuit of public interest aims with the requirements of the establishment and functioning of the common market. In case C-394/97 (Heinonen) the Court said that national legislation restricting imports of alcoholic drinks by travellers arriving from non-member countries in order to maintain public order is not, in principle, contrary to community law.

The French law, *Loi Evin*, bans direct or indirect television advertising for alcoholic beverages in France (Journal Officiel de la République Française 1991). In the infringement action (case C-262/02), the European Commission asked the Court to declare that the French rules are incompatible with the freedom to provide services guaranteed by the EC Treaty, on the ground that the *Loi Evin* creates obstacles to the retransmission in France of foreign sporting events. The reference for a preliminary ruling (case C-429/02) was based on the fact that Télévision Française TF1 requested Groupe Jean-Claude Darmon and Girosport, which was commissioned to negotiate on its behalf for television retransmission rights for football matches, to prevent the appearance on screen of brand names of alcoholic beverages. The Court stated that the French television advertising rules seek to protect public health and that they are appropriate to ensure that this objective is achieved. The rules restrict the situations in which advertising

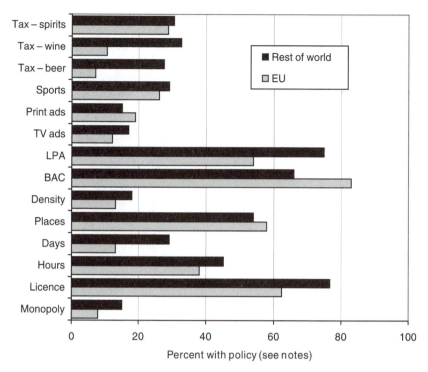

Figure 11.11   Proportion of EU countries with policy area, compared with the rest of the world

Notes:

Tax: % is for WHO 'high' tax band (> 30% of retail price for beer and wine; > 50% for spirits)

Sports: % is for legal restrictions (partial or complete) on beer sponsorship of sports events

Ads: % is for legal restrictions (partial or complete) for beer advertisements

LPA: % is for an on-premise minimum age of at least 18 for beer

BAC: % is for drink-driving limit (through blood alcohol concentration – BAC) of 50mg% or less

Density, places, days and hours: % is for off-premise restriction for any beverage

Source: World Health Organization (2004a)

hoardings for alcoholic beverages can be seen on television and, as a result, are likely to restrict the broadcasting of such advertisements, thereby reducing the occasions on which television viewers might be encouraged to consume alcoholic beverages.

Trade and alcohol policies

One of the core principles of trade agreements is that participating countries have to extend the best treatment that is afforded to domestic buyers and sellers equally to buyers and sellers from other countries. This ensures that internal tax and regulatory measures are applied equally to imported and domestic products so there is no protection for domestic production.

A central pillar of EC law is that quantitative restrictions or equivalents are not allowed. For alcohol, this has been seen most prominently in the *Cassis de Dijon* case (C-120/78). Germany refused to allow entry of French exports that did not meet German minimum alcohol content (to stop the proliferation of low-alcohol drinks in Germany), but this prohibition was overturned by the Court. Since then, the courts have interpreted this as meaning that any beverage that can be marketed in one EU state can also be marketed in the others.

The treatment of foreign and domestic goods on equal terms raises the question of what should be construed as 'like commodities'. The issue is whether beverages are 'like commodities', and thus need to be treated the same in terms of taxation, usually in terms of the equitability of the tax treatment of different imported and local alcoholic beverages. The European Court of Justice has dealt with this question several times as it relates to alcoholic beverages (Lubkin 1996). For example, the Court ruled that France's extra tax on grain-based (whisky) as opposed to grape-based (cognac) drinks was illegal (C-168/78). In other words, 'the tax policy of a member state must not crystallize existing consumer habits so as to be biased in favour of the competing national industries'. More recently, the Commission has sent a 'reasoned opinion' to Sweden to end tax discrimination against wine in comparison to beer (15/7/04). Currently, a litre of beer with 10 per cent alcohol by volume will bear 14.7 SEK in excise duties, whereas a litre of wine of exactly the same strength will be taxed at 22.08 SEK. The Commission argues that this violates Article 90 that forbids member states to impose higher taxes on products from other member states compared to competing domestic products.

Trade agreements also constrain the activities of state enterprises and monopolies. In the original European Community Treaty (Treaty of Rome, Article 31), it was agreed that monopolies can be maintained in the European common market as long as they are changed to fit the ideal of non-discrimination within Europe (Holder *et al.* 1998). The Manghera case at the European Court of Justice, which found that exclusive import rights are incompatible with the Treaty of Rome (C-59/75), ultimately led to Finland and Sweden abandoning their import, export, wholesale and production monopolies on joining the EU. What was left was a non-discriminatory off-licence retail monopoly. Nevertheless, it took the Gundersen (E-1/97) and Franzen (C-189/95) cases for the European Court of Justice to show that retail monopolies can be sustained. In one case, a shopkeeper applied for a licence and was turned down (Gundersen; for wine when beer was allowed), while in the other case, Franzen was prosecuted for actually selling wine in his store. The existence of the retail monopolies still cannot be assured however; as of July 2004 the Commission is taking Sweden to the Court for maintaining a ban on Swedish consumers using independent intermediaries to import alcoholic drinks for their private use into Sweden from other member states (even if they pay Swedish excise duties). The Commission considers that such an absolute ban imposed on all consumers is disproportionate and cannot be considered an integral part of the operation of the retail monopoly.

Alcohol taxes

There is great variation in alcohol excise levels across EU member states, with a zero tax on wine in six countries in southern and central Europe, and relatively high taxes in the United Kingdom, Ireland and the Nordic countries (Österberg and Karlsson 2004). This is the situation, despite the fact that the EU has made repeated attempts in the last 30 years to harmonize the alcohol taxes of its member states on the grounds that different taxes in member countries interfere with the efficient operation of the single market. In 1987 the Commission proposed that uniform alcohol excise duties should be adopted in all member states. In 1992, a target rate was adopted for distilled spirits and minimum rates for all alcoholic beverages. The minimum rate for wine was, however, set at zero. By accepting a wide divergence in taxes, the directive effectively puts pressure on high-tax jurisdictions to lower their alcohol excise duties, but does not pressure low-tax jurisdictions to raise them. A common structure for excise duties in the EU, adopted in 1993, also means that it is impossible to put a special tax on a beverage causing special harm. Beverages within each of the four alcoholic beverage categories – beer, wine, 'intermediate products' and spirits – have to be treated the same.

Since the harmonization of alcohol excise duties across the EU was not yet a reality, new proposals were made in 2001. Tax harmonization in the EU is a good example of the length of time these processes usually take. The EU also illustrates that once a topic is put on the agenda, the process has a tendency to proceed, however slowly. For instance, when the harmonization of alcohol excise duties seemed to be impossible through administrative decisions, the EU Commission tried to let market forces harmonize alcohol excise duties by increasing the rights of travellers to take alcoholic beverages across borders within the EU, thereby putting pressure on countries with higher-tax neighbours to lower their excise duty levels. As a general rule, EU citizens are allowed to take with them 10 litres of spirits, 20 litres of intermediate products, 90 litres of wine and 110 litres of beer from other EU member countries without paying tax on them when entering their home country.

When market forces put pressure on neighbouring countries to harmonize their alcohol excise duties in order to decrease the border trade in alcoholic beverages, taxes tend to gravitate towards the lowest levels of excise duties. For instance, to counter the effects of the low excise taxes in Germany, Denmark decreased excise duties on beer and wine by half in the early 1990s. As a consequence, Sweden decreased its excise duties on beer and wine to counter the pressure from Danish prices (Holder *et al.* 1998).

Currently, intra-EU transfers (mainly alcohol) are taxed in the purchase country for private use, or in the destination country if purchased for commercial use. The Commission, as of 2004, proposes that private users buying at distance (i.e. beverages transported on their behalf) should be taxed in the acquisition country and that the 'indicative' limits should be abolished.

Agriculture

Wine production has a special position as a part of the Common Agricultural Policy in the EU (Österberg and Karlsson 2004). Wine has made, and indeed still makes, a considerable contribution to the value of agricultural output in several EU member states. For instance, in the late 1990s the value of the output of wine accounted for about 17 per cent of the value of the total agricultural output in Portugal, about 14 per cent in France, about 10 per cent in Italy, about 7 per cent in Luxembourg, about 6 per cent in Austria and about 5 per cent in Spain. In many EU member states the wine-growing sector also appears to play a very important part in agricultural activity and the economy at certain regional and local levels. In many southern European regions wine production covers as much as 20 or even 30 per cent of the value of total agricultural output.

Despite the decrease in wine production inside the EU, the vineyards of the EU member states still account for approximately 45 per cent of the areas of vines in the world, and the EU member states produce about 60 per cent of all wine globally. Furthermore, the EU member states account for almost 60 per cent of global wine consumption.

For the year 2002 as much as €44,505 million was allocated to agricultural support from the EU budget. This was 45.2 per cent of the EU budget. In the market year 2001/2 altogether €1392 million was budgeted for the wine sector, half of this for production measures and a third for the restructuring measures.

The common market organization of the EU in the wine sector dates back to the early 1960s. This organization has been adapted to gradually allow the wine sector to respond to changes in production techniques and market trends in an attempt to reach a balance between wine supply and demand. The basic aims of the common wine policy have been to secure the survival of small family wine farms and to ensure a fair standard of living to wine farmers as well as to guarantee the supply of wine to consumers at reasonable prices. The common market organization for wine has been among the most complex and broadest within the Common Agricultural Policy. In addition to the traditional measures within the Common Agricultural Policy it has also covered other more technical matters which are specific to the wine sector only.

The Uruguay Round Agreement, which is one of the General Agreement on Tariffs and Trade (GATT) treaties, came into force on 1 July 1995, and radically changed the EU's trading system for wine, making it possible to import into the EU low-priced wine from third countries. Before July 1995, wine produced in the EU member states was protected by a minimum price for imported wine and the enforcement of customs duties, and, if necessary, the introduction of compensatory taxes.

The regulation establishing a new common organization for the wine market was adopted by the Agricultural Council as part of the Agenda 2000 reform on 17 May 1999, and it came into force on 1 August 2000 (Council regulation 1493/1999). The aim of the reform was to improve competitiveness and make full use of the new opportunities in the world market. In order to achieve these aims production is being directed from table wines to quality wines by compensating for the income losses and material costs caused by the change in the grape varieties as well as supporting the relocation of old vineyards and the development of production methods. In 1999 the Community contributed for the first time to the financing of wine sales promotion campaigns directed at third countries under Council regulation 2702/1999. The EU covered 60 per cent of the costs of the campaigns, and the Community funds granted for this purpose total a little under €3 million to be used within three years.

Thus far, many alcohol control measures, such as minimum age limits, public information campaigns, school-based alcohol education programmes and setting blood alcohol limits for driving have not been affected by international trade or common market agreements, although this may change with current discussions on a services agreement. The Commission is proposing to allow free movement of services, with general derogations allowed for services that are prohibited on the grounds of public health and temporary derogations if public health and protection of minors requires it (COM (2004/2001)).

Conclusions

Although alcohol consumption and alcohol-related harm are decreasing in Europe, they remain the highest in the world, and are at risk of increasing if economic growth increases. Alcohol is responsible for over 9 per cent of the total burden of ill health and premature death, and for a significant proportion of health inequalities within countries. Alcohol's social cost is an enormous drain on socioeconomic development and Europe's overall competitiveness.

For the individual, alcohol increases the risk of a wide range of harms in a dose-dependent manner. This is offset by a reduction in risk of coronary heart disease, although the exact size of the reduction is still disputed. Up to the age of 35, there is no level of alcohol consumption that is free of risk. After the age of 65, moderate drinking, defined as up to 10g of alcohol a day, might be risk-free in terms of overall mortality.

For societies, the more alcohol is consumed, the greater the harm. Reducing alcohol consumption for all European countries will bring health and economic benefits.

There are a wide range of alcohol policies available that are cost-effective, and which have a considerable impact in reducing the ill health and premature death caused by alcohol. Although alcohol policies have been strengthened over the last 50 years, compared to the rest of the world, Europe still lags behind, particularly in terms of regulatory and taxation policies. Countries that strengthen their alcohol policies are those that have had the largest reductions in alcohol consumption. Maintaining the status quo is inadequate as this is currently associated with increasing alcohol consumption.

Alcohol policy in Europe is a balance between policies designed to protect and promote public health and policies designed to serve European economic interests, particularly those related to trade and agriculture. At present, the balance appears to be in favour of trade. In the long run, if this balance is not corrected, it is likely to be to the detriment of the well-being of European citizens, as well as the socioeconomic development of the European region as a whole.

References

Academy of Medical Sciences (2004) *Calling Time: The Nation's Drinking as a Major Public Health Issue*, www.acmedsci.ac.uk.

Anderson, P. (2003) The risk of alcohol. Ph.D. thesis. Nijmegen: Radboud University.

Anderson, P. and Baumberg, B. (2006) *Alcohol in Europe*. London: Institute of Alcohol Studies.

Babor, T.F., Caetano, R., Casswell, S., Edwards, G. *et al.* (2003) *Alcohol: No Ordinary Commodity. Research and Public Policy*. Oxford: Oxford University Press.

Baltussen, R., Adam, T., Tan Torres, T., Hutubessy, R., Acharya, A., Evans, D.B. and Murray, C.J.L. (2004) *Generalized Cost-effectiveness Analysis: A Guide*. Geneva: World Health Organization.

Barefoot, J.C., Grønbæk, M., Feaganes, J.R., McPherson, R.S., Williams, R.B. and Siegle, I.C. (2002) Alcoholic beverage preference, diet, and health habits in the UNC Alumni Heart Study, *American Journal of Clinical Nutrition*, 76(2): 466–72.

Baum-Baicker, C. (1987) The psychological benefits of moderate alcohol consumption: a review of the literature, *Drug and Alcohol Dependence*, 15(4): 305–22.

Brown, S.A., Goldman, M.S., Inn, A. and Anderson, L.R. (1980) Expectations of reinforcement from alcohol: their domain and relation to drinking patterns, *Journal of Consulting & Clinical Psychology*, 48(4): 419–26.

Bruun, K., Edwards, G., Lumio, M., Mäkelä, K. *et al.* (1975) *Alcohol Control Policies in Public Health Perspective*. Helsinki: Finnish Foundation for Alcohol Studies.

Bushman, B.J. (1997) Effects of alcohol on human aggression: validity of proposed mechanisms, in M. Galanter (ed.) *Recent Developments in Alcoholism*, Vol. 13, *Alcohol and Violence*. New York: Plenum Press.

Caetano, R. and Cunradi, C. (2002) Alcohol dependence: a public health perspective, *Addiction*, 97(6): 633–45.

Chisholm, D., Rehm, J., Van Ommeren, M. and Monteiro, M. (2004) Reducing the global burden of hazardous alcohol use: a comparative cost-effectiveness analysis, *Journal of Studies in Alcohol*, 65(6): 782–93.

Collaborative Group on Hormonal Factors in Breast Cancer (2002) Alcohol, tobacco and breast cancer–collaborative reanalysis of individual data from 53 epidemiological studies, including 58,515 women with breast cancer and 95,067 women without the disease, *British Journal of Cancer*, 87(11): 1234–45.

Corrao, G., Rubbiati, L., Bagnardi, V., Zambon, A. and Poikolainen, K. (2000) Alcohol and coronary heart disease: a meta-analysis, *Addiction*, 95(10): 1505–23.

Darkes, J. and Goldman, M.S. (1993) Expectancy challenge and drinking reduction: experimental evidence for a mediational process, *Journal of Consulting & Clinical Psychology*, 61(2): 344–53.

Edwards, G., Anderson, P., Babor, T.F., Casswell, S. *et al.* (1994) *Alcohol Policy and the Public Good*. New York: Oxford University Press.

Fillmore, K.M, Golding, J.M., Graves, K.L., Kniep, S. *et al.* (1998a) Alcohol consumption and mortality: I. Characteristics of drinking groups, *Addiction*, 93(2): 183–203.

Fillmore, K.M., Golding, J.M., Graves, K.L., Kniep, S. *et al.* (1998b) Alcohol consumption and mortality: III. Studies of female populations, *Addiction*, 93(2): 219–29.

Fuchs, F.D., Chambless, L.E., Folsom, A.R., Eigenbrodt, M.L. *et al.* (2004) Association between alcoholic beverage consumption and incidence of coronary heart disease in whites and blacks – the Atherosclerosis Risk in Communities Study, *American Journal of Epidemiology*, 160(5): 466–74.

Gorinstein, S., Caspi, A., Goshev, I., Asku, S. *et al.* (2003) Structural changes in plasma ciculating fibrinogen after moderate beer consumption as determined by electrophoresis and spectroscopy, *Journal of Agricultural and Food Chemistry*, 51(3): 822–7.

Greenfield, T.K., Rehm, J. and Rodgers, J.D. (2002) Effects of depression and social integration on the relationship between alcohol consumption and all-cause mortality, *Addiction*, 97(1): 29–38.

Hart, C.L., Smith, G.D., Hole, D.J. and Hawthorne, V.M. (1999) Alcohol consumption and mortality from all causes, coronary heart disease and stroke: results from a prospective cohort study of Scottish men with 21 years of follow-up, *British Medical Journal*, 318: 1725–9.

Heather, N. (2001) Pleasures and pains of our favourite drug, in N. Heather, T.J. Peters and T. Stockwell (eds) *International Handbook of Alcohol Dependence and Problems*. Chichester: Wiley.

Hemström, Ö. (2001) The contribution of alcohol to socioeconomic differentials in mortality – the case of Sweden, in T. Norström (ed.) *Consumption, Drinking Patterns, Consequences and Policy Responses in 15 European Countries*. Stockholm: National Institute of Pubic Health.

Holder, H.D., Kühlhorn, E., Nordlund, S., Österberg, E. *et al.* (1998) *European Integration and Nordic Alcohol Policies: Changes in Alcohol Controls and Consequences in Finland, Norway and Sweden, 1980–1997*. Aldershot: Ashgate.

Journal Officiel de la République Française (1991) *Loi Evin* (Article L 3323).

Kessler, R.C., Nelson, C.B., Mcgonagle, K.A., Delund, M.J. *et al.* (1996) Epidemiology of co-occurring addictive and mental disorders: implications for prevention and service utilization, *American Journal of Orthopsychiatry*, 66(1): 17–31.

Klatsky, A.L. (1999) Moderate drinking and reduced risk of heart disease, *Alcohol Research and Health*, 23(1): 15–22.

Leino, E.V., Romelsjo, A., Shoemaker, C., Ager, C.R. *et al.* (1998) Alcohol consumption and mortality: II. Studies of male populations, *Addiction*, 93(2): 205–18.

Lemmens, P.H. (2001) Relationship of alcohol consumption and alcohol problems at the population level, in N. Heather, T.J. Peters and T. Stockwell (eds) *International Handbook of Alcohol Dependence and Problems*. Chichester: Wiley.

Lubkin, G. (1996) *Is Europe's Glass Half-full or Half-empty? The Taxation of Alcohol and the Development of a European Identity*. Jean Monnet Center, Working Paper 96/7. Cambridge, MA: Harvard University.

Mäkelä, K. (1970) Dryckegångernas frekvens enligt de konsumerade drykerna och mängden före och efter lagreformen [The frequency of drinking occasions according to type of beverage and amount consumed before and after the new alcohol law], *Alkoholpolitik*, 33: 144–53.

Mäkelä, P. (2002) Whose drinking does a liberalization of alcohol policy increase? Change in alcohol consumption by the initial level in the Finnish panel survey in 1968 and 1969, *Addiction*, 97(6): 701–6.

McKee, M. and Sholnikov, V. (2001) Understanding the toll of premature death among men in eastern Europe, *British Medical Journal*, 323: 1051–5.

McKee, M., Sholnikov, V. and Leon, D.A. (2001) Alcohol is implicated in the fluctuations in cardiovascular disease in Russia since the 1980s, *Annals of Epidemiology*, 11(1): 1–6.

McKenzie, C. and Eisenberg, P.R. (1996) Alcohol, coagulation, and arterial thrombosis, in S. Zakhari and M. Wassef (eds) *Alcohol and the Cardiovascular System*. Bethesda, MD: National Institutes of Health, National Institute on Alcohol Abuse and Alcoholism.

Murray, C.J.L., Evans, D.B., Acharya, A. and Baltussen, R.M.P.M. (2004) *Development of WHO Guidelines on Generalised Cost-Effectiveness Analysis*. Geneva: World Health Organization.

Norström, T. (2001) *Consumption, Drinking Patterns, Consequences and Policy Responses in 15 European Countries*. Stockholm: National Institute of Public Health.

Österberg, E. and Karlsson, T. (eds) (2004) *Alcohol Policies in EU Member States and Norway: A Collection of Country Reports*. Helsinki: STAKES.

Peele, S. and Grant, M. (eds) (1999) *Alcohol and Pleasure: A Health Perspective*. Washington, DC: International Center for Alcohol Policies.

Pliner, P. and Cappell, H. (1974) Modification of affective consequences of alcohol: a comparison of solitary and social drinking, *Journal of Abnormal Psychology*, 83(4): 418–25.

Ramstedt, M. (2001) Per capita alcohol consumption and liver cirrhosis mortality in 14 European countries, *Addiction*, 96, Supplement 1, S19–34.

Reeder, V.C., Aikens, M.L., Li, X.-N. and Booyse, F.M. (1996) Alcohol and the fibrinolytic system, in S. Zakhari and M. Wassef (eds) *Alcohol and the Cardiovascular System*. Bethesda, MD: National Institutes of Health, National Institute on Alcohol Abuse and Alcoholism.

Regier, D.A., Farmer, M.E., Rae, D.S., Locke, B.Z. *et al.* (1990) Comorbidity of mental disorders with alcohol and other drug abuse: results from the Epidemiologic Catchment Area (ECA) study, *Journal of the American Medical Association*, 264(9): 2511–18.

Rehm, J., Room, R., Monteiro, M., Gmel, G. *et al.* (2003) Alcohol as a risk factor for global burden of disease, *European Addiction Research*, 9(4): 157–64.

Rehm, J., Room, R., Monteiro, M., Gmel, G. *et al.* (2004) Alcohol, in WHO (ed.) *Comparative Quantification of Health Risks: Global and Regional Burden of Disease Due to Selected Major Risk Factors*. Geneva: WHO.

Rehn, N., Room, R. and Edwards, G. (2001) *Alcohol in the European Region – Consumption, Harm and Policies*. Copenhagen: World Health Organization Regional Office for Europe.

Rodgers, B., Korten, A.E., Jorm, A.F., Christensen, H., Henderson, S. and Jacomb, P.A. (2000) Risk factors for depression and anxiety in abstainers, moderate drinkers and heavy drinkers, *Addiction*, 95(12): 1833–45.

Sierksma, A. (2003) Moderate alcohol consumption and vascular health, Ph.D. thesis, Utrecht University.

Skog, O-J. (1991) Drinking and the distribution of alcohol consumption, in D.J. Pittman and H. Raskin (eds) *White Society, Culture, and Drinking Patterns Reexamined*. New Brunswick, NJ: Alcohol Research Documentation.

Skog, O-J. (1996) Public health consequences of the J-curve hypothesis of alcohol problems, *Addiction*, 91(3): 325–37.

Szucs, S., Sarvary, A., McKee, M. and Adany, R. (2005) Could the high level of cirrhosis in central and eastern Europe be due partly to the quality of alcohol consumed? An exploratory investigation, *Addiction*, 100(4): 536–42.

Thom, B. (2001) A social and political history of alcohol, in N. Heather, T.J. Peters and T. Stockwell (eds) *International Handbook of Alcohol Dependence and Problems*. Chichester: Wiley.

Thun, M., Peto, R., Lopez, A.D., Monaco, J. *et al.* (1997) Alcohol consumption and mortality among middle-aged and elderly US adults, *New England Journal of Medicine*, 337: 1705–14.

Wannamethee, S.G. and Shaper, A.G. (1999) Type of alcoholic drink and risk of major coronary heart disease events and all-cause mortality, *American Journal of Public Health*, 89(5): 685–90.

White, I.R., Altmann, D.R. and Nanchahal, K. (2002) Alcohol consumption and mortality: modelling risks for men and women at different ages, *British Medical Journal*, 325: 191–8.

World Health Organization (1992) *The ICD-10 Classification of Mental and Behavioural Disorders: Clinical Descriptions and Diagnostic Guidelines*. Geneva: World Health Organization.

World Health Organization (2002a) *The World Health Report 2002 – Reducing Risks, Promoting Healthy Life*. Geneva: World Health Organization.

World Health Organization (2002b) *The World Mental Health (WMH2000) Initiative.* Geneva: Assessment, Classification, and Epidemiology Group, WHO.

World Health Organization (2004a) *Global Status Report on Alcohol Policy.* Geneva: World Health Organization.

World Health Organization (2004b) *WHO-CHOICE Cost-effectiveness Analyses.* Geneva: World Health Organization.

World Health Organization (2004c) *Health for all Database.* Copenhagen: World Health Organization Regional Office for Europe.

chapter twelve

Housing and employment

Robert Anderson, Richard Wynne and David McDaid

This chapter focuses on measures to address the housing and employment difficulties of people with mental health disorders; little attention is paid to a lack of housing or unemployment problems as causes of mental ill health. Given the main themes, the chapter primarily deals with adults of working age (18–64), even though housing and homelessness problems also affect younger and older age groups. We will assess research, policy and practice where the key population is adults with mental disorders but not those whose primary problems relate to substance abuse, dementia or learning disabilities. Similarly, lessons from research and practice dealing with general problems of unemployment and homelessness are not drawn upon except where adults with mental illnesses are a main target group.

The populations of people with mental illness in different research studies are themselves very different – reflecting not only the diversity of mental health problems, but also the diversity of experiences, circumstances and requirements of people with complex and often multiple needs. European policy perspectives on the situation of people with multi-faceted and interlinked disadvantages are often framed in terms of the risk and experience of 'social exclusion' (European Commission 2003d). People with mental illness may be caught in a cycle of deprivation (Social Exclusion Unit 2004) – a downward spiral of ill health, poverty, family breakdown, unemployment and homelessness. Discrimination can seriously impair the ability of people with mental illness to maintain housing or employment (Public Health Alliance Ireland 2004). Poor housing and homelessness may exacerbate illness, making it difficult to gain access to adequate housing, employment and even health care in the future. However, the availability of adequate housing is evidently a key element in any strategy to provide care and support in the community.

The vast majority of people with mental illness are living in the community, and therefore are in need of a place to live, opportunities to work and adequate conditions for developing and maintaining social relationships. However, many of those with mental illness are disadvantaged in several respects and the

European Commission's report on social inclusion (European Commission 2003d) highlights the situation of people with mental illness in the new member states. In these countries, for example, it appears that those with mental health problems are among the most likely to live below the poverty line, to receive inadequate social benefits and to be isolated from the workplace (European Commission 2003a). There is a lack of measures in place to combat this deprivation and although, for example, new European Union (EU) initiatives to combat discrimination will address employment, neither EU measures nor national legislation, particularly in the new member states, adequately tackle discrimination in access to housing (European Commission 2003b).

The plans of the new member states to combat social exclusion (Joint Inclusion Memoranda) all refer to improving the situation of people with disabilities, but there are few, if any, references specifically to people with mental illness. Only a few of these countries (e.g. Malta and Slovenia) report special attention being given to the housing needs of disabled persons and people with mental health problems. This 'invisibility' of people with mental illness is also reflected in policy documents which have adopted a mainstreaming approach to disability, shifting away from disability-specific programmes (e.g. European Commission 2003c).

The EU's strategy to combat social exclusion has consistently put employment at its centre and in recent years has also emphasized access for all to decent and sanitary housing. Of course, employment and housing are linked – access to housing is fundamental to enabling people to take up job opportunities – and, for example, the support needs of many homeless people can make labour market reintegration inappropriate.

The *Joint Report on Social Inclusion* (European Commission 2003d) calls for the development of a truly multidimensional approach to meet the needs of disadvantaged groups, and echoes demands for more integrated approaches to tackling homelessness (Edgar *et al.* 2002) and unemployment (Pillinger 2001). The *Social Inclusion* report gives a new prominence to increasing access to services for people with mental illness; although deinstitutionalization has been a common feature of the last two decades and more in the EU, the availability and quality of support services has been very variable (Quilgars 1998; Freyhoff *et al.* 2004). Much of the rest of this chapter will be concerned with emphasizing and illustrating how community-based care services for people with mental illness must be developed and coordinated with other sectors such as housing and employment.

Policy and professional perspectives

The Council of Ministers at Nice in 2002 urged policy-makers and service providers to adapt to the needs of people suffering from social exclusion and to ensure that front-line staff would be sensitive to these needs (European Council 2003). However, housing and employment have often been seen, if at all, as marginal to the objectives of health and care services, with a lack of clear responsibilities for vocational and housing outcomes. Fakhoury *et al.* (2002)

argue that, historically, mental health services have distanced themselves from housing which they considered more as a 'social care' than a 'treatment' issue, while Watson and Tarpey (1998) identify a change, in the United Kingdom at least, in the early 1990s when the significance of housing became more fully recognized by policy-makers. In the United States, too, it seems that much mental health policy and practice has not considered housing as a key component of the system of mental health care (Newman 2001).

In recent years the concepts and language of partnership, coordination, localism and services tailored to individual needs have set the strategic directions for service reform. However, translating these concepts into practice has been a major challenge (EFILWC 2003). Partnerships between public authorities, health and other service providers have been slow to form, in part because of a lack of administrative and financial structures to integrate services (European Commission 2003d). The report of the Social Exclusion Unit in the United Kingdom (2004) underlines the continuing need to reinforce working together by government departments and agencies but a lack of resources is an obvious barrier to the development of more comprehensive and integrated services. Quilgars (1998, 2000) also points to the tendency for health and social services to concentrate on the provision of crisis, high-need interventions while housing providers may not have the capacity to provide housing-related services to people with mental illness living unsupported in ordinary housing.

There appears to be a lack of focus among policy-makers in the housing and employment fields, who have paid relatively little attention to the specific needs of people with mental illness. Recognition of the significance of ill health as a key factor in exclusion from employment has grown only recently at European level, particularly in initiatives to promote employment activity rates of people receiving disability benefits and measures to extend working life. In many countries traditional practices have sought to promote the protection of people with disabilities rather than active measures to combat discrimination or other obstacles to employment.

People with mental illnesses may experience stigma and discrimination from providers in housing and employment services (ONS 2000). They may be viewed as difficult clients, as unreliable due to health crises or hospital admissions and as unpredictable tenants. Clearly, the attitudes of professional workers in different sectors are key to the social integration of people with mental illness, but the values and beliefs of the most marginalized groups may often be markedly different from those of people in established medical and social organizations (SMES-Europa 2002), or in housing and employment sectors. Clients, for example, may prefer more independent living arrangements and privacy while staff prefer more structured environments; there may be tensions between moves to greater user control and flexibility and the administrative or managerial needs of service providers (Pillinger 2001).

Housing

Over the last decades policies to support people with mental illness have increasingly been oriented to life in the community, outside long-stay institutions, and to a life lived as independently as possible. This has led to the provision of various forms of housing, with or without support, as well as efforts to maintain within or return people to the family home. The challenge for people with mental health problems is illustrated in a recent survey report by the National Disability Authority in Ireland, quoted by the Public Health Alliance Ireland (2004). This survey found that only 30 per cent of respondents were fully comfortable with people who have mental health difficulties living in their neighbourhood, compared with 49 per cent for people with intellectual difficulties and 53 per cent for people with physical disabilities. Perhaps it is not surprising then that many people with severe mental illness are concentrated in deprived areas, often in inner cities, where they themselves fear harassment or intimidation (Sainsbury Centre for Mental Health 1998; SMES-Europa 2002).

Three main housing measures are examined below: retention of accommodation in the individual or family home; reintegration within the community through supported/sheltered accommodation in hostels, group homes, or supported tenancies; and responses to homelessness.

Housing as an issue

There is a profound lack of systematic information on the housing situation, problems and preferences of people with mental illness, and no existing European overview. Clearly any description of the housing situation must specify the population covered as the needs of people at different stages in the life cycle or with different severities of health problems correspondingly will be very different. So, too, the responses to housing needs will vary enormously across the EU, reflecting not only variations in resources and policy priorities for people with mental illness, but also the marked country differences in the structures of housing ownership. The availability of public sector or rented housing varies by a factor of 20 or more across the EU and equally there are major differences in the standards of private accommodation (EFILWC 2004). In general, there is a lack of good housing in the new member states and shortages of quality social housing in particular (European Commission 2004).

The housing situation of people with mental illness, to some extent, will reflect national differences in tenure and housing quality. Most people with mental illness are living in the community and in mainstream housing even if exact data are missing (Newman 2001; Social Exclusion Unit 2004). However, their housing situation may be vulnerable (Edgar *et al.* 2002) because of low income and a lack of affordable accommodation, discrimination, family breakdown and specific needs.

One survey in the United Kingdom (Office for National Statistics 2002) provides a detailed analysis of the circumstances of adults aged 16–74 with disorders such as neurosis, psychosis and alcohol and drug dependency. People with these disorders were more likely than the general population to be single, divorced or separated, and more likely to be living alone. More of those with mental health problems were living in rented accommodation and among people with 'probable psychosis' half were living in accommodation rented from a local authority or housing association. People with mental disorders experienced higher rates of unemployment and absence from work due to illness, and were more likely to fall into arrears with payment of rent and utilities. Altogether, the population with mental health problems were more likely than the general population to express dissatisfaction with their accommodation, to mention specific housing problems and to describe the state of repair of their accommodation as 'poor'. On the other hand, the main problems encountered were much the same for people with and without mental health disorders – financial difficulties; short-term leases; domestic problems; and problems with the landlord or estate agent.

People with mental illness face the same set of housing issues as other groups in the community – availability, adequacy, appropriateness and affordability. However, their situation may be especially insecure or precarious, and access to adequate, affordable housing may be especially critical to recovery from illness and to maintaining good mental health (Mental Health Commission 1999). Several research studies have demonstrated that living in poor quality or inappropriate housing increases risks of deterioration in functioning, reduced quality of life and readmission to hospital (Fakhoury *et al.* 2002). Housing costs may exacerbate other financial stresses, associated, for example, with paying for treatment, and may lead to overcrowding, inability to heat or maintain a property and unsustainable tenure.

Most people with mental illness do not suffer loss of housing due to their illness but some do, and the most important reason appears to be hospitalization for an acute episode (Mental Health Commission 1999). Severe mental illness is associated with homelessness, but this can reflect both becoming homeless due to ill health and becoming ill due to homelessness. Although there are narrower and broader definitions of 'homelessness', one review reports that between 30 and 50 per cent of people sleeping in night shelters, in hostels or on the street have some form of severe mental disorder (Sainsbury Centre for Mental Health 1998). A recent study in Cork, Ireland, reported that 40 per cent of hostel dwellers had a serious mental illness (Public Health Alliance, Ireland 2004). Homelessness is a major problem especially for those who do not engage with mental health services, and the development of sensitive strategies to reach these groups is part of a more integrated approach to their housing problems.

People with housing problems and mental illness have complex needs demanding a variety of responses. In many cases recovery requires specific housing arrangements that combine support for everyday living (including perhaps support in employment) with quality accommodation and a suitable social environment. The development of appropriate community-based housing and services is considered shortly but the next section begins by examining approaches to 'prevent' housing problems.

Maintenance in mainstream housing

The goal of retaining people with mental illness in their own homes and avoiding housing problems would appear to be very attractive. In most EU countries this is regarded as the preferred approach (Edgar *et al.* 2000) but it has received relatively little policy attention. When the Cochrane Library (Chilvers *et al.* 2003) sought to establish the value of regular visits by professional outreach workers to people with severe mental disorders living in 'ordinary' private or rented accommodation they were unable to identify any acceptable randomized or quasi-randomized trials. Likewise, the Centre for Housing Policy in York (England) reports (Quilgars 2000) that there has been little consideration of the value of low intensity services to enable people to live independently in ordinary housing. However, these critiques are to some extent research problems as a range of authorities have been developing more and less intensive support schemes, 'tenancy sustainment services', 'community resettlement teams' or other forms of support in housing – albeit many appear to be local initiatives.

Watson *et al.* (2003) have examined the planning and development of the United Kingdom's 'Supporting People' initiative between 1998 and 2003. This initiative commenced in April 2003 with the aim of providing housing related support to vulnerable tenants and households, specifically including people with mental health problems. This support involves helping individuals to obtain suitable accommodation, to sustain their accommodation and to develop skills and self-confidence as required. Local authorities, housing associations, health bodies and voluntary agencies contribute as strategic partners in developing and providing services. A wide range of services is funded by Supporting People including: community-based advice centres (mediation and dispute resolution, form-filling and benefit entitlement); visiting people at risk of homelessness; and drop-in centre support to combat isolation.

The identification and involvement of people at risk of exclusion or housing difficulties is a major issue, with an important role for primary care personnel in referral – assuming housing difficulties are seen as relevant. Supportive or 'benevolent' landlords can also make an important contribution, working in a public/private sector partnership with local agencies. In one example, the landlord agrees to provide and maintain accommodation in return for rent guarantees and management of support (Watson *et al.* 2003); there are examples where this has worked well for people with long-term mental health problems. In New Zealand (Mental Health Commission 1999), the 'benevolent' landlord concept entails the owner or primary tenant of a dwelling providing advice, security, materials and services; however, there was concern about whether the funding of such schemes should be a health or housing sector responsibility.

Support to people living in their own private accommodation has attracted less attention than the experience of people in rented accommodation (Social Exclusion Unit 2004). There are, of course, specific issues about finding a mortgage and insurance cover, as well as dealing with mortgage arrears. In the new member states very many people are owner-occupiers but the issue is about funds to maintain and repair properties (EFILWC 2004). In some cases there may be issues about charging for or means-testing support services to people who own their own homes – and some such owner-occupiers may be reluctant or concerned about the stigma of being drawn into the support 'system' (Watson *et al.* 2003).

Ill health or long periods in care may diminish the individual's capacity for self-care or application of basic skills for living independently. Support may be required to develop skills in shopping and budgeting, paying rent and bills on time, cooking, hygiene and clothing – or services will need to manage this provision. In her review of low-intensity support services Quilgars (2000) identifies such direct practical support as one of three main types alongside support to move into accommodation and sustain tenancies and emotional or social support, including home visiting, befriending and telephone support services. Although this review of the literature again highlights deficiencies in the research evidence, a number of substantively important messages were reported including: how the way in which a service is delivered (timing, attitudes of staff) influences the likelihood of a tenancy being successful; users consistently valued the support of a worker or volunteer, often in preference to more formal service interventions; and there was limited success in increasing users' social networks and activities. On the whole, whatever the specific caveats, users felt that these low-intensity support services helped them to approach life in a more positive way but it was difficult to establish the extent to which the services prevented tenancies breaking down.

In one other detailed review (Newman 2001) of the relationship between housing and mental illness – and notwithstanding the research and methodological problems – the strongest finding was that living in independent housing was associated with greater satisfaction with accommodation and the neighbourhood.

Accommodation in supported housing

In the messy world of real services, equivocal conclusions about the effectiveness of different interventions are the norm. It is rare to enjoy the luxury of randomized controlled trials, and the situation of client groups involves too many complex factors to isolate the evaluation of one element of an intervention. It is also often difficult to specify what exactly the constituents of the intervention are. 'Supported housing' is an example of this dilemma as its conceptualization and the corresponding diversity of service provision is so broad (Fakhoury et al. 2002); the inconsistent use of terminology makes it almost impossible to compare schemes, processes and outcomes.

A recent review of supported housing (Rog 2004) defined it broadly as independent housing in the community that is coupled with the provision of community mental health and support services. At low intensity levels of support this blurs the distinction with the previous discussion of supported tenancies. At medium and high levels of support the distinction is clearer, as the availability of professional support increases from being on call, to being on site, to being available on site at all hours. Perhaps the most useful distinction between support 'in (mainstream) housing' and 'supported housing' lies with the ownership and control of the accommodation. Most supported housing is run by the organizations (public, private and voluntary) or services providing or managing the support to people with mental illness. The dwellings range from larger, more institutional hostels or group homes to small, shared or self-contained units; and provision is evolving in the latter direction.

The supported accommodation offered by the Estuar Foundation in Bucharest comprises four ordinary flats in different areas of the city. Each of the flats can accommodate three tenants, all of whom have individual bedrooms with their own keys. The flats have been fully furnished by Estuar to create a normal domestic environment. The tenants have mental health problems and are supported by trained workers who help with social activities and domestic tasks, and offer counselling to develop coping skills. The tenants are permanently supported in their learning processes and in their efforts to manage everyday life (Freyhoff *et al.* 2004).

In many EU countries, public policies have strongly supported the development of supported housing, leading to a significant change in the amount, type and range of housing support options. The European Commission's *Joint Report on Social Inclusion* (2003d) highlights developments in Denmark, France, Germany, the Netherlands, Sweden and the United Kingdom, although there also appears to be a concentration of such options in urban areas (Edgar *et al.* 2002) or in the big cities in new member states (European Commission 2004). Fakhoury *et al.* (2002) report that in Berlin the number of places for mentally ill people in supported housing rose threefold in the 1990s, and in the United Kingdom numbers in supported housing appear to have increased 'enormously' (Priebe and Turner 2003), although precise data on numbers and duration are largely not available.

New Zealand's Mental Health Commission assessed the need for supported housing as being relatively low (6–7 per cent) among the whole population of users of mental health services; but the numbers appear to be increasing in Europe. In a review of both European and non-European experience – and acknowledging the limited level of research – it seems that residents in supported housing are likely to be older, less educated and unemployed compared with those living in independent or semi-supervised settings; they are more likely to include people with schizophrenia but less likely to include people with behavioural problems including violence and antisocial behaviour (Fakhoury *et al.* 2002).

The benefits of supported housing were identified by Middleboe (1997) for a group of long-term mentally ill people in group homes in Copenhagen. Over a period of a year, 83 per cent of individuals remained in the programme and showed a significant improvement across the dimensions of subjective quality of life, social integration and hospitalization. Fakhoury *et al.* (2002) likewise conclude that supported housing can improve functioning, facilitate social integration and offer a more satisfactory environment for residents than hospital care. It appears that most people prefer the more independent living arrangements and less restrictive regimes, and appreciate the privacy offered. Many reports refer to a lack of suitable supported housing in the community. However, concerns also have been voiced about the possible isolation and loneliness of more independent living, of risks of dependence on professional support (Chilvers *et al.* 2003), of reinstitutionalization (Priebe and Turner 2003), and of failure to promote independence over time, while others have pointed to the high costs and the need for a well trained workforce (Sainsbury Centre for Mental Health 1998).

Altogether, there is a lack of systematic information on the factors affecting the outcomes of supported housing and the necessary skills or resources for success. However, it has developed widely as a model both to prevent homelessness and to reintegrate those who have been excluded from community life.

Responses to homelessness

However 'homelessness' is defined (European Commission 2003d), mental health problems are prevalent among an important proportion of those without accommodation; and homelessness causes a set of other difficulties with, for example, access to health services, education or employment. It is a multi-dimensional problem. Measures to combat social exclusion emphasize the challenge to develop appropriate integrated responses both to prevent and address homelessness. However, housing supply is only part of the problem; discrimination and the letting practices of both public and private sector landlords can lead to exclusion (Edgar et al. 2002).

The risk of homelessness has been associated with deinstitutionalization and discharge from long-stay psychiatric hospitals, but it is also raised by hospital admission for acute episodes of mental illness. Altogether, homelessness is more likely among people with mental health problems for a variety of reasons including affordability, conflicts and unsafe living environments (Mental Health Commission 1999) – even among those in contact with mental health services. Of course, for many homeless persons the first challenge is to enable access to appropriate services. The SMES-Europa (2002) report offers a number of examples of initiatives to provide health and social care, often involving volunteers.

In Athens, a non-governmental humanitarian organization (Doctors without Borders) offers medical and social help to homeless people with psychosocial problems, drug addicts, alcohol addicts, refugees, immigrants and ex-prisoners. Paid employees comprise just a quarter of the staff, the remaining 75 per cent being professionals who volunteer their assistance (doctors, psychologists and social workers). Component services include psychological support and social care, a mobile unit and needle exchange programme. Users are recruited through self-demand as well as referral from social and health services and the police. The project collaborates with other similar projects to meet the multiple needs of these users (SMES-Europa 2002).

The need for interdisciplinary teams or more integrated services to meet complex and multiple needs has led to the introduction of a range of one-stop-shop type provision – for example, the services of housing officers, benefit staff, social workers, specialist mental health workers and voluntary organizations (Mental Health Commission 1999; Pillinger 2001). The engagement of homeless mentally ill people with services often takes time and perseverance, and demands that services go to where the homeless persons are – thus, the development of street-outreach services or mobile outreach teams.

Homeless people with mental illness are contacted in a range of accommodation settings from emergency and temporary hostels to long-term sheltered accommodation and supported housing. Emergency accommodation in hostels is available across Europe in urban areas and provides an essential safety net. In general, such hostels have beds immediately available, and impose no referral or treatment requirements. Many offer free assistance with clothing and provide a meal as well as access to laundry facilities. The large direct access hostel is still the prevalent model across the EU although SMES-Europa (2002) reports the development of smaller, more homely shelters as well as the emergence of specialized shelters for groups such as young people. The quality of emergency hostels is very variable, as are their financial and staff resources (Edgar *et al.* 2000). However, all member states describe efforts in place to improve emergency reception and temporary housing of homeless persons (European Commission 2003d).

In principle, emergency hostels are intended for a short length of stay, but there is a widespread lack of longer-term, safe and suitable move-on accommodation. Temporary housing in bed and breakfast accommodation is not very suitable, but the Social Exclusion Unit (2004) found that stays of five years and more were now common in temporary accommodation in London. Many homeless people with severe mental illness are in need of long-term shelter and rehabilitation, and emergency hostels are not well equipped to help with resettlement or longer-term health care. Developments in longer-term residential care embrace a wide range of care philosophies ranging from an explicit focus on treatment and rehabilitation to accommodation free of any specific therapeutic goal. Again, to take an example from the report of SMES-Europa (2002: 24) – the Lunghezza project in Rome:

> It provides care for homeless ex-psychiatric hospital patients. Twenty places are available in a number of apartments. It is part of a care and treatment programme of the Rome B Local Area Health Authority. Its users are patients suffering from serious and enduring mental illness, some of whom come from long-term stays in psychiatric hospitals or clinics and who have neither family support nor fixed abode. Other patients have come from difficult family situations.

Many such projects aim to help residents to develop skills to live more independently – time management, financial prudence, interpersonal skills – but move-on rates appear to be low. Nevertheless, they can provide a relatively secure environment although there may be a lack of meaningful daily activity.

Research on the effects of providing supported housing to formerly homeless people with serious and persistent mental illness indicates that long-term residential stability can be achieved for many (Lipton *et al.* 2000) and cognitive functioning can be improved (Seidman *et al.* 2003). In Lipton's study older age was associated with longer tenure and a history of substance abuse with shorter tenure; referrals from a state psychiatric centre had a higher risk of shorter tenure. Other research (e.g. Dickey *et al.* 1996) has underlined the housing disruption caused to formerly homeless people when they are admitted to psychiatric care.

Summing up

The housing needs of people with mental illness have been a relatively low priority of policies in both the mental health and housing fields. Increasing recognition of the importance of decent and stable housing and of the nature and scale of housing problems calls for the development of more defined policies and integrated approaches, as well as the provision of new services and facilities. Although such provision is widely regarded as under-resourced, particularly in view of decades of deinstitutionalization, this chapter has presented some positive initiatives and practices from EU member states. These examples demonstrate the importance of strategies for the prevention of housing problems and homelessness, but also of the need for health, social protection, employment or other daytime activity, and other services to provide comprehensive and coordinated support in the face of multi-faceted needs. At the same time, the responsibilities of different services must be clear and well defined (Pillinger 2001).

Housing policies are, and should be, principally concerned with the availability of permanent homes in both mainstream and supported developments (Social Exclusion Unit 2004); but there are needs for better temporary and rental accommodation, as well as important issues concerning the protection of tenure and improving the quality of accommodation. Housing quality in the enlarged Europe is a growing problem, especially in rural areas.

Various authors have argued for more choice and flexibility in housing provision for people with mental illness. Watson *et al.* (1998, 2003) have argued for more development of self-contained flats and networks of flats or houses, reflecting the need for some forms of purpose-designed housing and also the need to access support services. In general, there is a need to combat discrimination in access to housing and, in a complementary manner, to avoid segregation of people with mental illness, whether in mainstream housing or in supported accommodation – for example, for people who have been homeless. Perhaps, in new developments, consideration could be given to allocating one or two units to people who have been discharged from mental health services.

What do people with mental illness want or prefer for housing? For the vast majority it will be to live in their own home, with their family, without stigma or social isolation. Evidently, support in housing, if required, is the most attractive strategy for most people – and for their families who need support – to prevent the hospital admissions or loss of income or failure to manage a tenancy that precipitate a housing crisis. Among people with more severe mental illness there is some suggestion that people enjoy better outcomes in settings with fewer occupants (Newman 2001) and that most people will choose to live as independently as possible, perhaps because sharing accommodation with others who have mental illness can seem institutional or lacking in privacy (Chilvers *et al.* 2003).

Housing and services for people with mental illness are being provided by public, private and non-governmental or voluntary organizations. Civil society and housing associations appear to have played an important role in the development of innovative housing schemes (Edgar *et al.* 2002) and in the provision of accommodation and services to particularly disadvantaged groups (SMES-Europa 2002). However, the numbers of people with mental illness who live in ordinary housing underlines the need to be attentive to mainstream provision, and its maintenance, in the public and private sectors. In the case of private rented housing the potential for further public-private partnerships, as in the case of 'benevolent landlord' schemes, bears further examination.

In this context of increasingly diverse housing and services provision there is a growing need to monitor standards and quality assurance (Pillinger 2001). In particular, the growth in personalized services increases demands upon coordination of services (and networking with volunteers), and the development of interdisciplinary teams. More integrated approaches underline the importance of comprehensive needs assessment, including appropriate measures of housing need. Finally, the placing of the client at the centre of service provision calls for more attention to the rights, needs and contribution of the person with mental illness (Disability Legislation Consultation Group 2003).

Strategies to remove barriers to services must address any discrimination against people with mental illness, including that of service providers. The net effect of these trends is increasing demand for appropriately skilled and sensitive staff. The absolute numbers of staff may be less important than the ways in which they are organized and managed (Quilgars 2000). The key to good provision is likely to be the way in which services are delivered (Sainsbury Centre for Mental Health 1998; Quilgars 2000); for example, in dealing with homeless people with mental illness, attitudes and respect are regarded as more important than a specific technique (SMES-Europa 2002). In assessing and responding to complex and changing needs, nevertheless, staff need training – which currently is underdeveloped, for example, in some aspects of supported housing (Fakhoury *et al.* 2002). Volunteers also are very often highly valued but also need training. New services and ways of delivering them, for example involving service users, may challenge the values and preferences of both professionals and volunteers who, themselves, need support and sensitive development. Therefore, there is a need for more attention to strengthening the supply of well-qualified staff capable of working in stressful environments.

The quality of life of people with mental illness is, like all the population, profoundly affected by the availability and quality of their home. It is remarkable, then, that research and reporting on housing and accommodation issues for people with mental illness is so inadequate (Mental Health Commission 1999; Priebe and Turner 2003). Of course there are many complexities concerning the concepts and classification of housing but there is little information on the housing or social situation of most people with mental illness – those living in mainstream housing in the community without service support (Newman 2001). Such information could contribute to developing preventive strategies. More generally, there appears to be a lack of research and assessment to understand the housing needs of different groups; this is a particularly urgent need in the new member states of the EU where, for example, there is a lack of information on homelessness (European Commission 2004). Systematic research into, and information on, the effectiveness of different housing solutions for people with more severe mental illnesses is poorly developed (Chilvers *et al.* 2003) and there appears to be a need for substantial improvements in research methodologies (Quilgars 2000) as well as clearer conceptualization of policy-relevant outcomes.

Employment

Work is an essential part of life. For the individual it provides an opportunity to earn wages, which in turn provides greater financial security and increases the opportunities to acquire material wealth. It also provides social status and identity, a sense of achievement and a means of structuring one's time (Jahoda 1981). It is important for mental health, as secure employment can help promote or restore good mental well-being and independence, but it is also true that the demanding nature of the modern workplace can increase the risks of mental health problems, most often recognized as occupational stress, which can be a significant contributor to high levels of absenteeism and long-term disability across Europe.

This section of the chapter is thus concerned with two aspects of work and mental health. The first part focuses on how mental health issues are dealt with within the workplace, with what might be termed workplace mental health management, while the second is concerned with what happens outside the workplace to people with mental health disorders, i.e. the various measures which may be taken to return people to employment. As discussed in Chapter 3 of this volume, this group are particularly vulnerable to being excluded from entering or returning to the workforce.

Approaches to workplace mental health

There are basically three main approaches to dealing with health issues in the workplace. These are:

- occupational safety and health;
- workplace health promotion;
- rehabilitation/reintegration.

Occupational safety and health (OSH) is usually the only workplace health practice that is legislated for. The practitioners of OSH are legally obliged to prevent and protect against hazards to health or well-being that emanate from the workplace. In addition, they are expected to promote good OSH practice among the workforce. The definitions of the scope of good practice of OSH emphasize, *inter alia*, the concerns that OSH has for the whole spectrum of health and well-being of the worker. To the extent that mental health problems are caused, or exacerbated, by workplace factors, OSH practice could, in theory, address activity towards this issue. However, in practice, OSH tends to focus heavily on physical hazards in the workplace and also to focus on accident prevention rather than on health and well-being. Even to the extent that it does address health issues, these tend to be confined to the known list of occupational diseases rather than the emergent concept of occupation-related disease (i.e. illnesses which are not exclusively caused by occupational factors, but in whose aetiology occupational factors play a role). There is one growing exception to this general approach and that is the case of occupational stress, which is dealt with below.

Workplace health promotion (WHP) is a relatively new approach to dealing with general health issues in the workplace (as opposed to the narrower focus of occupational health in practice). Initially developed in the United States in the late 1970s and early 1980s, it has now developed its own specific character in Europe (see the work of the European Network for Workplace Health Promotion, www.enwhp.org). Unlike OSH legislation and practice, which emanated from concerns over working conditions and their effects on health, WHP has its origins in public health, where concerns about the major causes of mortality led to the development of, initially, health education approaches in the 1970s, and more recently to a more comprehensive health promotion approach. Within the field of health promotion, the concept of settings, i.e. physical milieu, where people spend significant parts of their lives and in which health and well-being may either be influenced positively or negatively, is central to the approach. One of these settings is the workplace.

WHP in Europe (unlike in the United States) emphasizes both the importance of the individual and of the workplace in relation to the generation of health and the creation of damage to health and well-being. It focuses its actions on the attitudes, skills and behaviours of the individual workers, while at the same time acting on the characteristics of the work environment (defined in its broadest sense) that contribute to the generation of health. Thus, it is not untypical to see WHP programmes that deal with issues as diverse as manual handling techniques, machine design and teamworking. WHP is usually driven by employee-defined health improvement needs, and in this context the issue of occupational stress often comes to the fore.

Despite the efforts of occupational health services and WHP, which are essentially focused on prevention and promotion, many workers succumb to illness or accident, be it caused by workplace factors or otherwise. In this situation, where workers have been absent from work for extended periods, many workplaces have in place a set of policies that are designed to promote the reintegration of the ill or injured worker. These policies, sometimes known as disability management policies, are targeted towards the safe and early return to work of the employee, either into the employee's former job or certain types of modified or alternative jobs. These policies are usually implemented by some combination of the human resource management function and occupational health, sometimes alongside training departments, since the effective return to work of a worker who is absent long term depends not only on the health status of the individual, but also on the process of reintegration, on the nature of the work to be performed and on the residual skills and abilities of the worker. Although disability management procedures can be relatively successful in returning people to work, they are not yet widespread, they tend to be more successful with workers who have physical illnesses or injuries and they are generally confined (though not exclusively so) to members of the workforce who have become ill or been injured.

A variation on this latter type of health intervention concerns the integration of people with a disability into the workplace. Generally, though not exclusively, these procedures are targeted at people who have a long-standing disability, perhaps from birth, and they are often targeted at people who have never worked in the open labour market. Workplaces themselves may adapt or use their procedures for disability management when engaging an employee with a disability who has never worked for them, but the challenge to the service providers and to the individuals is generally greater than is the case for a person who has acquired a disability at some time in their working career. Here, the difficulties are essentially those of employability; that is, they relate to the complement of skills and knowledge that the person has and their capacity to undertake work in the open labour market. Crucially, individuals in this situation do not have a relationship with a specific employer and from the employers' perspective they face the problems of hiring individuals who have been long-term unemployed as well as those associated with their disability.

In practice, this group of people has proved to have the lowest success rate in competing on the open labour market and despite regulations in many countries, that for example apply minimum quotas to the employment of people with disabilities, employment levels among this group remain very low. In part, (especially for those with a mental illness), this is also a consequence of the widespread stigma and discrimination that is just as likely to be found in employers and in potential fellow workers as in the general population. Some approaches to help return individuals with long-term mental health problems to the workforce – for example, supported employment schemes – have been more successful than others, and are discussed later in the chapter.

Mental health issues in the workplace

There are two main approaches to treating the issue of mental health in the literature. The first stems broadly from the epidemiological approach; that is, where studies have sought to identify factors existing in the workplace which impact upon mental health. This type of research can be described as falling within the health and safety tradition, i.e. in identifying workplace hazards to mental health it seeks to provide the basis for the control of these hazards using the tools of occupational health and safety.

However, there are a number of features of this type of research that should be borne in mind. Firstly, it generally does not focus on clinical diagnoses of psychiatric conditions; rather it more often focuses on general measures of mental well-being. Secondly, its focus is generally on the identification and measurement of workplace factors and mental well-being, rather than on all of the factors that may contribute to an individual's state of well-being. This research is therefore of limited utility when addressing the broader issues of mental health in a number of respects – it can be difficult to relate its findings to general psychiatric diagnoses and also many of its findings have limited relevance to the treatment or rehabilitation of people with psychiatric disorders.

The second type of treatment of workplace and mental health issues can be found in the rehabilitation literature. Here the main concern is with identifying and improving methods of rehabilitation and with seeking to integrate people with psychiatric problems into the workplace. The starting point in this literature (and the practice of rehabilitation in reality) is the psychiatric diagnosis and the measures that may be taken in relation to treatment and rehabilitation. This literature is notable for the fact that often it is not explicitly concerned with enabling the person with the psychiatric disability to re-enter the labour market; rather it is concerned with ensuring that the person has the skills and attitudes which enable them to function personally and socially.

Though these are generalizations, and there is some recent work that breaks these boundaries, the two general approaches typify the main practical approaches to dealing with mental health issues and work. Within the health and safety tradition, it can be argued that the focus of practice is mainly on occupational disease and occupation-related disease, rather than on general health *per se*. It is seen more as a means of meeting legal obligations not to harm workers' health and well-being, rather than as an instrument of public health. As the links between workplace factors and psychiatric illness have not been demonstrated to be strong, from the perspective of health and safety and that of employers, psychiatric illness is something of a non-issue.

Equally, it might be argued that from the perspective of clinical practitioners and rehabilitation professionals, this lack of an explicit and clear workplace link to the major psychiatric disorders has meant that there is a limited focus on reintegrating people with psychiatric illnesses into the workplace.

However, recent decades have seen the emergence of a phenomenon that does not neatly fit into this generalization – the issue of stress, and particularly occupational stress, has come to occupy the attention of both workplace health professionals and non-professional actors.

Occupational stress and mental health

There has been a large and growing research effort into occupational stress over the past 25 years. It is beyond the scope of this chapter to review this work in detail but a short summary of some of the major findings is presented below. For more detail on occupational stress and mental health, an ongoing EU research project has undertaken detailed literature reviews in the area of stress and mental health – see D'Amato and Zijlstra (2003), Joensuu and Lindstrom (2003), Van den Bossche and Houtman (2003) and Clarkin and Wynne (2003). A good general overview of the area of occupational stress is provided by Cox *et al.* (2000).

Occupational stress has been found to be a multi-faceted phenomenon. Workplace factors associated with higher levels of stress include:

- high job demands;
- low levels of control;
- ambiguity and lack of clarity about work roles;
- having responsibility for people;
- lack of participation in decision-making;
- quantitative and qualitative work overload;
- managerial style, e.g. lack of feedback of performance, persistent negative feedback;
- poor workplace communications;
- long or irregular work hours;
- job insecurity.

In addition to these factors, the relationship between job stress and mental well-being is moderated by a number of important factors. These include the level of social support at work, the coping style of the individual worker, the occupational grade of the worker and socioeconomic status.

Stress at work has been demonstrated to be related to a number of indicators of mental well-being. These include symptoms of anxiety, depression and various elements of mood. At its most extreme, where stress can be characterized as severe and traumatic, post-traumatic stress disorder may result.

Of course, stress generally and occupational stress in particular may impact on other aspects of well-being apart from mental health – there are well demonstrated relationships with a range of physical health measures (e.g. the cardiovascular system, the digestive system, the immune system, and the endocrine system) and with a range of workplace indicators such as 'on the job' performance, job satisfaction, absenteeism and workforce morale.

Workplace interventions for occupational stress

Stress at work is a multi-dimensional phenomenon with implications for both the individual in terms of health, well-being and work performance, and for the workplace in terms of the organization of work, levels of performance at work and ultimately such indicators as absenteeism and productivity. The multi-faceted nature of the problem can lead to interventions in the workplace which have been designed for multiple purposes – they may, for example, simultaneously seek to improve the organization of work as well as improve the health and well-being of the individual. Equally, interventions which are designed to address only one aspect of the problem may have effects on other areas. This point is important, as most interventions are designed for reasons other than the improvement of mental health (e.g. to meet health and safety requirements, to reduce absenteeism figures, to improve productivity). However, because of the inter-relatedness of the effects of stress, such interventions may have positive effects on mental health.

Interventions for dealing with stress may be broadly categorized as worker-oriented and workplace-oriented. In addition, they may also be categorized on the basis of whether they are primary, secondary or tertiary in their focus. Table 12.1 describes some of the major interventions that may be made using this categorization.

In theory, workplace interventions to ameliorate stress and improve mental health should include activities at all three levels, and should also address both the workplace and the individual worker. However, in practice it is relatively rare to find such integrated interventions, and most are still directed at the worker and are often only secondary or tertiary in nature (Van den Bossche and Houtman 2003). However, more comprehensive approaches have been described (e.g. see Kompier and Cooper 1999).

Table 12.1 Types of workplace stress intervention

Level	Worker focused	Workplace focused
Primary		Reduction, elimination or changing sources of stress at work
Secondary	Prevention of workers showing signs of stress from becoming ill	Providing protective systems in the workplace, e.g. training in job skills or coping skills
Tertiary	Treatment, rehabilitation and return to work of workers who have become ill, e.g. use of public health services	Provision of worksite-based treatment, e.g. stress debriefing, counselling, occupational health based treatment

The effectiveness of workplace stress interventions

The effectiveness of workplace stress interventions is a subject of much current interest. However, the numbers of evaluation studies in the area are quite small and most of these address only the least complex interventions. Most evaluation research has been undertaken with respect to individually-focused interventions, most of which have the aim of assessing therapeutic approaches. Evaluation studies of integrated interventions are quite rare, in part due to the difficulty of designing such studies in complex settings and also because they are expensive to conduct.

The findings from evaluations of intervention studies reveal that a range of therapeutic interventions have positive effects on workers' experience either of stress or its symptoms, at least in the short to medium term. A range of relaxation techniques, such as progressive relaxation, meditation and yoga, have been found to have positive effects on psychological functioning and mental well-being, and in some cases on organizational performance. In addition, cognitive-behavioural approaches such as rational emotive therapy and stress inoculation training have also been found to be effective in improving mental well-being.

Other interventions have sought to help the interaction between individual workers and their work environment. In particular, the aim of these interventions was to improve levels of social support at work. However, there are few studies of this type and their effectiveness results are inconclusive. Similarly, evidence from studies seeking to alter the work environment is mixed. In general, organizational-level interventions would seem to have positive, if weak, effects on mental well-being.

Workplace mental health promotion

Recent years have seen an increase in interest in using the workplace as a setting for the promotion of mental health. Two broad approaches may be distinguished. The first comes from within the tradition of health education and seeks to provide workers with information about the nature of, and strategies for the prevention of mental health problems. Examples of this type of intervention would include information campaigns about depression or schizophrenia. These initiatives seek to inform the worker about the general phenomena associated with these illnesses and generally do not seek to establish any causal link to the workplace. Further examples of this type of initiative may be found in a EU-wide study by Kuhn and Henke (2003).

The second type of initiative recognizes that workplace factors have an influence on mental well-being, even if they do not claim that workplace factors are the sole cause of mental illness. This approach generally seeks to control workplace factors that are associated with deficits in mental well-being. The initiative comes from within the tradition of occupational stress and the specific nature of such interventions has been informed by more general approaches to health and safety at work – prevention, protection and treatment.

The reintegration of workers with stress-related disorders

Recent years have seen the rise of long-term absenteeism due to stress-related disorders in many countries. For example, in the United Kingdom stress is now the single most significant cause of absence, accounting for approximately 30 per cent of all absence, while there is evidence from the Nordic countries of similar trends (Stress Impact 2006). Although studies in this area do not make clear what precisely is meant by stress-related disorders, the term is generally taken to refer to mental health problems such as depression or anxiety, or to less well-defined forms of disruption to mental well-being. Whatever the precise diagnoses involved, the issue of returning to work for people with these problems is moving up the agenda, not least because of the finding that they tend to be absent from work longer, that they tend to be less successful in returning to work and also because the costs of maintaining people on long-term disability payments are rising in an era of social welfare reforms (Jarvisalo *et al.* 2005).

Therefore, there has been a growth of interest in the area of return to work for employees with stress-related disorders. This has been assumed to be more difficult than would be the case of returnees with physical disorders, not least because the conditions and organization of work may be contributory factors to the absence. However, a recent study by the Health and Safety Executive in the United Kingdom (Thomson *et al.* 2003) undertook 12 case studies of good practice in the area, with the aim of trying to identify elements of good practice in organizational responses to workers who have become absent because of stress.

Among the factors associated with a successful return to work were early intervention, having a detailed and accurate diagnosis and ensuring the availability of appropriate treatments. Within the employing organization a number of factors such as having appropriate policy, designating clear responsibilities for managing the return to work process and applying case management techniques, were associated with effective return to work practices.

Return to work for people with severe mental illness

The previous discussion has dealt largely with the efforts made to maintain people in work or to return those people to work who have developed a mental health problem relatively recently. These people still have a more or less strong link with the workplace and with their employer and the labour market generally.

However, there is a group of people for whom this link has been broken – they have mental illnesses of such severity that they have been absent from work for long periods (at least for 12 months), often with conditions such as schizophrenia or bi-polar disorder. Indeed, they may never have entered the labour market. Looking at people with schizophrenia, for example, who tend to have lower employment rates than many other severe mental health problems, one recent review of the situation in Europe reported rates of employment ranging from just 10 to 30 per cent (Marwaha and Johnson 2004).

Measures taken to help people with severe mental illness to return to work are quite different to those taken in relation to people who maintain a link to their former workplace or with the wider labour market. The services and approaches available share much in common with people who have been long-term physically disabled. They face many of the same problems of obtaining work that this group does, as well as a number of obstacles that are specific to people with mental illnesses, including stigma, ignorance and discrimination. One study in Germany, for instance, reported that there were strong negative responses to people with schizophrenia returning to their place of employment (Schulze and Angermeyer 2003). The Social Exclusion Unit report in England (2004) noted that public sector employers could do much more to employ people with mental health problems. Changes in the nature of work in recent decades also present challenges; there is now less emphasis on manual labour and more on the high technology and service sectors. Consequently, individuals with severe mental health problems who have a poor job history and a lack of appropriate social skills and qualifications may find it increasingly difficult to find employment. Recent research in England suggests that individuals with mental health problems have up to a 40 per cent lower chance of obtaining employment compared with other disability groups (Berthoud 2006).

Systems that have been set up to try to integrate the long-term disabled into work have evolved over many years and some, in practice, may constitute an alternative, or are parallel to, the open labour market. Experience has demonstrated that movement between these parallel systems is very difficult for people with disabilities, be they physical or mental in nature. Indeed, many of these alternative approaches were not set up with any intention of getting individuals back into the open labour market. Although estimates vary as to their effectiveness, it is clear that perhaps no more than 10 to 20 per cent of people with disabilities move through these vocational systems to compete on the open labour market. The rates for obtaining open employment for people with severe mental illnesses are generally no higher than those observed for people with physical disabilities and in many instance may be lower.

What then are the approaches taken to return people with severe mental illnesses to work? These may be categorized into two main types: pre-vocational training and supported employment. Pre-vocational training is the older of the two approaches and encompasses a range of interventions which have evolved in line with developments in general psychiatric treatment over past decades (e.g. the move away from hospital-based to community-based care). It may include any approach to vocational rehabilitation that involves a period of training or work experience prior to seeking work in the competitive labour market. The aim is to ultimately encourage clients to compete on the open job market, but in some cases the activities of pre-vocational training do not necessarily focus on returning the person to such work environments; rather, they are seen as an integral part of the treatment and rehabilitation process. Return to work may also be achieved through some kind of graduated process eventually moving, for example, from sheltered work schemes or clubhouse programmes to open employment supported by training and perhaps other interventions.

Sheltered employment typically refers to an intervention that arose from the old tradition of hospital-based workshops that provided structured and segregated employment. These workshops aimed to place people in open employment after a period of pre-vocational training, but without much success (5–10 per cent). The clubhouse movement represents one alternative type of pre-vocational training that originated in, and is predominantly found in, the United States (Macias *et al.* 1999) but increasingly can be seen in some parts of Europe, particularly in Scandinavia and the Baltic states. It began in the 1950s and moved away from hospital-based services to seek to foster independent living and employment. There are two separate activities of preparation – the work-ordered day and transitional employment. In the work-ordered day clients join a work crew operating in the clubhouse, while transitional employment involves working outside of the clubhouse (but controlled by it) in a structured way. Current evidence suggests that rates of employment are lower than those reported for people in supported employment (Schneider 2005).

The distinction between the pre-vocational training and supported employment approaches has been characterized in terms of 'train and place', where training is provided prior to competing on the open labour market for the former, and 'individual placement and support' (IPS) where open employment is found and training and other supports are provided on-the-job for the latter. The concept of supported employment evolved in the mid-1980s, being originally developed for people with learning disabilities, and subsequently expanding to other client groups. This approach is based on criticisms that pre-vocational training encourages dependency and does not foster work-related skills. In supported employment clients can for instance receive support from job coaches which may involve some element of training. A major influence on supported employment has been the development of the IPS framework (Becker and Drake 1993). This framework has synthesized some of the key concepts connected with supported employment, including the principle of obtaining paid work in a normal setting where the majority of employees are unlikely to have any disability. It also implies that the choice of job should be that of the client rather than that of any agency or professional, and furthermore, there is no specified time limit for support that individuals may receive following employment. Another key feature of IPS is the emphasis on close links between rehabilitation, employment and mental health services.

Effectiveness of pre-vocational and supported employment schemes

What do we know about the effectiveness of these approaches? There is in fact a growing body of evidence, but it should be noted that much of this evidence comes from the United States, with comparatively little evaluation conducted in Europe. It is important to bear in mind that the context in which interventions are delivered, such as the system of disability benefits, access to health care, anti-discrimination legislation and the level of stigma towards those with mental health problems, will all have an impact on effectiveness. Careful evaluation of interventions shown to be effective in the United States, to determine whether they will work in different European contexts, is still required.

A Cochrane review of vocational rehabilitation for people with severe mental illnesses (Crowther *et al.* 2003) provides a good overview of the research literature in the area, contrasting the effectiveness of pre-vocational training and supported employment approaches in terms of their success in achieving employment in the open labour market. The review points to a consistent finding across five studies which indicates that supported employment is more effective than different types of pre-vocational training in terms of achieving and maintaining employment, with a greater number of hours worked and higher average earnings. More recently, Marshall (2005) updated Crowther's review to include one additional meta-analysis and an additional randomized controlled trial comparing supported employment with pre-vocational training. Again the findings of the meta-analysis were consistent with those of the Cochrane review, while this additional review reported that in a two-year follow-up 27 per cent of those who had participated in a supported employment programme were still in employment compared with just 7 per cent of those who had been enrolled in pre-vocational training (Lehman *et al.* 2002).

Bond (2004) also conducted a review of supported employment interventions and concluded that the evidence base for these was strong, with a number of randomized controlled trials demonstrating that supported employment was effective in getting individuals back into work, and that the rates of employment were superior to vocational rehabilitation programmes. Another review undertaken by Schneider (2005) which looked at both rigorous evidence from meta-analyses and randomized controlled trials, as well as less rigorous evaluation methods, again concluded that supported employment interventions that adopted the principles of IPS were most effective in helping individuals to obtain employment. It also found no evidence that sheltered workshops were effective; indeed there was evidence that such workshops were detrimental.

One potential way of strengthening further the effectiveness of supported employment schemes may be through the improved integration of clinical and vocational rehabilitation, but little research has been undertaken in this area. One exception is the work undertaken by Cook *et al.* (2005) who reported that supported employment schemes that combine clinical and vocational rehabilitation programmes had more favourable employment outcomes compared with usual supported employment. Some studies have suggested that IPS-type supported employment was no more successful than vocational rehabilitation when looking at the length of time that individuals kept their jobs (Drake *et al.* 1996; Lehman *et al.* 2002). There is also some evidence suggesting that the quality of support for individuals while in the workplace can make a difference to long-term retention of employment. One evaluation of a workplace fundamental skills module which provided training in social and workplace skills for people with mental health problems that had obtained employment reported a lower level of job turnover compared with those individuals who received standard IPS-type support alone (Wallace and Tauber 2004).

While the evidence on effectiveness for supported employment interventions seems strong, it is difficult to generalize any findings on their cost-effectiveness in comparison to other types of intervention because these are highly context-specific and most analyses have focused on individuals with learning disabilities (Schneider 2003). Indeed the costs of IPS interventions may often outweigh the gains in terms of benefit payments avoided, or income tax payments made, as for instance shown in one recent study in Australia (Chalamat *et al.* 2005). It is important however to consider broader measures of outcome as well as narrow measures such as rate of return to employment. In comparison to other interventions higher rates of employment can be associated with other benefits such as increased levels of social inclusion and improved quality of life.

Although the evidence on most sheltered workplaces suggests that they are not effective in getting individuals into mainstream employment, one emerging area where further careful evaluation is required is that of social firms or social cooperatives (Schneider 2005). These companies are created for the employment of disabled people, and typically at least 30 per cent of the workforce has some disability. Some qualitative analysis suggests that important factors in the success of social firms in ultimately improving the chances of open employment include the participation of employees in the firm's development, wages above the minimum wage rate, genuine opportunities for employees to develop their potential and the involvement of local agencies in firm development (Secker *et al.* 2003). Certainly there has been some growth in social firms across Europe. Most are to be found in Italy, with more than 8000 employing in total 60,000 people and Germany where there are 520 firms employing 16,500 people (Seyfried and Ziomas 2005). The Confederation of European Social Firms, Employer Initiatives and Social Cooperatives (CEFEC) now has organizational members in 14 countries in both western and eastern Europe. One mapping in the United Kingdom suggested there were 118 full or emerging social firms with more than 1500 employees of which more than 900 places were filled by people with disabilities. People with mental health problems formed the largest single group accounting for more than 30 per cent of these 900 jobs (Baker 2005).

Financial disincentives to employment

We have already noted that many studies have been undertaken in the United States where the welfare system is somewhat different to that found in most European countries. This makes it difficult to generalize findings to a European context where disability benefits appear to act as a significant disincentive to a return to work in many countries. This is in contrast to the situation in the US where regulations governing access to disability benefits can allow individuals to retain high levels of benefit even when their income from employment may be substantial. In one recent study of 12 countries, including 10 in western Europe, expenditure on disability benefits was negatively associated with the participation of people with schizophrenia in the labour force (Kilian and Becker 2006).

In European countries with advanced economies, these disincentives are perhaps greatest in the United Kingdom and least problematic in Italy (Warner 2000). There are also bureaucratic regulations to be overcome – for instance, if an individual returns to work but then loses his or her job it may take a considerable period of time to reclaim disability benefits, during which time significant hardship may be endured (OECD 2003). Many national financial support systems in Europe require reshaping to tackle this 'benefit trap' and encourage more people to return to work while safeguarding the quality of life and income of those who cannot obtain employment. One ongoing attempt to address some of these barriers is the Pathways to Work initiative in England. This has involved a proactive programme of support and advice on how to return to work, training to enhance skills, as well as support while at work. In many respects it is an approach consistent with IPS. In addition, in an attempt to counter the benefit trap, a system of tax credits and additional return to work credits paid as a supplement to earnings during the first year of work have been introduced. Recent qualitative analysis suggests that this financial support, if effective, is of key importance in getting people back to work; when payments are delayed or not claimed financial problems occur quickly (Corden and Nice 2006). Further evaluation of this initiative and of those elsewhere in Europe that address both the financial disincentive to work as well as some of the more cumbersome aspects of entitlement regulations is required.

Conclusion

In conclusion, a number of points seem to be clear with regard to how mental health issues are treated in the workplace. In general terms, mental health is still not perceived to be an important workplace health issue by most workplace stakeholders when compared to occupational health and safety. This is particularly true in relation to mental health problems with no causative association with the workplace.

Nevertheless, occupational stress and its effects on mental well-being are gaining an increasing level of attention. This is occurring in two main contexts, that of occupational health and safety, where preventing and managing stress is obligatory under legislation, and also with respect to the return to work of workers with stress-related disorders. Most workplace interventions that affect mental well-being focus on occupational stress and most focus on the individual worker. However, there is also a rise in workplace-based health education programmes in relation to mental illness. In contrast, public health and rehabilitation services, which deal with people with psychiatric illness, tend to have weak links with the workplace. However, mental health issues are likely to become more important to workplace stakeholders in the coming years;

these conditions are becoming more common and are an increasing cause of workplace absenteeism, leading to losses of productivity and an increased burden on social welfare systems.

With respect to measures to help integrate or reintegrate people with mental health problems into the workplace, very different approaches are adopted which are similar to those used to help people with physical disabilities. Recent meta-analyses and systematic reviews indicate that supported employment schemes appear to be the most effective in helping individuals return to work, although evidence in a European context remains limited. Nevertheless, employment rates for those with severe mental health problems remain low, reflecting, in part, the changing nature of work and also the high level of stigma and prejudice still to be found in the open labour market.

The employment rates of both those with less and more severe mental health problems will also be influenced to some extent by entitlement to, and level of, disability benefits and social welfare payments across Europe; further research is required to fully understand what influence such benefits have on the willingness to return to and/or seek employment.

References

Baker, K. (2005) *Mapping the Social Firm Sector 2005*. Redhill: Social Firms UK.

Becker, D.R. and Drake, R.E. (1993) *A Working Life: The Individual Placement and Support (IPS) Program*. Concord, NH: Dartmouth Psychiatric Research Center.

Berthoud, R. (2006) *The Employment Rates of Disabled People*. London: Department of Work and Pensions, Research Report 298.

Bond, G.R. (2004) Supported employment: evidence for an evidence-based practice, *Psychiatric Rehabilitation Journal*, 27(4): 345–59.

Chalamat, M., Mihalopoulos, C., Carter, R. and Vos, T. (2005) Assessing cost effectiveness in mental health: vocational rehabilitation for schizophrenia and related conditions, *Australian and New Zealand Journal of Psychiatry*, 39: 693–700.

Chilvers, R., Macdonald, G.M. and Hayes, A.A. (2003) Supported housing for people with severe mental disorders (Cochrane Review), *Cochrane Database Systematic Review CD 000453*, http://www.cochrane.org/reviews.

Clarkin, N. and Wynne, R. (2003) *Vocational Rehabilitation and Work Resumption. Stress Impact Project*. Dublin: Work Research Centre.

Cook, J.A., Leff, H.S., Blyler, C.R., Gold, P.B. *et al.* (2005) Results of a multisite randomized trial of supported employment interventions for individuals with severe mental illness, *Archives of General Psychiatry*, 62(5): 505–12.

Corden, A. and Nice, K. (2006) *Incapacity Benefit Reforms Pilot: Findings from the Second Cohort in a Longitudinal Panel of Clients*. London: Department of Work and Pensions, Research Report 345.

Cox, T., Griffiths, A. and Rial-Gonzales, E. (2000) *Research on Work Related Stress*. Bilbao: European Agency for Safety and Health at Work.

Crowther, R., Marshall, M., Bond, G. and Huxley, P. (2003) Vocational rehabilitation for people with severe mental illness (Cochrane review), in *The Cochrane Library*, Issue 3. Oxford: Update Software.

D'Amato, A. and Zijlstra, F. (2003) *Occupational Stress: A Review of the Literature Relating to Mental Health. Stress Impact Project*. Guildford: University of Surrey.

Dickey, B., Gonzalez, O., Latimer, E., Powers, K., Schutt, R. and Goldfinger, S. (1996) Use of mental health services by formerly homeless adults residing in group and independent housing, *Psychiatric Services*, 47: 152–8.

Disability Legislation Consultation Group (2003) *Equal Citizens: Proposals for Core Elements of Disability Legislation*. Dublin: National Disability Authority.

Drake, R.E. *et al.* (1996) The New Hampshire study of supported employment for people with severe mental illness: vocational outcomes, *Journal of Consulting and Clinical Psychology*, 64: 391–9.

Edgar, B., Doherty, J. and Mina-Coull, A. (2000) *Support and Housing in Europe*. Bristol: The Policy Press.

Edgar, B., Doherty, J. and Meert, H. (2002) *Access to Housing: Homelessness and Vulnerability in Europe*. Bristol: The Policy Press.

European Commission (2003a) *The Social Protection Systems in the 13 Candidate Countries*. Country reports at: http://europa.eu.int/comm/employment_social/soc-prot/social/index_en.htm.

European Commission (2003b) *Equality, Diversity and Enlargement: Report on Measures to Combat Discrimination in Acceding and Candidate Countries*. Brussels: European Commission.

European Commission (2003c) *Communication on Equal Opportunities for People with Disabilities: a European Action Plan*. Brussels: European Commission.

European Commission (2003d) *Joint Report on Social Inclusion*, COM (2003) 773 final. Brussels: European Commission.

European Commission (2004) *Social Inclusion in the New Member States: A Synthesis of the Joint Memoranda on Social Inclusion*. Brussels: European Commission.

European Council (2003) Resolution of 15 July 2003 on promoting the employment and social integration of people with disabilities, *Official Journal of the European Union*, C 175/1 (24 July).

European Foundation for the Improvement of Living and Working Conditions (EFILWC) (2003) *Access to Employment for Vulnerable Groups. Foundation Paper No. 2*. Luxembourg: Office for Official Publications of the European Communities.

European Foundation for the Improvement of Living and Working Conditions (EFILWC) (2004) *Quality of Life in Europe*. Luxembourg: Office for Official Publications of the European Communities.

Fakhoury, W.K.H., Murray, A., Shepherd, G. and Priebe, S. (2002) Research in supported housing, *Social Psychiatry and Psychiatric Epidemiology*, 37(7): 301–15.

Freyhoff, G., Parker, C., Voué, M. and Greig, N. (eds) (2004) *Included in Society: Results and Recommendations of the European Research Initiative on Community-based Residential Alternatives for Disabled People*, www.community-living.info.

Jahoda, M. (1981) Work employment and unemployment: values theories and approaches in social research, *American Psychologist*, 36: 184–91.

Jarvisalo, J., Andersson, B., Boedeker, W. and Houtman, I. (eds) (2005) *Mental Disorders as a Major Challenge in the Prevention of Work Disability: Experiences in Finland, Germany, the Netherlands and Sweden*. Helsinki: The Social Insurance Institution, Finland.

Joensuu, M. and Lindstrom, K. (2003) *Sickness Absence and Stress Factors at Work. Stress Impact Project*. Helsinki: Finnish Institute of Occupational Health.

Kilian, R. and Becker, T. (2006) Macroeconomic indicators and labour force participation of people with schizophrenia, *Journal of Mental Health*, forthcoming.

Kompier, M. and Cooper, C. (1999) *Preventing Stress, Improving Productivity; European Case Studies in the Workplace*. London: Routledge.

Kuhn, K. and Henke, N. (2003) *Mental Health Promotion in Europe: Final Report – Working Adults*. Dortmund: Federal Institute for Occupational Safety and Health.

Lehman, A.F., Goldberg, R., Dixon, L.B., McNary, S. *et al.* (2002) Improving employment outcomes for persons with severe mental illnesses, *Archives of General Psychiatry*, 59(2): 165–72.

Lipton, F.R., Siegel, C., Hannigan, A., Samuels, J. and Baker, S. (2000) Tenure in supportive housing for homeless persons with severe mental illness, *Psychiatric Services*, 51(4): 479–86.

Macias, C., Jackson, R., Schroeder, C. and Wang, Q. (1999) What is a clubhouse? Report on the ICCD 1996 survey of USA clubhouses, *Community Mental Health Journal*, 35(2): 181–90.

Marshall, M. (2005) *How Effective are Different Types of Day Care Service for People with Severe Mental Disorders? Health Evidence Network Synthesis Report*. Copenhagen: World Health Organization.

Marwaha, S. and Johnson, S. (2004) Schizophrenia and employment: a review, *Social Psychiatry and Psychiatric Epidemiology*, 39(5): 337–49.

Mental Health Commission (1999) *Housing and Mental Health: Reducing Housing Difficulties for People with Mental Illness – A Discussion Paper*. Wellington, New Zealand: Mental Health Commission.

Middleboe, T. (1997) Prospective study of clinical and social outcome of stay in small group homes for people with mental illness, *British Journal of Psychiatry*, 171: 251–5.

Newman, S.J. (2001) Housing attributes and serious mental illness: implications for research and practice, *Psychiatric Services*, 52(10): 1309–17.

Office for National Statistics (2000) *Survey of Psychiatric Morbidity Among Adults Living in Private Households*. London: The Stationery Office.

Office for National Statistics (2002) *The Social and Economic Circumstances of Adults with Mental Disorders*. London: The Stationery Office.

Organization for Economic Cooperation and Development (2003) *Transforming Disability into Ability: Policies to Promote Work and Income Security for Disabled People*. Paris: OECD.

Pillinger, J. (2001) *Quality in Social Public Services*. Luxembourg: Office for Official Publications of the European Communities.

Priebe, S. and Turner, T. (2003) Reinstitutionalization in mental health care, *British Medical Journal*, 326: 175–6.

Public Health Alliance Ireland (2004) *Health in Ireland – An Unequal State*, www.publichealthallianceireland.org.

Quilgars, D. (1998) *Supporting People with Mental Health Problems in Ordinary Housing*. York: Joseph Rowntree Foundation.

Quilgars, D. (2000) *Low Intensity Support Services: A Systematic Literature Review*. York: Joseph Rowntree Foundation.

Rog, D.J. (2004) The evidence on supported housing, *Psychiatric Rehabilitation Journal*, 27(4): 334–44.

Sainsbury Centre for Mental Health (1998) *Keys to Engagement: Review of Care for People with Severe Mental Illness who are Hard to Engage with Services*. London: SCMH.

Schneider, J. (2003) Is supported employment cost effective? A review, *International Journal of Psychosocial Rehabilitation*, 7: 145–56.

Schneider, J. (2005) Getting back to work: what do we know about what works? In B. Grove, J. Secker and P. Seebohm (eds) *New Thinking about Mental Health and Employment*. Oxford: Radcliffe Publishing Limited.

Schulze, B. and Angermeyer, M.C. (2003) Subjective experiences of stigma: a focus group study of schizophrenic patients, their relatives and mental health professionals, *Social Science and Medicine*, 56(2): 299–312.

Secker, J., Dass, S. and Grove, B. (2003) Developing social firms in the UK: a contribution to identifying good practice, *Disability and Society*, 18(5): 659–74.

Seidman, L.J., Schutt, R.K., Caplan, B., Tolomiczenko, G.S., Turner, W.M. and Goldfinger,

S.M. (2003) The effect of housing interventions on neuropsychological functioning among homeless persons with mental illness, *Psychiatric Services*, 54(4): 905–8.

Seyfried, E. and Ziomas, D. (2005) Pathways to social integration for people with mental health problems: the establishment of social cooperatives in Greece, discussion paper prepared for Peer Review in the Field of Social Inclusion Policies Meeting, Athens, Greece 5–7 October 2005. Available at www.peer-review-social_inclusion.net/peer/pdf_pool/05_EL_agenda_en_050912.pdf.

SMES-Europa (2002) *To Live in Health and Dignity*. Brussels: SMES-Europa.

Social Exclusion Unit (2004) *Mental Health and Social Exclusion*. London: Office of the Deputy Prime Minister.

Stress Impact (2006) *Impact of Changing Social Structures on Stress and Quality of Life: Individual and Social Perspectives*. Guildford: Department of Psychology, University of Surrey.

Thomson, L., Neathey, F. and Rick, J. (2003) *Best Practice in Rehabilitating Employees Following Absence Due to Work Related Stress*. London: Health and Safety Executive.

Van den Bossche, S. and Houtman, I. (2003) *Work Stress Interventions and their Effectiveness: A Literature Review. Stress Impact Project*. Hoofddorp: TNO, Work and Employment.

Wallace, C.J. and Tauber, R. (2004) Supplementing supported employment with work-place skills training, *Psychiatric Services*, 55(5): 513–15.

Warner, R. (2000) *The Environment of Schizophrenia: Innovations in Practice, Policy and Communication*. Philadelphia, PA: Brunner-Routledge.

Watson, L. and Tarpey, M. (1998) *Pick and Mix: Developing Flexible Housing Choices in Community Care*. Coventry: Chartered Institute of Housing.

Watson, L., Tarpey, M., Alexander, K. and Humphreys, C. (2003) *Supporting People: Real Change? Planning Housing and Support for Marginal Groups*. York: Joseph Rowntree Foundation.

thirteen

Developing mental health policy: a human rights perspective[1]

Camilla Parker

Introduction

This chapter considers the development of mental health policy – and the legislation required to support such a policy – from a human rights perspective. It is
argued that such an approach not only reinforces the arguments for moving
from institutional care to the provision of good quality community-based care
for people with mental health problems, as advocated by the World Health
Organization (WHO) (2001), but also demonstrates that the essential goal of
mental health policy must be to ensure that such individuals can participate
in society as equal citizens. Crucially, it also places the individuals receiving
mental health services at the heart of the planning, development and implementation of such policies.

Scope of this chapter

In 1948 the United Nations (UN) adopted the Universal Declaration of Human
Rights (UDHR). This sets out a range of civil, cultural, economic, political and
social rights. Since then numerous and wide-ranging human rights instruments
have been introduced (see Boxes 13.1 and 13.2). While it is beyond the scope of
this chapter to provide a comprehensive analysis of all of these documents, the
first part provides an overview of the international human rights instruments
and explains their relevance to mental health. The second part considers how
human rights principles can assist in the development and implementation of
mental health policy and identifies areas in which legislation is required to
support the policy.

Nor has it been possible, within the confines of one chapter, to address the specific issues relating to particular groups of people receiving mental health care, such as people with intellectual disabilities, children and young people, older people and offenders with mental health problems. However, many of the general issues that are explored will be relevant to these groups of people.

Box 13.1   United Nations international human rights: key treaties

- International Covenant on Civil and Political Rights (ICCPR), 1966.
- International Covenant on Economic, Social and Cultural Rights (ICESCR), 1966.
- Convention on the Elimination of All Forms of Racial Discrimination (CERD), 1965.
- Convention on the Elimination of All Forms of Discrimination against Women (CEDAW), 1979.
- Convention Against Torture and Other Cruel, Inhuman or Degrading Treatment or Punishment (CAT), 1984.
- Convention on the Rights of the Child (CRC), 1989.

For details of which states have ratified these treaties see: www.unhchr.ch/pdf/report.pdf

---

Box 13.2   The Council of Europe and human rights: key treaties

- The European Convention on Human Rights (ECHR), 1950: sets out a range of civil and political rights. It has been ratified by 45 of the 46 member states.
- European Social Charter 1961 (revised 1996): protects fundamental social and economic rights, including the right to work, the right to protection of health and the right to social security. The revised Charter includes the right to housing. The European Social Charter has been ratified by 26 states and 19 states have ratified the revised Charter.
- European Convention on the Prevention of Torture and Inhuman or Degrading Treatment or Punishment, 1987: establishes the European Committee for the Prevention of Torture and Inhuman or Degrading Treatment or Punishment (the CPT) which by means of visits examines 'the treatment of all categories of persons deprived of their liberty by a public authority, including persons with mental health problems' (CPT Standards, para. 25). It has been ratified by 45 states.

For further information on Council of Europe treaties see: http://convention.coe.int

Terminology

A variety of terms are used in relation to people who have been diagnosed as having a mental illness. Many people with such a diagnosis consider the term 'mental illness' pejorative and stigmatizing. Accordingly, this chapter refers to 'people with mental health problems or 'service users'. However, human rights instruments use terms such as 'mental illness' and 'mental disorder' in addition to 'disabled people' or 'people with disabilities' (which include people with mental health problems and/or intellectual disabilities in addition to individuals with physical and/or sensory impairments), and these terms will be used where relevant. Another term which is commonly used is 'mental disability'. This term includes both people with mental health problems and people with intellectual disabilities.

International human rights and mental health: overview

Human rights instruments cover a broad range of areas, often divided into 'civil and political rights' and 'economic, social and cultural rights'. Civil and political rights include the rights to liberty, private and family life and freedom from torture, inhuman or degrading treatment, or punishment. Economic, social and cultural rights include the right to work, education and the highest attainable standard of physical and mental health. However, increasingly it is recognized that these two categories of rights are related and interdependent (JCHR 2004: 21). The right to health illustrates this point. It is closely related to, and dependent upon, the realization of other human rights such as rights to food, housing, work, education, human dignity, life, non-discrimination, equality, the prohibition of torture, privacy, access to information and the freedoms of association, assembly and movement (ICESCR GC 14 2000: para. 3). Both categories of rights are of equal importance to the development of mental health policy.

General issues

States' obligations under international human rights instruments

All of the human rights instruments in Box 13.1 (UN) and Box 13.2 (Council of Europe) are legally binding. Thus, states that ratify any of these treaties are required to implement the provisions of that treaty within their jurisdiction. Accordingly, governments must ensure that the development and implementation of mental health policies and legislation to support such policies comply with their obligations under these treaties.

Monitoring compliance with the international human rights treaties

While it will be up to each state to decide what legislative and other measures should be adopted in order to give effect to the rights recognized under the treaties, their compliance with the treaty obligations will be subject to some form of scrutiny.

UN human rights treaty system

The main UN monitoring mechanism is periodic reporting. Each of the UN treaties has a monitoring body responsible for examining the implementation of the relevant treaty and states are required to submit periodic reports (ranging from every two to every five years) to them, outlining their compliance with that treaty (O'Flaherty 2002: 1).

The treaty-monitoring bodies publish 'General Comments' which highlight the issues that states are expected to address in their periodic reports and also provide general interpretations of the treaty provisions (Alston and Crawford 2000: 22; O'Flaherty 2002: 7).

While four of the treaties (ICCPR, CERD, CAT and CEDAW – see Box 13.1) enable the monitoring bodies to consider complaints from alleged victims of violations of the relevant treaty, this procedure is subject to the state's acceptance of the procedure. Furthermore, the treaty-monitoring bodies have no means of enforcing their findings on such complaints (O'Flaherty 2002).

European Convention on Human Rights (ECHR)

Individuals alleging that their rights under the ECHR have been violated can pursue a complaint to the European Court of Human Rights, once they have exhausted domestic remedies. Where the complaint is upheld, the state is required to take remedial action (see Starmer 1999: Ch. 30). Thus, the ECHR is of major significance as it can have a direct impact on government law and policy: 'it is the only international Treaty in the history of humankind that guarantees the right of an individual to make a complaint that is capable of resulting in a binding judgment enforceable against a member state' (Clements and Read 2003: 17).

European Social Charter

States are required to submit annual reports to the European Committee of Social Rights on how they are implementing the Charter and the Committee publishes its 'conclusions' on each state's compliance. Although individuals cannot pursue complaints to the Committee, since 1998 certain organizations, for example employers' organizations and trade unions in the country concerned and non-governmental organizations enjoying participatory status within the Council of Europe, may lodge complaints against those states which have accepted this 'collective complaints procedure'. The state may be asked to take specific measures in order to comply with the Charter. However, Churchill and Khaliq (2004: 454) point out that given only about a third of the states which are parties to the Charter have accepted the collective complaints system, it is still 'very much a minority option'.

European Union and human rights

The protection and promotion of human rights is described as one of the defining principles of the European Union (EU) (Council of the European Union 2002: 1). Since the formulation of the 'Copenhagen Criteria' for membership of the EU in 1993, which included 'stability of institutions guaranteeing democracy, the rule of law, human rights and protection of minorities', human rights issues have been 'at the forefront of the accession process' (Williams 2004: 64–5).

Directives on non-discrimination

Article 13 of the Treaty of Amsterdam 1999 authorizes the EU to take action to combat discrimination based on a range of grounds, including disability. Two directives to promote equal treatment were adopted in 2000 (see below).

EU Charter of Fundamental Rights 2000

This Charter covers a range of economic, social and cultural rights, and civil and political rights. Although not legally binding, it is suggested that the European Court of Justice would be able to use the Charter as a guide to general principles of Community law 'thus conferring on it legal status of sorts through the back door' (Quinn 2001: 872). If the EU Constitution for Europe (which incorporates the Charter) comes into force, the Charter will become legally binding. Thus, EU institutions and bodies will be required to comply with the Charter, as will member states when implementing EU legislation, while the European Court of Justice will ensure adherence to the Charter (European Communities 2004: 10). However, at the time of writing the process of ratification (all member states must adopt the Constitution) has been, at the very least, delayed in the light of the results of the referenda in France and the Netherlands, with both countries rejecting the text of the Constitution.

European Union Agency for Fundamental Rights

In June 2005 the European Commission issued a proposal to establish an EU Agency for Fundamental Rights. The Agency is to be an independent centre which can provide assistance and expertise on fundamental rights issues to EU institutions and the member states: 'in order to support them when they take measures or formulate courses of action within their respective spheres of competence to fully respect fundamental human rights' (Commission of the European Communities: 2005). The proposal suggests that the Agency should become operational on 1 January 2007.

Mental health

All of the rights set out in the international human rights treaties apply to people with mental health problems. The universality of human rights is stressed by *Enable*, the UN website dedicated to disability and human rights: 'All international human rights instruments protect the rights of persons with disabilities, as they apply to all persons. This principle of universality is reinforced by the principles of equality and non-discrimination, which are included in human rights instruments (*Enable* 2005).

Mental health, disability and human rights

In their report to the UN on human rights and disability Quinn *et al.* (2002: 1) note that the process of ensuring that disabled people enjoy their rights is 'slow and uneven' but that the shift to a human rights perspective has been authoritatively endorsed by the UN, the best example being the UN Standard Rules on the Equalization of Opportunities for Persons with Disabilities ('the Standard Rules').

The Standard Rules and the Mental Illness Principles

The Standard Rules seek to ensure that all disabled people, 'as members of their societies, may exercise the same rights and obligations as others'. For example, they provide that states should include disability issues in all relevant policy-making and national planning; that the needs and concerns of disabled people are incorporated into general development plans; and that organizations of disabled people are included in the decision-making process. The Standard Rules make clear that the term 'disability' includes mental health problems (para. 17). A Special Rapporteur monitors the implementation of the Standards Rules, reporting yearly to the UN Commission for Social Development.

The Principles for the Protection of Persons with Mental Illness ('the MI Principles'), adopted by the UN in 1991 play a particularly important role in raising awareness about the human rights of people with mental health problems. They provide guidance on areas such as the procedures for involuntary admission to mental health care facilities and standards of care. While some of the provisions offer weaker protection than other human rights instruments, the MI Principles highlight some key issues that governments must address when developing mental health policies and legislation, particularly in relation to the provision of care in psychiatric facilities (United Nations 2003: para. 13).

Although referring to 'people with mental illness' the scope of the MI Principles is much wider as they include all persons admitted into a mental health facility (MI Principle 24). This is important given that in central and eastern Europe it is still common practice for people with mental health problems and intellectual disabilities to be placed in the same facilities.

The Standard Rules and MI Principles are examples of 'soft law', described as such because, although not legally binding, they can provide a useful guide to the implementation and interpretation of the legally binding treaties.

Other relevant documents

In September 2004, the Committee of Ministers of the Council of Europe adopted Recommendation No. REC(2004)10 ('REC(2004)10') which provides guidelines 'concerning the protection of the human rights and dignity of persons with mental disorder' together with an Explanatory Memorandum (Council of Europe 2004).

The WHO has issued a range of documents on mental heath legislation and human rights; the most recent publication draws on its previous work and provides guidance on developing mental health legislation (WHO 2003). (The WHO *Resource Book on Mental Health, Human Rights and Legislation* was in preparation at the time of writing this chapter and has since been published – WHO 2005c.) In January 2005, government representatives from 52 countries in the WHO European region adopted the mental health *Declaration* and *Action Plan* for Europe. These documents call for the development of comprehensive mental health policies which include actions to: 'tackle stigma and discrimination, ensure the protection of human rights and dignity and implement the necessary legislation in order to empower people at risk or suffering from mental health problems and disabilities to participate fully and equally in society' (WHO 2005a: 3).

An ad hoc committee of the UN is considering proposals for a specific convention to promote and protect the rights and dignity of disabled people (General Assembly Resolution 56/168 2001).

Emerging key principles

The following are examples of principles, common to many of the human rights instruments, which can be used as a basis for the development of mental health policy and related legislation.

Protection against discrimination

This is a fundamental right recognized by all major international treaties. In order to ensure that everyone benefits from the right to non-discrimination, states may be required to take affirmative action to counter existing discrimination against certain parts of the population. Provided that this is necessary to correct the discrimination, preferential treatment will be considered a legitimate differentiation (ICCPR GC 18 1989; ICESCR GC 5 1994). Recommendation REC(2004)(10) paragraph 40 states:

> the term 'discrimination' is understood to mean 'unfair discrimination'. In particular, the principle cannot prohibit positive measures that may be implemented with the aim of re-establishing a balance in favour of those at a disadvantage on the grounds of their past or present mental disorder. Hence, special measures undertaken to protect the rights or secure the advancement of persons with mental disorder should not be regarded as discriminatory.
>
> (Council of Europe 2004)

Equality and social inclusion

Quinn *et al.* (2002: 16) consider that 'human equality' is 'central to the system of basic freedoms postulated by human rights law'. As the Standard Rules illustrate, the equalization of opportunities and full inclusion within societies of disabled people is a key goal for the UN. Governments should take steps to remove the barriers preventing disabled people from exercising their rights and freedoms and making it difficult for them to participate fully in the activities of their societies (Standard Rules, para. 15). Article 25 of the EU Charter provides for the integration of disabled people: 'The Union recognizes and respects the right of persons with disabilities to benefit from measures designed to ensure their independence, social and occupational integration and participation in the life of the community'.

Promoting personal autonomy and independence

Promoting individuals' independence and ensuring they are given the opportunity to make decisions about their own care and treatment are key features of the MI Principles and the Standard Rules. The European Court of Human Rights considers that the right to self-determination and the notion of personal autonomy are inherent to the right to private and family life under Article 8 of the ECHR (*Pretty* v. *United Kingdom* 2002).

Least restrictive alternative/proportionality

Individuals with a mental illness have the right to live and work in the community (MI Principle 3) and to be treated and cared for in the community in which they live (MI Principle 7) so far as possible. They also 'have the right to be treated in the least restrictive environment and with the least restrictive or intrusive treatment appropriate' to their health needs and the need to protect others (MI Principle 9(1)). This is similar to the principle of 'proportionality' under the ECHR. Even where it is clear that there is a legitimate reason for restricting a right guaranteed by the ECHR, the restriction must not exceed what is strictly necessary to achieve that purpose. The action taken will not be considered to be proportionate if a less restrictive, but equally effective, alternative is available (Starmer 1999: 4.37–55). This principle is particularly relevant to decisions about the level, and type, of care and treatment provided to individuals and should be reflected in legislation relating to detention and treatment without consent.

Provision of care on the basis of individual needs

The importance of providing care and support to meet the individual's needs is emphasized by both the Standard Rules (para. 26) and the MI Principles (Principle 8). The MI Principles state that individuals' treatment and care shall be based on an individually prescribed plan which is discussed with the patient and regularly reviewed, revised as necessary and provided by qualified professional staff (Principle 9). Furthermore, the treatment must be suited to the person's cultural background (Principle 7(1)).

Participation in policy development

The involvement of service users and relatives who provide informal care is generally accepted as being a crucial component to the development and implementation of mental health policy (WHO 2001: 100). However, this is not simply a matter of good practice. Involving disabled people and their families in policy-making and national planning is a key theme of the Standard Rules. The treaty-monitoring body for the ICESCR considers that individuals' participation in decision-making on matters such as governments' plans to address the right to the highest attainable standard of physical and mental health is essential (ICESCR GC 14 2000: 54).

The role of legislation in protecting and promoting human rights

That legislation has a major role in protecting and promoting the rights of individuals is emphasized by both the ICESCR Committee (ICESCR GC 3 1990: para. 3) and the Human Rights Committee, which monitors the ICCPR (ICCPR GC 31 2004: para. 7). In relation to the use of compulsory powers (such as involuntary admission to mental health facilities and treatment without consent) legislation 'must ensure that these powers may only be exercised in strictly defined circumstances and that adequate safeguards are included in order to prevent arbitrary interference with individuals' rights and freedoms' (Jenkins *et al.* 2002: 42).

Action to support the implementation of legislation

While its introduction is a crucial step towards ensuring the enjoyment of the rights and freedoms set out under human rights instruments, legislation, in itself, will not be enough to achieve this goal (ICESCR GC 3 1990: para. 4; ICCPR GC 31 2004). Additional measures are required to maximize the effectiveness of legal safeguards, including raised awareness, training and guidance, and effective and accessible remedies.

The Human Rights Committee stresses the importance of states raising awareness of the ICCPR, not only among public officials, but also among the population at large (ICCPR GC 31 1990: para. 7). The Committee responsible for monitoring the implementation of the ICESCR notes that legislation will not always be the most effective means of seeking to eliminate discrimination. This is why the Standard Rules place particular emphasis on the need for states to 'take action to raise awareness in society about persons with disabilities, their rights, their needs, their potential and their contribution' (ICESCR GC 5 1994: para. 11).

States must also provide details of the instruction and training given to personnel involved in the custody and treatment of detainees and how Article 7 ICCPR (prohibition of torture and inhuman or degrading treatment) 'forms an integral part of the operational rules and ethical standards to be followed by such persons' (ICCPR GC 20 1992: para. 10).

Lastly, states must ensure that effective remedies are available to any individual whose rights and freedoms are violated. The Human Rights Committee (ICCPR GC 31 2004: para. 15) states that available remedies 'should be appropriately adapted so as to take account of the special categories of person, including, in particular, children'. While such comments are welcome, the limited access to justice for many disabled people is an area that, to date, seems to have received little attention from the monitoring bodies. Prohibitive rules for those individuals considered to lack capacity to make decisions for themselves, lack of adequate advocacy, lack of legal aid and lack of access to lawyers (Clements and Read 2003: 41–6), in addition to the fear of complaining against those responsible for providing care, are all serious obstacles to seeking redress. For those subject to guardianship (discussed below) and/or incarcerated in remote institutions, the barriers to accessing the legal process can be insurmountable. Unless these major barriers are addressed the remedies provided by legislation will be rendered meaningless in practice.

The importance of independent monitoring

While they are no substitute for ensuring that individuals have access to effective legal remedies, mechanisms for ensuring compliance with human rights standards must also be established. REC(2004)10, the CPT Standards and the MI Principles all highlight the importance of introducing such mechanisms. These should include systems for the inspection of mental health care facilities and investigation of complaints. These are discussed in more detail below.

Applying human rights principles to mental health policy

This part of the chapter considers the following four areas, highlighting the human rights perspective and the role of legislation in protecting and promoting the human rights of people with mental health problems:

- addressing the barriers to social inclusion;
- providing community-based care;
- defining the circumstances justifying compulsory care and treatment; and
- safeguarding the rights of individuals receiving care in psychiatric facilities.

Addressing the issues raised in these areas will involve a wide range of individuals, organizations and government sectors, in addition to service users and their families, mental health professionals, mental health non-governmental organizations (NGOs) and the health ministry. The government sectors that will have an interest in these areas include social welfare, housing, education, employment and social security. Other stakeholders include employers, schools and the media (Jenkins *et al.* 2002: 25).

Addressing the barriers to social inclusion

Although the provision of community-based services will be a crucial component of a comprehensive mental health policy, as the Parliamentary Assembly of
the Council of Europe points out, this alone will not ensure that service users
can enjoy the same rights as other members of society:

> The right to receive support and assistance, although essential to improving
> the quality of life of people with disabilities is not enough. Guaranteeing
> access to equal political, social, economic and cultural rights should be a
> common political objective for the next decade. Equal status, inclusion, full
> citizenship, and the right to choose should be further promoted and
> implemented.
>
> (Council of Europe 2003: 1)

Stigma and discrimination

Many people with mental health problems face significant and pervasive barriers
to social inclusion (Sayce 2000). The stigma attached to, and prejudice against,
'the mentally ill' is one such example. This can be manifested in a range of
misconceptions about people with mental health problems, such as potential
employers believing that they are not competent to work; officials assuming
that they lack the capacity to vote in public elections; and local communities
arguing that they should not be allowed to live in the neighbourhood because
the 'mentally ill' are dangerous. Such discriminatory attitudes and beliefs pose
a serious threat to the ability of people with mental health problems to enjoy
their civil, political, economic, social and cultural rights, such as the right to
work and to found a family. They also represent a major obstacle to the successful implementation of key aspects of mental health policies such as the development of community-based alternatives to institutional care (Sayce 2000: 42) and
mental health promotion (Jenkins *et al.* 2002: 70).

Guardianship

In some jurisdictions individuals considered to be 'incapacitated' are placed
under 'plenary guardianship', giving the appointed guardian wide-ranging
powers with little or no safeguards for the individual concerned (United Nations
2003: para. 15). Such individuals may be prevented from making a range of life
choices such as whether to marry or be employed, while the guardian will have
control over the person's finances and have the power to decide where the
person should live (Lewis 2002a: 300–1; Inclusion Europe 2003). Such powers
give rise to serious human rights violations; for example, the circumvention of
laws governing admission to a mental health facility (UN Report 2003: para. 15).
Rosenthal and Sundram (2003: 48) explain how this might happen: 'Once a
family member or the director of a psychiatric facility is declared an individual's
guardian, he or she may "voluntarily" commit a person to a psychiatric facility –
without ever asking that person what he or she really wants and, in fact, over
the active objection of the person'.

Combating stigma and discrimination: the role of legislation

The introduction of anti-discrimination legislation will be an important step in promoting the social inclusion of people with mental health problems. Both the ICCPR (Article 26) and the ICESCR (Article 2) support the need for such legislation.

At the European level, the EU Directive on equal treatment in employment requires member states to make discrimination unlawful on the grounds of religion or belief, disability, age or sexual orientation in the areas of employment and occupation (Council Directive 2000/43/EC). A second Directive requires member states to make discrimination on the grounds of racial or ethnic origin unlawful in a wide range of areas including employment, education and access to health care (Council Directive 2000/78/EC). Disability advocates are also campaigning for a further EU Directive requiring states to introduce measures to combat discrimination on the basis of disability in a range of additional areas, such as health care, education and access to goods and services (European Disability Forum 2003).

Recognizing that anti-discrimination legislation cannot, in itself, change attitudes and behaviour, the EU has introduced an action programme to 'improve understanding of the factors giving rise to discrimination, to develop better ways of combating them and to help create the conditions for a fairer society' (European Commission 2003: 22).

Raising awareness is also a key strategy. The World Health Organization (2001: 98) stresses the importance of public awareness campaigns in the development of mental health policy:

> Tackling stigma and discrimination requires a multilevel approach involving education of health professionals and workers, the closing down of psychiatric institutions which serve to maintain and reinforce stigma, the provision of mental health services in the community, and the implementation of legislation to protect the rights of the mentally ill. Fighting stigma also requires public information campaigns to educate and inform the community about the nature, extent and impact of mental disorders in order to dispel common myths and encourage more positive attitudes and behaviours.

Protecting the rights of people who may lack capacity: the role of legislation

Those involved in developing mental health policy must consider how to protect the rights of people who are thought to lack capacity to make certain decisions for themselves (this is likely to include a number of different client groups, such as older people, people with intellectual disabilities and some people with mental health problems). An essential step would be to introduce legislation to provide a framework for decision-making on behalf of people who lack the capacity to make decisions for themselves in relation to personal welfare (including health) and financial matters.

The Council of Europe's recommendation on *Principles Concerning the Legal Protection of Incapable Adults* (1999) provides a useful guide for legislators. For example, it states that the 'legislative framework should, so far as possible, recognize that different degrees of incapacity may exist and that incapacity may vary from time to time'. In order to comply with the principles of the least restrictive alternative/proportionality and personal autonomy/independence, such legislation should provide that decisions can only be made on behalf of others if the person concerned lacks capacity to make that particular decision for him or herself (United Nations 2003: para. 46). The UN report envisages that it will be for a court to determine whether or not the person has capacity and if the person needs assistance in relation to some areas of decision-making: 'the judge should always choose an option which, in accordance with the principles of autonomy and proportionality, best accommodates the needs of the person concerned'. Decisions made in connection with a person's legal capacity should be subject to periodic review (Council of Europe 1999; United Nations 2003: para. 46).

Safeguards to protect individuals who lack capacity from abuse and exploitation should also be included in such legislation; for example, by establishing an independent body with the authority to investigate cases where there are concerns that substitute decision-making powers are being exercised inappropriately. States must also provide appropriate safeguards for people who lack capacity to consent to their placement in mental health care facilities (REC(2004)10; *HL* v. *United Kingdom* 2004).

Providing community-based care

Community-based treatment and care is described by the WHO as the 'ultimate goal' for mental health policy. Such a goal is underpinned by the principles of least restrictive alternative, equality and social inclusion (although, as discussed above, this cannot be achieved simply by shifting the location of care from institutions into the community), and the promotion of personal autonomy and independence. The planning and development of community-based care should involve service users and their families (principle of participation) and care plans delivered on the basis of individuals' assessed needs (Freyhoff *et al.* 2004: 61).

Institutional care versus community-based care

As Chapter 10 points out, for the last 20 years there has been a broad consensus in western European countries on the need to close the large, isolated and long-stay institutions and focus on the provision of community-based services. Concerns about the ill-treatment and neglect of the residents of these institutions were a major factor in this shift in policy (Carrier and Kendall 1997: 12). However, remote and oppressive institutions are still prevalent in central and eastern Europe and recent reports on the serious human rights abuses within them highlight the importance and urgency of introducing similar reforms in these countries (Amnesty International 2003; Mental Disability Advocacy Center 2003).

In addition to the failings in care and unacceptable conditions, residents are segregated from society. The US Supreme Court held in *Olmsted* v. *LC* (1999) that the unjustified institutional isolation of disabled people amounted to unlawful discrimination. This was not only evidenced by the restrictions placed on the rights of those confined in the institutions, but also by the fact that 'institutional placement of persons who can handle and benefit from community settings perpetuates unwarranted assumptions that persons so isolated are incapable or unworthy of participating in life'.

Subject to factors such as available resources and the equitable use of such resources for those in need of services, the Court held that where individuals are assessed as being able to receive support in the community and do not wish to remain in institutional care, public authorities are required to provide for such individuals in community settings.

In the European context, such a case could constitute a violation of Article 8 (respect for private and family life) in combination with Article 14 (freedom from discrimination in relation to the rights under the ECHR) of the ECHR (Clements and Read 2003: 67).

Community-based care and the ECHR

The European Court of Human Rights has alluded to the link between the justification for detention under Article 5 (the right to liberty) and the availability of alternative community-based support when stating that individuals should not be detained unless other less severe measures are considered insufficient to safeguard the interests of that individual or the public (*Witold Litwa* v. *Poland* 2001).

To date, the European Court of Human Rights has not considered to what extent, if any, states are required to make community-based services available in order to avoid the need for detention. However, the development of case law concerning Article 8 (respect for private and family life) may provide greater opportunities for arguing that states are required to develop community-based services as alternatives to institutional care. This is because in certain limited circumstances Article 8 can place positive obligations on a state to adopt measures to secure respect for private and family life. For example, in *Kutzner* v. *Germany* (2002) the removal of children from parents with mild intellectual disabilities was held to have breached Article 8 on the basis that there were insufficient reasons for such a serious interference with the parents' family life. A significant factor in the Court's decision was the concern that the authorities had given insufficient consideration to providing additional measures of support as an alternative to the 'extreme measure' of separating the children from their parents.

The Explanatory Memorandum to REC(2004)10 (para. 75) stresses the importance of providing services in order to avoid the need for compulsory powers: 'Involuntary placement and involuntary treatment are measures that involve a significant restriction of the rights of the individual concerned. They should be a last resort ... Article 10 emphasizes the need to develop alternatives to involuntary treatment, in accordance with the principle of least restriction'.

Providing a legal framework for community-based care

Legislation could provide a framework for the planning and delivery of services to meet the needs of service users living in the community; for example by including the following:

- Powers and responsibilities of the relevant agencies (such as central and local government, public bodies, service providers (including non-governmental organizations).
- Financial mechanisms for the commissioning and provision of services.
- Procedures for ensuring that individuals receive appropriate care and support. For example, by requiring:
  - the comprehensive assessment of individuals' needs for health and social care and other support (such as accommodation);
  - services (such as housing and social support) to be appropriately tailored to the individual's assessed needs;
  - service users to be involved fully (with support from an independent advocate if necessary) in the procedures for assessing their needs and developing (and reviewing) their care plan – subject to issues of confidentiality, families and friends who provide informal care should be involved in this process as well.
- Complaints procedures.
- Provision of information to service users about the procedures involved in the assessment of their needs and decisions on the services to be provided and how to make a complaint.

Defining the circumstances justifying compulsory care and treatment

The circumstances in which the state is justified in detaining individuals and/or treating them without their consent raise 'a plethora of human rights concerns' which will need to be addressed by mental health policy and legislation (Davidson *et al.* 2003: 12).

Both the ICCPR and the ECHR allow for the detention of individuals in certain circumstances. Article 9 of the ICCPR states that everyone has the right to 'liberty and security of person', with no one being subjected to arbitrary arrest or detention nor deprived of their liberty 'except on grounds and in accordance with such procedures as are established by law'. Article 5 includes similar provisions, but specifies an exhaustive list of circumstances in which individuals may be deprived of their liberty. These include the 'lawful detention . . . of persons of unsound mind . . .'.

In 2002, an analysis of the legislation of the then 15 EU member states, relating to compulsory admission and treatment provisions (the Salize Report) found that the conditions for detention varied as follows: six states required the existence of a mental disorder and 'danger'; three required the existence of a mental disorder and a need for treatment; and six required the existence of a mental disorder and either a need for treatment or a 'danger' criterion to be satisfied.

The application of the 'danger' criteria differs between the states, with some countries including only public threats while others also include self-harm (but the report suggests that suicidal behaviour would be covered by need for treatment in any event) (Salize *et al.* 2002: 1.10).

Determination of mental disorder

While all the relevant human rights instruments stress the need to protect individuals from arbitrary detention, no clear definition of 'mental disorder' is provided. Although pointing out that 'the detention of a person simply because his views or behaviour deviate from the norms prevailing in a particular society' is not permitted, the European Court of Human Rights considers that no definitive interpretation should be given to 'unsound mind' as the meaning of this term is continually evolving (*Winterwerp* v. *the Netherlands* 1979: 37). REC(2004)10 suggests that 'mental disorder' should be defined 'in accordance with internationally accepted medical standards' such as ICD-10 (set out in Chapter V of the WHO's 2006 *International Statistical Classification of Diseases and Related Health Problems*).

The Salize Report found that while all the legislation stipulated a given and confirmed mental disorder as a major condition for detention, diagnostic criteria are rarely mentioned and when they are 'very global concepts are used' (1.11).

Detention and the MI Principles

The MI Principles provide for the detention ('involuntary admission') of individuals with a 'mental illness' in mental health facilities, setting out the conditions for such detention (Rule 16), the review of the decision to detain (Rule 17) and relevant procedural safeguards (Rule 18). However, commentators have raised concerns about the level of protection offered by the MI Principles criteria for detention (Rosenthal and Sundram 2003: 65) and it has been suggested that these need to be reviewed (United Nations 2003: para. 47).

Detention and the ECHR

ECHR case law relating to Article 5 has established some key requirements for the lawful detention of persons on the basis of 'unsound mind'. These are summarized below.

Lawfulness of the detention. In addition to conforming to the substantive and procedural rules of national law, save in emergencies, the following conditions must be satisfied (*Winterwerp* v. *the Netherlands* 1979):

- objective medical evidence must demonstrate to a competent national authority that the person is of 'unsound mind';
- the mental disorder must be of a kind or degree which warrants compulsory confinement;
- the validity of the continued confinement depends on the persistency of such a mental disorder.

Emergency cases. While the emergency detention 'of persons capable of presenting a danger to others' would justify detention for a short duration, continued detention is subject to objective medical evidence confirming that the conditions set in *Winterwerp* v. *the Netherlands* (above) are met (*X* v. *UK* 1981).

Reasons for detention. The individual must have a mental disorder warranting 'compulsory confinement'. While the detention must be in a 'suitable therapeutic environment', it can be justified either because the person needs treatment to cure or alleviate the condition, or the person needs control and supervision to prevent harm to self or to other persons (*Reid* v. *UK* 2003).

Least restrictive alternative. Detention is only justified where other less severe measures have been considered and found to be insufficient to safeguard the individual or public interest, which might require that the person be detained (*Witold Litwa* v. *Poland* 2001).

Detention must be in an appropriate institution. The detention of an individual on the basis of his or her mental disorder will only be lawful if it is in a hospital, clinic or other appropriate facility (*Ashingdane* v. *UK* 1985).

Provision of Information. The reasons for the detention must be given promptly to the detainee, in a language that the person can understand (Article 5(2)).

Review of the decision to detain. A regular periodic review by a 'court' (a judicial body which is independent of the executive and the parties concerned) must consider the conditions which are essential for the lawful detention of persons of unsound mind and have the power to discharge if the conditions for detention no longer apply (Article 5(4); *X* v. *UK* 1981). The initial review should take place soon after the detention – a period of just under eight weeks did not meet the requirements for the lawfulness of the detention to be considered 'speedily' (*E* v. *Norway* 1994). Relevant case law suggests individuals have a right to legal representation before the review hearings and that this is not dependent on the individual concerned requesting such legal representation (*Megyeri* v. *Germany* 1992; see also Thorold 1996: 627–8; Clements and Read 2003: 57) and the legal assistance provided must be adequate (*Pereira* v. *Portugal* 2002; see Lewis 2002b: 299).

Deferring discharge. Where the conditions for detention no longer exist, discharge from detention may be deferred in order to make arrangements for the individual's aftercare. However, the discharge must not be unreasonably delayed (*Johnson* v. *UK* 1999).

Providing a legal framework for detention on the basis of mental disorder

The substantive and procedural safeguards, suggested by ECHR case law and outlined above will need to be addressed when drafting legislation providing for the detention of individuals on the grounds of mental disorder. REC(2004)10 provides further guidance which will be of assistance to legislators. Article 17(1) sets out the conditions which must be met (save in an emergency) if a person is to be subject to 'involuntary placement':

- the person has a mental disorder;
- the person's condition represents a significant risk of harm to his or her health or to other persons;

- the placement includes a therapeutic purpose;
- no less restrictive means of providing appropriate care are available; and
- the opinion of the person concerned has been taken into account.

Article 17(2) provides that individuals may be subject to involuntary placement in order to determine whether they have a mental disorder if they present a risk of serious harm to self or others. Article 20 states that the decision to subject a person to involuntary placement should be taken by a court or 'another competent body' (which is defined as 'an authority, or a person or body provided by law which is distinct from the person or body proposing an involuntary measure, and that can make an independent decision'). Paragraph 151 of the Explanatory Memorandum states: 'The underlying principle is that a party that is independent of the person or body proposing the measure takes an independent decision. The body that takes the decision must be satisfied that the criteria in Article 17 are met'.

Treatment: capacity, consent and involuntary treatment

Neither the ICCPR nor the ECHR make specific reference to treatment without consent, save that Article 7 of the ICCPR prohibits medical or scientific experiments without the individual's free consent. While an analysis of human rights instruments suggests a general consensus that treatment without consent can be given only in exceptional circumstances, in most of the instruments these circumstances are either not described or are ill-defined.

Consent to treatment and UN human rights instruments

The treaty-monitoring body for the ICESCR states that compulsory treatment can be given for mental illness in exceptional cases but such interventions should be subject to specific and restrictive conditions which comply with 'best practices' and 'applicable international standards', including the MI Principles (ICESCR GC 14 2000: para. 34). However, it is not clear what is meant by either 'best practice' or 'applicable international standards'.

Furthermore, the MI Principles have been criticized for providing inadequate protection in this area. While the MI Principles state that treatment should not be given without the individual's consent, what might appear to be a right to consent to (and accordingly, refuse) treatment is subject to a range of exceptions that 'appear to be more a long enumeration of authorized restrictions that can be imposed on this right, than as an expression of a true intention to recognize the right' (Gendreau 1997: 277). Rosenthal and Sundram (2003) note that under MI Principle 11 an 'independent authority' may order the compulsory treatment of detained patients, but the MI Principles neither define what would constitute such a body nor provide for any procedural protections for people whose decisions have been overridden by this body. The UN Report (2003: para. 45) notes that the MI Principles do not include an explicit right to refuse treatment for individuals detained in psychiatric facilities and that 'the generous exceptions to this right contained in principle 11 deprive it of real meaning'.

Consent to treatment and Council of Europe human right instruments

Bioethics Convention
Issues relating to consent to treatment are addressed by the Convention for the Protection of Human Rights and Dignity of the Human Being and Medicine: Convention on Human Rights and Biomedicine 1997 ('the Bioethics Convention'). It states, as a 'general rule' that a health intervention may only be carried out after the person concerned has given free and informed consent to it (although the personal representative of an individual who lacks capacity to make treatment decisions may consent to treatment on that person's behalf). However, Article 7 provides that individuals may be given treatment without their consent if they have a mental disorder of a serious nature, the intervention is aimed at treating the mental disorder and without treatment serious harm is likely to result in the person's health. Furthermore, Article 26 allows individuals to be treated without their consent if, for example, this was considered necessary to 'protect other people's rights and freedoms'. Paragraph 151 of the Explanatory Report to the Bioethics Convention explains: 'A person who may, due to his or her mental disorder, be a possible source of serious harm to others may, according to the law, be subjected to a measure of confinement or treatment without his or her consent'.

Although the Bioethics Convention states that the circumstances in which compulsory treatment is given for a mental disorder must be subject to safeguards, none are specified. It is also worrying that there is no requirement for safeguards to be provided in relation to compulsory treatment on the basis of protecting others under Article 26. Any such intervention would have to be justified under Article 8 of the ECHR (the right to private and family life). This is discussed below under the heading 'The ECHR and compulsory treatment for mental disorder'.

CPT Standards and REC(2004)10
The CPT states that all individuals in psychiatric institutions should have the opportunity to refuse treatment and that 'any derogation from this fundamental principle should be based upon law and only relate to clearly and strictly defined exceptional circumstances'; but provides no further explanation. However, REC(2004)10 offers more detailed guidance on the circumstances in which treatment without consent will be justified. Article 18 states that a person should be subject to involuntary treatment only if the individual has a mental disorder which 'represents a significant risk of serious harm to his or her health or to other persons', less intrusive means of providing appropriate care are not available and 'the opinion of the person concerned has been taken into consideration'. Article 20 requires that the decision to provide treatment without consent is taken by a court or 'competent body', save that if the person is detained, the decision may be taken by a doctor 'having the requisite competence and experience, after examination of the person concerned and taking into account his or her opinion'. The recommendations set out various procedural requirements such as providing the person with information (verbally and in writing) about their rights and remedies open to them (Article 22) and

ensuring that individuals can exercise their right to appeal against such decisions (Article 25).

Treatment without consent and detention – separate issues?

Both the UN Report 2003 (para. 45) and the CPT Standards distinguish between decisions concerning detention and those relating to treatment without consent. For example, the CPT Standards state that 'the admission of a person to a psychiatric establishment on an involuntary basis should not be construed as authorizing treatment without his consent' (para. 41).

However, the WHO states that this remains a controversial area, with some arguing that two separate procedures could act as a barrier to, or delay, treatment (WHO 2003: 3.1.5). Paragraph 150 of the Explanatory Memorandum to REC(2004)10 states that the procedures for detention and treatment without consent should be considered separately, although 'the fact that both types of measure might be considered at the same time is not excluded', adding, 'Thus, in administrative terms, a decision on involuntary placement and a decision on involuntary treatment may be combined in a single administrative or judicial decision and subject to a single appeal procedure'.

The Salize Report (Salize *et al.* 2002: 1.22) notes that seven of the 15 EU member states studied have separate procedures for 'involuntary placement and involuntary treatment', and comments that such a distinction may increase awareness for safeguarding patients' rights when applying coercive interventions.

In relation to 'compulsory outpatient treatment', only four of the states include this in their legislation but this may be because 'the efficacy of coercive outpatient treatment has not yet been confirmed by research (Salize *et al.* 2002: 1.27). ECHR case law suggests that such powers do not, *per se*, breach rights under the ECHR but that the manner in which they are exercised may do so (Davidson *et al.* 2003).

ECHR and compulsory treatment for mental disorder

Although it has not as yet adjudicated on this issue, when considering the provision of treatment for a physical disorder, the European Court of Human Rights commented: 'the imposition of medical treatment, without the consent of a mentally competent adult patient, would interfere with a person's physical integrity in a manner capable of engaging the rights protected under Article 8 § 1 of the Convention' (*Pretty* v. *United Kingdom* 2002).

Compulsory treatment issues may engage other ECHR articles in addition to Article 8. For example, in *Herczegfalvy* v. *Austria* (1992), the European Court considered whether the treatment given to the complainant amounted to a breach of Article 3 (freedom from torture, inhuman and degrading treatment or punishment). Although finding that a measure which is of therapeutic necessity cannot be regarded as inhuman or degrading, the Court stressed that the medical necessity for such treatment must be convincingly shown to exist.

A recent case before the English courts has highlighted the relevance of the ECHR to the issue of compulsory treatment for mental disorder. Although finding in this particular case that treatment could be given to the patient despite his or her competency to refuse it, the Court considered that the compulsory treatment of a competent patient has the potential to breach Articles 8 and 3, even if the proposed treatment complies with the legislative requirements. In deciding whether treatment could be given in these circumstances, the Court considered factors such as the consequences of the patient not receiving the proposed treatment, its possible side-effects and whether there were any other less invasive treatments (*R on the application of PS and others* 2003).

Consent to treatment: issues for legislators

Given the lack of consensus on the circumstances in which treatment without consent may be given, this issue will need to be explored at national level before legislation is introduced. Such dialogue should take into account that treatment without consent relates to two different situations.

Incapacity
The individual concerned lacks the capacity to decide whether to accept or refuse the treatment, but it is proposed to give the treatment in the absence of the person's consent. In such situations the following questions are relevant:

- How is the person's capacity to make treatment decisions determined and who should be involved in this decision?
- On what basis can the treatment be given and who should be involved in making this decision? For example, will this apply to all treatment or just treatment for mental disorder?
- Will there be any restrictions on the types of treatment that can be given or any special safeguards for certain treatments? For example, providing that psychosurgery cannot be given without consent, specifying in what circumstances (if any) electroconvulsive therapy (ECT) can be given without consent and prohibiting 'unmodified' ECT.
- Will an 'advance directive' (also referred to as a 'psychiatric will') be respected? The Salize Report (Salize *et al.* 2002: 3.4) describes this term as 'the predefined instructions of a patient about the preference or refusal of certain treatments or interventions in the event of any later incapacity to decide due to their mental state', but definitions may vary. If included in legislation, a clear definition of the term must be provided, in addition to the conditions which must be met in order for such a directive to be valid.

Competent refusal
The individual has the capacity to make decisions about treatment and is refusing such treatment, but it is proposed to give the treatment despite the individual's refusal. In such situations the following questions are relevant:

- Will the compulsory treatment provisions only apply to treatment for mental disorder?
- In what circumstances can the individual's refusal be overridden? For example, where there is risk to others? Risk of harm to self? The person presents a suicide risk? Or risk to the health of the individual (for example, the person's health will deteriorate if not given the treatment)?

- As discussed under 'Incapacity', will there be any restrictions on the types of treatment that can be given or any special safeguards for certain treatments?
- As discussed under 'Incapacity', will an 'advance directive/refusal' be respected?

The legislation must ensure that the limited circumstances in which treatment can be given without consent are clearly set out and such provisions are accompanied by appropriate safeguards. Legislation should also provide a definition of 'consent' so that it is clear that consent is only valid when it is freely given and 'informed', which would include requirements such as the patient understanding 'the purpose, nature, likely effects and risks of the treatment including the likelihood of its success and any alternatives to it' (DH 1999: 15.13). The WHO (2005b: 7) calls upon states to consider introducing legal rights for people subject to involuntary care to choose their independent advocate.

Safeguarding the rights of people receiving care in psychiatric facilities

In addition to considering general guidelines for the provision of mental health care, specific safeguards will be required in order protect individuals receiving care in psychiatric facilities, particularly those who are detained, as they will be especially vulnerable to abuse. Key issues to be addressed when developing legislation, policies and guidance on standards of care and other measures to safeguard individuals' rights are outlined below.

General issues

REC(2004)10 sets out a range of areas which should be considered in relation to the provision of mental heath care. For example:

- *Health service provision (Article 10)*. Taking into account available resources, states should take measures to provide a range of services of appropriate quality to meet the mental health needs of persons with a mental disorder, and ensure equitable access to such services. Alternatives to detention and compulsory treatment should be as widely available as possible.
- *Treatment plans (Article 12)*. Treatment and care should be provided to individuals with a mental disorder by adequately qualified staff and based on an appropriate individually prescribed treatment plan. Wherever possible the treatment plan should be prepared in consultation with the person concerned. His or her opinion should be taken into account and the plan regularly reviewed and revised if necessary. (The need for individuals to have their own care plan, which is based on their particular needs and regularly reviewed is also emphasized by the MI Principles and the CPT standards.)
- *Confidentiality and record-keeping (Article 13)*. All personal data (such as medical records, which should be maintained for individuals receiving treatment for a mental disorder) relating to individuals with a mental disorder should be treated as confidential: 'Such data may only be collected, processed and

communicated according to the rules relating to professional confidentiality and personal data protection'.

- *Quality assurance and monitoring (Articles 36–7).* States should ensure compliance with the standards set out in REC(2004)10 and mental health law. Monitoring should include conducting visits and inspections of mental health facilities and ensuring that complaints procedures are provided, and that complaints are responded to in an appropriate way. Monitoring systems should involve a range of individuals including mental health professionals and individuals with mental disorders. The CPT standards recommend that there should be an effective complaints procedure, with arrangements for formal complaints to be lodged with a clearly designated body, and for patients to be able to communicate on a confidential basis with an appropriate body outside the establishment.

Conditions of detention, care and treatment

Environment
Governments must ensure that the conditions of detention are suitable. In *Aerts* v. *Belgium* (1998) the European Court of Human Rights held that the failure to provide either medical attention or a therapeutic environment breached Article 5 of the ECHR (the right to liberty). The CPT Standards highlight the importance of creating a 'positive therapeutic environment'; for example, providing sufficient living space for each patient and maintaining the state of repair and hygiene requirements. In addition, respect for the privacy and dignity of patients must be ensured by providing lockable space for patients to keep their possessions and ensuring that sanitary facilities allow the patients some privacy.

Provision of care
The CPT Standards stress that irrespective of resources, basic necessities, including adequate food, heating, clothing and appropriate medication must be provided for both voluntarily- and involuntarily-placed patients. There should also be adequate numbers of staff with the necessary qualifications, training and experience.

Protecting the rights of detainees

States must ensure that detainees are 'treated with humanity and with respect for the inherent dignity of the human person' and are not subjected to any hardship or constraint other than that resulting from the deprivation of liberty (Article 10, ICCPR 1992 and ICCPR GC 21 1992).

Both the ECHR and the ICCPR prohibit the arbitrary interference in individuals' private and family lives. An interference with Article 8 (right to respect for private and family life) will only be justified if certain criteria are met – for example, that the interference complies with national law, its purpose is to protect one of the specified interests such as the protection of health, and the interference does not exceed what is strictly necessary to achieve that purpose (the principle of proportionality).

Article 8 covers a broad range of areas relevant to detainees, such as the administration of medical treatment, personal searches, receiving and sending correspondence, mixed-sex wards and/or bathroom facilities, access to health and personal records, contact with family and friends and the duty of confidentiality (staff must be required to keep personal information relating to detainees confidential).

The CPT Standards recommend that individuals in mental health facilities should be able to send and receive correspondence, to have access to a telephone, and to receive visits from family and friends. They should also be able to have confidential access to a lawyer. REC(2004)10 seeks to reflect these points, stating that individuals' rights to communicate with their lawyers, representatives or appropriate authority should not be unreasonably restricted. The Explanatory Memorandum to REC(2004)10 makes clear that any such restrictions should only be in exceptional circumstances, such as to prevent a criminal offence.

Given that people confined in institutions are particularly vulnerable to abuses of their basic rights, the CPT has recommended that regular visits should be made to psychiatric establishments by an independent outside body. REC(2004)10 has adopted some specific recommendations of the CPT in relation to such monitoring. Thus, Article 37 states that those involved in monitoring should be able to meet privately with individuals who are subject to the provisions of mental health law and receive confidential complaints from such individuals.

The CPT also recommends that detainees and their families should be given an introductory brochure setting out the psychiatric facility's routine and the patients' rights.

Protection of life and prevention of ill-treatment

Given the vulnerable position of detainees, authorities are under a duty to protect them from harm. For example, the CPT Standards state that appropriate procedures must be in place to protect patients from other patients who may cause them harm and there should be adequate numbers of staff present at all times.

Case law under the ECHR has established that states have a duty to protect the health of detainees (*Hurtado* v. *Switzerland* 1994) and that the lack of medical treatment may amount to treatment contrary to Article 3 (prohibition of torture and inhuman and degrading treatment and punishment) (*Ilhan* v. *Turkey* 2002). Furthermore, Article 2 (the right to life) can impose a duty to take preventative measures to 'diminish the opportunities of self-harm' (*Keenan* v. *United Kingdom* 2001). An independent investigation must take place where a person has died in circumstances which might amount to a breach of Article 2 or has an arguable claim that the individual has been seriously ill-treated in breach of Article 3. Such an investigation must be capable of leading to the identification and punishment of those responsible (*Assenov & Others* v. *Bulgaria* 1998).

In *Keenan* v. *United Kingdom* (2001) the European Court of Human Rights held that there had been a lack of both effective monitoring and informed psychiatric input into the assessment and treatment of a 28-year-old prisoner, known to have a mental illness and be at risk of suicide. The failure to respond adequately to the prisoner's deteriorating condition amounted to inhuman and degrading treatment, and punishment within the meaning of Article 3 of the ECHR.

In determining whether punishment or treatment is 'degrading' the European Court usually considers whether there was any *intention* to humiliate or debase the person concerned. However, *Price* v. *United Kingdom* (2001) held that the police and the prison authorities were in breach of Article 3 due to their failure to provide adequate facilities for a woman with severe physical disabilities, even though there was no intention to humiliate or debase her. This is significant given that, as Rosenthal and Sundram (2003) observe, most mental health professionals would not intentionally cause harm or suffering to individuals.

Conclusion

As this chapter has sought to demonstrate, a human rights perspective to mental health policy should be integral to its development. The application of human rights principles not only enables governments to comply with their obligations under international human rights treaties but also assists in the development of mental health policy and the identification of areas in which legislation will be required to support the policy. For example, when considering the use of powers to detain individuals on the grounds of their mental disorder, a human rights approach requires not only that legislation ensures that such powers only apply in strictly defined circumstances, with appropriate safeguards in place to protect the rights of individuals subjected to such powers, but also highlights the need for legislation and policies that facilitate the provision of community-based services as alternatives to institutionalized care. Similarly, addressing the barriers to social inclusion is not only essential in protecting the rights of people with mental health problems, for example against unfair discrimination, but is likely to be necessary for the successful implementation of policies to develop community-based services.

More fundamentally, if mental health policy – and the legislation to support such a policy – is to make a real difference to the lives of people with mental health problems and those who care for, and about them, then a human rights approach must be central to its development and implementation. This is because a human rights perspective highlights the importance of enabling people with mental health problems to participate in society as equal citizens – and that must surely be the ultimate goal of any mental health policy.

Note

1   The author thanks Luke Clements, John Horne, Judith Klein and Arman Vardanyan for their helpful comments on earlier drafts of this chapter.

References

Alston, P. and Crawford, J. (2000) *The Future of UN Human Rights Treaty Monitoring.* Cambridge: Cambridge University Press.

Amnesty International (2003) *Bulgaria, Far from the Eyes of Society: Systematic Discrimination against People with Mental Disabilities.* London: Amnesty International.

Carrier, J. and Kendall, I. (1997) Evolution of Policy, in J. Leff (ed.) *Care in the Community, Illusion or Reality?* Chichester: Wiley.

Churchill, R. and Khaliq, U. (2004) The collective complaints system of the European Social Charter: an effective mechanism for ensuring compliance with economic and social rights? *European Journal of International Law*, 15(3): 417–56.

Clements, L. and Read, J. (2003) *Disabled People and European Human Rights: A Review of the Implications of the 1998 Human Rights Act for Disabled Children and Adults in the UK.* Bristol: The Policy Press.

Commission of the European Communities (2005) *Proposal for a Council Regulation Establishing a European Union Agency for Fundamental Rights.* Brussels: 30.06.2005, COM(2005)280 final, 2005/0124 (CNS) 2005/0125 (CNS).

Council Directive 2000/78/EC (2000) Establishing a general framework for equal treatment in employment and occupation, OJ L303/16.

Council Directive 2000/43/EC (2000) Implementing the principle of equal treatment between persons irrespective of race or ethnic origin, OJ L180/22.

Council of Europe (1999) *Recommendation No R(99)4 of the Committee of Ministers to Member States on Principles Concerning the Legal Protection of Incapable Adults.* Strasbourg: Council of Europe.

Council of Europe (2003) *Recommendation 1592: Towards Full Social Inclusion of People with Disabilities.* Parliamentary Assembly, Council of Europe. Strasbourg: Council of Europe.

Council of Europe (2004) *Recommendation No REC(2004)10 of the Committee of Ministers Concerning the Protection of the Human Rights and Dignity of Persons with a Mental Disorder and its Explanatory Memorandum.* Strasbourg: Council of Europe.

Council of the European Union (2002) *European Union Annual Report on Human Rights 2002.* Luxembourg: Office for Official Publications of the European Communities.

Davidson, G., McCallion, M. and Potter, M. (2003) *Connecting Mental Health and Human Rights.* Belfast: Northern Irish Human Rights Commission.

DH (Department of Health and Welsh Office) (1999) *Mental Health Act 1983 Code of Practice.* London: The Stationery Office.

Enable (2005) Overview of international legal framework for disability legislation, 2004, www.un.org/esa/socdev/enable/disovlf.htm (accessed 7 March 2005).

European Commission, Employment and Social Affairs (2003) *Annual Report on Equality and Non-discrimination 2003, Towards Diversity.* Luxembourg: Office for Official Publications of the European Communities.

European Communities (2004) *A Constitution for Europe, Constitution Adopted by Heads of State and Government – Presentation to Citizens.* Luxembourg: Office for Official Publications of the European Communities.

European Disability Forum (EDF) (2003) *The EDF Proposal for a Disability Specific Directive,* see www.edf-feph.org/en/policy/nondiscrim/nond_pol.htm (accessed 7 March 2005).

Freyhoff, G., Parker, C., Coué, M. and Grieg, N. (2004) *Included in Society – Results and Recommendations of the European Research Initiative on Community-based Residential Alternatives for Disabled People.* (Supported by the European Commission). Brussels: European Coalition for Community Living.

Gendreau, C. (1997) The rights of psychiatric patients in the light of the principles announced by the United Nations: a recognition of the right to consent to treatment? *International Journal of Law and Psychiatry*, 20(2): 259–78.

ICCPR GC 18 (1989) *International Covenant on Civil and Political Rights, General Comment 18, Non-discrimination.*

ICCPR GC 20 (1992) *International Covenant on Civil and Political Rights, General Comment 20, Article 7.*

ICCPR GC 21 (1992) *International Covenant on Civil and Political Rights, General Comment 21*, Article 9 (replaces general comment 9 concerning humane treatment of persons deprived of liberty) (Article 10).

ICCPR GC 31 (2004) *International Covenant on Civil and Political Rights, General Comment 31*, Article 2, Implementation at the national level.

ICESCR GC 3 (1990) *International Covenant on Economic, Social and Cultural Rights, General Comment 3*, The nature of states parties obligations.

ICESCR GC 5 (1994) *International Covenant on Economic, Social and Cultural Rights, General Comment 5*, Persons with disabilities.

ICESCR GC 14 (2000) *International Covenant on Economic, Social and Cultural Rights, General Comment 14*, The right to the highest attainable standard of health (Article 12).

Inclusion Europe (2003) *Justice, Rights and Inclusion for People with Intellectual Disability.* Brussels: Inclusion Europe.

JCHR (Joint Committee on Human Rights) (2004) *The International Covenant on Economic, Social and Cultural Rights*, 21st Report of Session 2003–4, HL Paper 183.

Jenkins, R., McCulloch, A., Friedli, L. and Parker, C. (2002) *Developing a National Mental Health Policy*. Hove: Psychology Press.

Lewis, O. (2002a) Mental disability law in central and eastern Europe: paper, practice, promise, *Journal of Mental Health Law*, 8 (December): 293–303.

Lewis, O. (2002b) Protecting the rights of people with mental disabilities: the European Convention on Human Rights, *European Journal of Health Law*, 9(4): 293–320.

Mental Disability Advocacy Center (MDAC) (2003) *Cage Beds, Inhuman and Degrading Treatment in Four Accession Countries*. Budapest: MDAC.

O'Flaherty, M. (2002) *Human Rights and the UN: Practice Before the Treaty Bodies*, 2nd edn. The Netherlands: Kluwer International.

Quinn, G. (2001) The European Union and the Council of Europe on the issue of human rights: twins separated at birth? *McGill Law Journal*, 46: 849.

Quinn, G. and Degener, T. with Bruce, A., Burke, C., Castellino, J., Kenna, P., Kilkelly, U. and Quinlivan, S. (2002) *Human Rights and Disability: The Current Use and Future Potential of United Nations Human Rights Instruments in the Context of Disability*, www.unhchr.ch/disability/hrstudy.htm.

Rosenthal, E. and Sundram, C.J. (2003)*International Human Rights and Mental Health Legislation*. Geneva: World Health Organization.

Salize, H., Drefsing, H. and Peitz, M. (2002) *Compulsory Admission and Involuntary Treatment of Mentally Ill Patients – Legislation and Practice in EU Member States*. Brussels: European Commission.

Sayce, L. (2000) *From Psychiatric Patient to Citizen – Overcoming Discrimination and Social Exclusion*. Basingstoke: Palgrave.

Starmer, K. (1999) *European Human Rights Law, The Human Rights Act 1998 and the European Convention on Human Rights*. London: Legal Action Group.

Thorold, O. (1996) The implications of the European Convention on Human Rights for United Kingdom mental health legislation, *European Human Rights Law Review*, 6: 619–36.

United Nations (2003) *Report of the Secretary-General: Progress of efforts to ensure the full recognition of the human rights of persons with disabilities*, A/58/181. New York: United Nations.

Williams, A. (2004) *EU Human Rights Policies – A Study in Irony*. Oxford: Oxford University Press.

World Health Organization (2001) *The World Health Report – Mental Health: New Understanding, New Hope*. Geneva: World Health Organization.

World Health Organization (2003) *Mental Health Policy and Service Guidance Package: Mental Health Legislation and Human Rights*. Geneva: World Health Organization.

World Health Organization (2005a) *Mental Health Declaration for Europe – Facing Challenges, Building Solutions*. Geneva: World Health Organization.

World Health Organization (2005b) *Mental Health Action Plan for Europe – Facing Challenges, Building Solutions*. Geneva: World Health Organization.

World Health Organization (2005c) *Resource Book on Mental Health, Human Rights and Legislation*. Geneva: World Health Organization.

World Health Organization (2006) *International Statistics Classification of Diseases and Related Health Problems*. Geneva: World Health Organization.

Cases

European Court of Human Rights

Aerts v. *Belgium* (1998) 29 EHRR 50

Ashingdane v. *United Kingdom* (1985) 7 EHRR 528

Assenov & Others v. *Bulgaria* (1998) 28 EHRR 652

E v. *Norway* (1994) 17 EHRR 30

Herczegfalvy v. *Austria* (1992) 15 EHRR 437

HL v. *United Kingdom* (2004) Application no. 45508/99, 5 October 2004

Hurtado v. *Switzerland* A/280-A (1994) (unreported)

Ilhan v. *Turkey* (2002) 34 EHHR 36

Johnson v. *United Kingdom* (1999) 27 EHRR 196

Keenan v. *United Kingdom* (2001) 33 EHRR 39

Kutzner v. *Germany* 46544/99; 26 February 2002

Witold Litwa v. *Poland* (2001) 33 EHRR 53

Megyeri v. *Germany* (1992) 15 EHRR 584

Pereira v. *Portugal* (2002) Application No. 44872/98

Pretty v. *United Kingdom* (2002) 35 EHRR 1

Price v. *United Kingdom* (2001) 34 EHRR 1285

Reid v. *United Kingdom* (2003) Application 50272/99

Winterwerp v. *Netherlands* (1979) 2 EHRR 387

X v. *United Kingdom* (1981) 4 EHRR 188

Other cases

Olmstead v. *LC* (1999) 527 US 581

R on the application of PS and others (2003) EWHC 2335

chapter fourteen

The user and survivor movement in Europe

Diana Rose and Jo Lucas

Introduction

This chapter explores the role of user involvement in mental health policy and practice both at a European level and across selected countries. The issues we seek to elucidate are: the history of the user movement; its activities (i.e. what groups do); and whether or not these groups are user-controlled. We then briefly comment on the role users can play in research and what influence they have, if any, on policy.

User involvement in mental health is one of the most exciting and innovative developments in the field of psychiatry. It empowers individual service users and enables them to organize collectively. Historically, users of mental health services did not have such a voice but this has been changing with involvement growing in a number of countries in recent years (Wallcraft *et al.* 2003; Rush 2004; Campbell 2005; Chamberlin 2005).

Clearly, moving towards greater user involvement is not without tensions with other stakeholders. When a disempowered group finds its voice and formulates a position from which to develop change, there will always be obstacles. While never underestimating the newly-found power of users, this chapter will also describe some of the hurdles that are still to be overcome.

In addition to the strong ethical and democratic imperatives for user involvement in the planning and delivery of activities, there is also an increasing, albeit still limited, body of evidence supporting the vital contribution that service users can make to mental health research. Indeed, service users may be better placed than professionals to assess how services address their needs (Thornicroft and Tansella 2005). It also has been shown, for example, that users report less satisfaction with services when interviewed by other service users (Simpson and House 2002). User involvement in research can also have benefits for the individuals involved, including the acquisition of new skills and knowledge, a sense of empowerment and being valued, and a better understanding and relation-ship with other researchers (Allam *et al.* 2004).

User involvement can take place at the European level as well as in individual countries. The mandate that the European Union (EU) has to intervene to pro-mote social inclusion, eliminate discrimination, protect human rights and promote good health and well-being (see Chapter 13) provides opportunities for active user involvement at a pan-European level. Unfortunately, user involve-ment at this level today exists mostly in the virtual realm due to a lack of funding, and more generally, user involvement across Europe is very unevenly developed. This is partly due to differing social, economic and political condi-tions in the various regions, and differs from the disability movement which seems to be more well accepted and active at an EU level (e.g. the European Disability Forum).

Another factor influencing the level and nature of user involvement is the way in which mental health services are provided. On the one hand, the transi-tion to community care appears to facilitate the rise of user groups. On the other, harsh involuntary treatment legislation and practice appears to give rise to sympathetic professionals, including lawyers, forming non-user initiated groups to change these practices. One exception to this pattern is the Nether-lands where there is a strong (albeit divided) user movement, even though men-tal health provision remains largely hospital-based.

These structural differences in the way groups are formed present challenges when seeking to map user groups across Europe. Those familiar with the situ-ation in the United Kingdom will know that a 'user group' is usually defined as a group whose members are users only and/or where the major decisions are taken by service users. This is not necessarily the case in all European countries. Groups may involve families (indeed they may be primarily groups of family members), sympathetic professionals and interested members of the general public. In the email survey for this chapter (see below) we included a question on whether or not groups were user-controlled, where this was defined as users controlling decision-making in an organization. Few groups outside the United Kingdom answered this question, which may indicate that this concept is not known to them.

Another challenge is that in most western European countries (but not all), groups are organized at both the national, regional and local levels. Such struc-tures are well developed, for instance in Sweden, Denmark, France and Austria among others, where local and regional groups are often affiliated to national organizations. The links in other countries are less clear. In many countries there also may be diagnosis-specific groups which again may be linked to national umbrella organizations. In France, for example, some diagnosis-specific groups are linked to the national French network of user organizations – FNAP PSY (Fédération Nationale des Associations de Patients et [ex] Patients 'PSY'). In the countries of eastern and central Europe there are no user groups with a national brief currently, although there are developments in both Lithuania and Georgia.

A final challenge in mapping the European scene is the sustainability and turnover of user groups. It is well known that user groups emerge and close down with some rapidity (Wallcraft *et al.* 2003). Even quite large organizations, such as FAPI (Forum Anti-Psychiatrischer Initiativen) operating in German-speaking countries, may not last forever. The main reason for closure would appear to be the struggle with long-term financial sustainability as groups are usually heavily reliant on public grants and support. However, it should be noted that some groups exist with no funding, relying solely on the goodwill, time and resources of volunteers.

It is important to end this introduction by briefly discussing terminology for those readers who are unfamiliar with the user movement. Terms used by groups and individuals reflect their philosophical stance towards psychiatry. 'User' tends to denote people who are still in receipt of services. 'Survivor' is used by those who feel that the psychiatric system is something to survive; one copes despite it, not because of it. Indeed, some people who are still 'users' nevertheless refer to themselves as survivors. When user groups are actually in a position to run and provide services they generally refer to people in receipt of these services as 'clients' or perhaps 'consumers' as these user-run services do offer a choice. In practice, words like 'client' or 'consumer' are rarely used. Many people still feel that psychiatric services within their own countries deny users choice. Poverty also can deny them the option of choosing private alternatives. 'Patient' is the least-used term, again as it is not associated with choice and also implies the use of the 'medical model' approach. In this chapter, these different terms will be used as the groups themselves use them.

Methods

The principal method used for gathering information for this chapter was largely through a search of internet resources, augmented by studies reported in the literature. The authors also relied on their personal knowledge. Diana Rose has been a member of the user/survivor movement in the United Kingdom since the mid-1980s. Jo Lucas is an independent consultant and former director of the Hamlet Trust. Mary Nettle, a British user board member of ENUSP (European Network of (ex) Users and Survivors of Psychiatry), was also interviewed and provided some documentation.

The key web resource used was that of ENUSP (www.enusp.org) and its two email lists. The website is mostly written in German but sections of it are accessible in English, Dutch, Finnish, French, Romanian and Spanish, with welcome screens in most other languages – although it is still advertising for users to translate parts of the site into other languages.

This diversity of languages is significant and has posed a difficulty in writing this chapter. While most professionals may accept that English is the international language of scientific and professional communication, this is not the case for users of mental health systems. Access to English language teaching or to opportunities to practise English learnt at school on an everyday basis is not common for many service users. In addition to this, native English speakers are well known to be lazy about learning other languages, making it difficult for us to understand information on websites such as that of ENUSP!

A further caveat lies in our emphasis on the internet. Access is likely to be denied to users in institutions or to those who live in poverty. User involvement activity may therefore go unrecorded because there is no internet participation. Indeed, although most of the local groups listed on the ENUSP website do now provide email access and often have websites, it is still true that for a significant minority only postal addresses are available.

Notwithstanding these limitations, information was initially gathered via a message posted on the ENUSP email list. This only generated three replies – from Sweden, the Netherlands and Bosnia and Herzegovina. Then, the ENUSP website was used. The website includes a list of user groups in all European countries who have provided details to the organization. This is not comprehensive and some countries have no entries. However, it appears to be the best source of information about user groups in Europe. Every national organization in each country was then emailed if they had an email address. Some regional and local groups were emailed as well. This strategy generated a much better response – from Sweden, Denmark, Norway, Germany, Switzerland, Spain, Lithuania and Georgia. Four groups seemed to have a non-working email address, which may indicate that they no longer exist.

The first author also relied on personal knowledge for the United Kingdom and the website information on France as this was comprehensive and comprehensible. The second author contributed information on central and eastern Europe to the chapter, relying on extensive knowledge gained while working in these countries, drawn largely from the experiences of one United Kingdom non-governmental organization (NGO).

There is also some literature upon which we can rely. For instance, Wallcraft *et al.* (2003) recently published a survey of the user/survivor movement in England; many of the issues discussed in their report are shared by users in other European countries. In addition, Peter Lehmann, former secretary of ENUSP, has written an unpublished report comparing user involvement in Austria, France, the Netherlands, Spain and the United Kingdom. There are also accounts of specific projects – for example, a project looking at the harassment of psychiatric service users – on the ENUSP website. Some groups, for example PSYCHEX in Switzerland, circulate their annual reports through the ENUSP email list.

History of the user movement in Europe

Although patient criticisms of psychiatric care go back at least to the nineteenth century, with the establishment by John Perceval of the Alleged Lunatics' Friends Society in 1845, the modern user movement in western Europe began to flourish in the 1960s and 1970s (Campbell 1996). It was linked to the anti-psychiatry writings of Laing (1959) and Szasz (1972) and appears to have been strongest in the Nordic countries, the Netherlands, the German-speaking countries and in the United Kingdom. Social upheavals, such as the protests of May 1968 in Paris and other cities around the world also played a role.

The oldest user groups started explicitly by users themselves emerged in the 1960s in Norway and Sweden. Denmark also has an NGO, which is not user-controlled but was started in similar circumstances around the same time. All of these groups welcomed supportive non-users as they developed. Today, the

Swedish organization RSMH (Riksforbundet for Social och Mental Halsa) has about 8000 members organized in 200 affiliated regional and local groups. The user groups in Sweden receive state funding, have salaried employees and provide services. User involvement in Norway is more dispersed, groups are smaller, but there is still state funding.

As noted above, even apparently well-established groups do not always survive forever. Networks such as the British Network for Alternatives to Psychiatry, active in the 1970s, were influenced by events in Italy where the Italian psychiatrist Basaglia made the first move to close down large institutions and provide community care. However, this gave way to the formation of user-only groups, prefigured by organizations like CAPO (Campaign Against Psychiatric Oppression) which were also active in the 1970s. Like the British Network, FAPI (Federation Antipsychiatrie) was a network critical of psychiatry in German-speaking countries. Established in 1989, it was involved in conferences and publishing but now only exists as an email list for individuals.

A further development was the establishment in the 1970s of Patients' Councils in hospitals in the Netherlands. Although the number of psychiatric beds in the Netherlands has recently declined, many users are still treated in hospitals for extensive periods of time. These Patients' Councils are now publicly funded. Some authors (Van Hoorn 1992) argue that this public funding and the associated legal framework have meant that the Patients' Councils have lost their radical edge. Nevertheless, historically speaking, the establishment of these Councils had a positive effect on the development of the user movement in the United Kingdom. In 1985, at a conference jointly organized by the World Federation of Mental Health and UK MIND, a representative of Patients' Councils from the Netherlands was instrumental in the establishment of the first such councils in England.

Over time, small local user groups also began to develop. The 1985 conference, for instance, was attended by a handful of the local user groups in existence in the United Kingdom at this time. Local user groups continued to emerge quickly as community care policies developed in the country. Indeed, groups often formed around the closure of specific hospitals and the resettlement policies for their residents. The group Survivors Speak Out was also formed. This national network, dedicated to the formation of independent user groups, in terms of today's user involvement activity in the United Kingdom, was politically radical, and it has been argued that the group was significant in ensuring that new actions were not all directed through large voluntary (non user-led) organizations (Campbell 2005). The group still exists, albeit in vestigial form.

The history of the user movement is somewhat different when turning to the countries of central and eastern Europe.[1] The history of mental health care in this region, and in the former Soviet Union in particular, is one of closed institutions (see also Chapter 17). Individuals who were different and could not fulfil the role of healthy workers were usually locked away either in hospitals or more often in social care homes (*internats*). Psychiatry was also subject to some political abuse, with mental illness being given as a reason for institutionalizing individuals with 'dangerous' political views. The high levels of stigma associated with poor mental health also meant that families often had no choice but to accept institutionalization as the best option. Given the history of purges and the movement of people in the former Soviet Union, it was often felt to be less risky for the whole family if the relative simply disappeared.

The practice of using caged beds in institutions remains common in many of these countries – even in the Czech Republic, Hungary and Slovenia, which have joined the EU. The report on such beds prepared by the Mental Disability Advocacy Centre (MDAC 2003) illustrated not only that they continue to exist but also that some professionals working in the mental health system (and politicians) do not see them as being problematic. In many of the countries of central and eastern Europe, the current system remains infused with a passive sense of acceptance of central control. However, this is beginning to change as individuals obtain improved access to information and resources, and realize that there are better alternatives.

In contrast to the long-standing emergence of user groups in western Europe, progress has been modest in the east. As we have noted, under the communist system that developed in many of these countries the very process of taking individual initiative, at best, was frowned upon. Consequently, this has meant that the local capacity to develop groups has been limited. Some international organizations have taken a role in trying to address this issue, including the Open Society Mental Health Initiative and the Hamlet Trust. This latter group was established in 1988 in the United Kingdom to work in a variety of ways with adults who have had mental health problems. The Trust aims to support the development of user-led and community-based alternatives to institutions and has prioritized the three areas of self-help, advocacy and employment as the foundations of this movement. The Trust was first invited to Poland around 1989, working with colleagues there to support the development of what became the Krakowska Fundacja Hamlet (KFH) in Krakow, the first member of the Hamlet's network. Over time, the Trust's network has expanded to involve some 52 NGOs in 18 countries. Of these, in 2004, around 8 were user-led or user-only while the rest involved users actively in a number of different roles.

User involvement at the European level

What of user involvement at a pan-European level? The first pan-European meeting of users and ex-users was held at Zandvoort in the Netherlands in 1991, funded jointly by the Dutch government and the European Commission. Forty-two representatives from 16 countries were present, mainly from northern Europe. The name of this organization at that point was the 'European Network of Users and Ex-Users in Mental Health', later to become ENUSP, the key group operating on a transnational basis (Hölling 2001). That meeting decided that the overall direction for the Network should lie with a bi-annual conference, with an elected board convening between conferences. A further feature of ENUSP was the creation of a 'European desk' serving as a point of information transmission. This was located first in the Netherlands and now in Germany. Extensive web and email forums arose from the work of the European desk.

Subsequent ENUSP conferences were held in Denmark (1994) and England (1997). By the time of the 1999 Luxembourg conference, 90 delegates were present, all of them (ex-) users and survivors, representing 26 European countries. In 1998 the network was legally incorporated, becoming a federation of *associations* of users and survivors. However, changes in rules governing NGO funding by the EU meant that between 1999 and 2004 no conferences were held. Under these rules ENUSP could only attract funding in partnership with other organizations and not simply to fund its own conferences. However, the organization continued to hold web-based board meetings and finally was able to hold its fifth congress in Denmark in July 2004.

The protection of human rights remains a fundamental concern of the user movement and ENUSP places human rights at the centre of its approach to mental health. The organization is committed to improving the status of people who are involuntarily detained and treated – i.e. coerced by the psychiatric system. The network campaigns for advanced directives or 'psychiatric wills'. These set out how an individual wishes to be treated in the event that they are unable to make clear their choices at the time of a future emergency, and have been shown in at least one randomized study to reduce the need for compulsory treatment and admission (Henderson *et al.* 2004). The ENUSP campaign has had some successes; for instance, users in Germany have succeeded in preventing new legislation that would have permitted compulsory treatment in the community.

Chapter 13 has set out some of the existing legal safeguards and international conventions applying to service users. The user movement, including ENUSP, devotes much energy to seeking to further tighten human rights legislation with respect to psychiatric service users. This includes not only the European Convention on Human Rights but also global treaties. However, some in the user movement regard the European Convention as a piece of hypocrisy when it comes to mental health. The Convention was drafted in the early 1950s and excludes 'persons of unsound mind' from many of its provisions.

One other principle activity for ENUSP and many of its constituent organizations is the development of anti-stigma and public education campaigns (see Chapter 3). This can be very difficult in countries where the majority of people using mental health services may be hidden away from view in large institutions.

It is important for all NGOs to have good lines of communication to a range of stakeholders. ENUSP has recognized the importance of effective communication with the media, having built up expertise in this area, and also with other stakeholder groups. This can be illustrated by the substantial presence of ENUSP and many of its member organizations at the 2002 Leipzig conference of the World Federation of Mental Health, a body representing psychiatrists from around the world.

ENUSP is affiliated to, or lobbies, many organizations at both the European and global levels. These include the European Commission, the NGO Mental Health Europe, the World Health Organization (WHO) Regional Office for Europe, the World Network of Users and Survivors of Psychiatry (WNUSP), the United Nations (UN) (Ad Hoc Committee Convention on Persons with Disabilities) and the WHO worldwide. However, ENUSP is constrained by limited resources in what it can do. It receives no funding from the above-mentioned international organizations, other than for special projects run in conjunction with these organizations. It is not a rich organization and relies on the dedication of a few individuals.

Activities of user groups

Turning now to the different organizations affiliated to ENUSP, as has already been mentioned, user involvement across Europe has developed very unevenly. Table 14.1 provides information on the number of groups known to ENUSP. Only seven countries in ENUSP have not reported any user groups, while much activity can now be seen in many of the countries of central and eastern Europe. France, the United Kingdom, the Netherlands and Spain provide the most links to groups.

Table 14.1 may, however, be biased because five of the countries with 11 or more groups were part of a specific study conducted by Peter Lehmann (who manages the website) and thus more information may have been collected from these locations. Another limitation of this analysis is that it cannot take account of the size of individual groups. Some countries, which have only a few groups (notably Sweden and Denmark), in fact have very high membership levels with thousands of members organized at national, regional and local level. Finally, the list is clearly far from comprehensive at least as far as local groups go; in England alone it has been reported that there are over 700 user-controlled groups (Wallcraft *et al.* 2003). One study in London alone identified 74 user groups in the city, with groups having between 5 and 200 members (Crawford *et al.* 2003).

User involvement can take place in a number of ways. Key identified activities of these groups include self-help, the provision of services outside the statutory sector, advocacy, anti-stigma and public education initiatives, creative activities

Table 14.1 Number of user groups known to ENUSP

Number	Countries
No Groups	Andorra, Croatia, Cyprus, Latvia San Marino, Serbia & Montenegro, Turkey
1	Albania, Azerbaijan, Belarus, Faroe Islands, Iceland, Liechtenstein, FYR Macedonia, Malta, Slovakia, Sweden
2–5	Armenia, Belgium, Bulgaria, Czech Republic, Denmark, Finland, Georgia, Greece, Hungary, Lithuania, Luxembourg, Moldova, Portugal, Russian Federation, Ukraine
6–10	Bosnia and Herzegovina, Estonia, Ireland, Norway, Poland, Romania, Slovenia
11–20	Austria, Germany, Italy, Switzerland
21–30	Netherlands, Spain
30+	France, United Kingdom

Source: ENUSP (2005)

and lobbying/political activism to influence policy and practice. They can also be involved as stakeholders in the planning and delivery of services by the statutory sectors. One final area where data was not collected, but which is important for user involvement, is that of research, where the United Kingdom would seem to be leading the way in service user-led research activities. Service user researchers may either be professional researchers or alternatively may be lay individuals who receive research training enabling them to undertake such work. This is discussed briefly later in the chapter.

Funding is of course a major determinant of what groups can do. Large groups such as those in the Nordic countries and the Netherlands receive substantial funding from their national governments. In the United Kingdom, groups are mostly funded through local government, in addition to support from charitable monies – for example, through grants from the National Lottery. This funding is often insufficient and insecure, with groups having to apply and reapply for money on an annual basis. Where the user movement is less developed, groups tend to be part of larger NGOs. Some groups, of course, have no funding at all and rely on the goodwill of volunteers.

Self-help and mutual support

The main activity of most user groups across the whole of Europe is self-help and mutual support, where users share their experiences and create a place to support each other, develop self-confidence, learn skills and ways of coping, and share knowledge. In the United Kingdom for instance, 69 per cent of user groups provide such activities (Wallcraft *et al.* 2003). Small self-help groups, where people meet regularly, can have a profound impact on their lives, and one advantage of this system is that it costs virtually nothing, even though finding the rent for a meeting space can be a problem for many such small groups. Larger organizations, for example in Sweden, may run drop-ins and social clubs. Forms of self-help may also be designed for people experiencing or recovering from crises. For instance, there is a 'runaway house' (*weglaufhaus*) in Berlin. This house, an antipsychiatric project which has received some public funding, provides an opportunity for people to live for up to six months in an environment not subject to psychiatric diagnosis or psychiatric drugs. One survey at the house reported that the overwhelming majority of house residents continued to reside in the community after leaving (Hölling 1999). Another example comes from Helsingborg, Sweden, where there is a well-appointed hotel, the Hotel Magnus Stenbock, run by the RSMH and funded by the Swedish government. It is a place where people recovering from crises or those who are homeless can stay as long as they like (Brown and Fleischmann 1999). The hotel is managed by a user-controlled council and some of the staff are service users.

Advocacy

In line with the human rights orientation of many European groups, advocacy is another activity practised by some. Individuals, particularly those living in institutions, may be vulnerable to having their rights curtailed, and may not always be able to express their preferences and needs. Advocacy can play an important role in filling this gap. The United Kingdom has a national group, the UK Advocacy Network (UKAN), a federation of organizations that are mainly advocacy-focused groups or Patients' Councils. Certainly, advocacy is a common activity for Patients' Councils in the Netherlands, although it should be stressed that in both countries these councils engage in other activities such as pressing for the improvement of conditions in hospitals.

There has been a major advance in the provision of advocacy services in England recently, through proposed, highly controversial changes in mental health legislation. While there has been almost unanimous opposition to much of this legislation, most users take it as an achievement that the legislation proposes that all detained and compulsorily-treated patients will now have an advocate by law.

Advocacy can also take new forms. In one part of Sweden there is a new project whereby users are allocated a *'personligt ombud'*. This roughly translates as 'personal ombudsman' and is a mixture of an advocate and the best forms of keyworking. Personal ombudsmen are professional workers, while in many forms of advocacy the advocates are service users themselves. Elsewhere, the Estonian Patient Advocacy Association began as a purely mental health organization but now works across the whole health field and is funded by central government. It tends to take a systemic approach to advocacy, focusing on campaigning for change nationally. An advocacy project in Georgia focuses more on individual problems, many of which have a legal basis, like access to housing and passports. This project employs both ex-users and professionals as advocates.

Anti-stigma work

In addition to advocacy, anti-stigma work is also very common and a key activity of many user groups in Europe. For instance, there may be concerns about social inclusion; thus, activities may take the form of training for work or setting up small businesses, often based on the model of a social firm, especially among better-funded groups. However, some users have criticized training schemes as, in effect, the equivalent of 'sheltered workshops', arguing that they do not promote social inclusion (see Chapter 12).

For many user groups, stigma and discrimination lead to, or compound, mental distress – and this is the message they wish to convey to the media and the public. Anti-stigma and public education campaigns thus can cause division between user groups and other stakeholders. For instance, while organizations such as the WHO engage in anti-stigma work, their campaigns tend to be based on a medical model, with mental illness seen as an illness like any other. For them, mental illness is a disease of the brain; many user groups see this as a counterproductive stance, as diseases of the brain also do not have a socially acceptable image.

Other activities

Some user groups provide creative activities revolving mainly around poetry, theatre and painting. In the United Kingdom, Survivors' Poetry puts on performance poetry events and has published several anthologies written by survivors. The Skane branch of RSMH in Sweden has a very successful theatre group run by a retired professional theatre director. This direction is much more common in the groups in central and eastern Europe, where a lot of energy goes into art, poetry and theatre. For example, KFH hold regular exhibitions of members' work in a commercial gallery in the town centre and many publish newsletters featuring poetry and art work.

In the more established user groups – for example, in Denmark, Sweden, France, the Netherlands and the United Kingdom – representatives consult with policy-makers. In the United Kingdom, 62 per cent of groups are engaged in consultation (Wallcraft *et al.* 2003). We will discuss this in more detail below, but suffice to say for now that this activity is not uncontroversial for some activists.

Specific issues in central and eastern Europe

For central and eastern Europe, the fall of the Berlin wall and the restored independence of the countries of the former Soviet bloc brought new access to information through the internet and the media, freedom to travel for those with an income, and a sense of freedom and the possibility of challenging past events and practices. However, as we have already indicated there remains a need to help build capacity among user groups. Established NGOs can play an important role supporting this process of capacity-building.

The Hamlet Trust often provided a role model for user involvement by inviting ex-user colleagues from the United Kingdom to events in central and eastern Europe; and it went on to involve ex-user trainers from other countries in the region. It has also supported the participation of people from central and eastern Europe at ENUSP conferences, promoting some positive Europe-wide networking. At the same time, there are opportunities for east-to-west learning. All of its programmes have focused on involving users, and while occasionally this has meant disagreeing with a professionally-run group's views and therefore stopping work in a specific town, on the whole, local organizations have recognized the importance of this approach. Some criticism has been levelled at the Trust for not involving users enough or for insisting on including them.

Slovenia is one country where a lot of work has been undertaken: in a country with a population of around 2 million there are seven or eight registered mental health NGOs, three of which have numerous regional branches. In contrast to many other countries in the region, the user movement started off quite early with the Committee for the Social Protection of Madness in the late 1970s. This reflects Slovenia's close ties with both Austria and Italy, and in particular the city of Trieste, where many of the activities around the Psyciatria Democratia movement took place. The Committee challenged the system by actually going into one of the social care homes, Hrastovic, and then opening the first community-based group home (with pump priming from Hamlet Trust's grant programme) for three people who had lived there for many years. These three now live quiet and contented lives in the community, but unfortunately the development of further group homes never took off. While there are now around 35 group homes in Slovenia, they only cater for people with short-term problems and until recently no one else had moved out of institutional care. As a mental health professional said, 'We seem to have lost the compass of user involvement here'. However, Hrastovic is now undergoing a complete transformation and many former residents now live, and sometimes work, in the community. One area where there is perhaps a better opportunity for change is in Bosnia and Herzegovina. The situation in this war-torn country is fairly unique, as many of its institutions were destroyed. Mental health services are now being rebuilt around a community alternative and, again with the help of the Hamlet Trust, the first user group was established in 1999. There are now seven groups meeting in different cantons in the country.

The issues that are, in a sense, unique to this part of Europe are as follows, and while they have a unique profile in each country, there are some common features:

- the impact of the Soviet system – primarily institutionalization and passivity or complete reliance on professionals, and above all, an assumption that people are better off in institutions;
- the impact of the abuse of psychiatry;
- the impact of immense social, cultural and political upheaval;
- the fact that each country's economy took a major downturn and they all experienced some kind of inflation, so that money to run services has been severely limited; and
- the influence of the World Bank and International Monetary Fund, which have insisted on the development of market economies, shifting each government's focus away from social developments.

Are groups user-controlled?

It is not enough just to describe the activities in which user/survivor groups are involved. The fundamental principle underpinning all of these activities is that users should have more control over their lives, both individually and collectively. This is still mostly a novel idea as traditionally nearly all aspects of users' lives were controlled by mental health professionals or by the state.

As mentioned earlier, we asked groups to indicate whether or not they were user-controlled, but many could not make sense of this question. We believe this indicates that they are not, in fact, user-controlled. There are wide discrepancies in western European countries on this issue. An example of a national group wholly user-controlled is Clientenbond in the Netherlands. On the other hand, in Austria, many local user groups are organized by Pro Mente, a non-user controlled NGO and mental health service provider.

In the West, there seem to be two historical trajectories at work exemplified by the United Kingdom on the one hand and Sweden on the other. In the United Kingdom, early national groups, including Survivors Speak Out, were not user-only groups as they admitted 'allies' as members. Gradually, the role of these allies diminished. Again, early local user groups in the United Kingdom tended to be alliances of users, families and professionals. Later, a 'user group' came to be defined as a group where decision-making is solely in the hands of users and indeed most user groups today are user-only. The main user group, RSMH in Sweden, can be used to illustrate a different pattern of development. The organization was founded by users in the 1960s. It quickly admitted sympathetic professionals as members and there were many of these as a result of the revolutionary events of May 1968. Subsequently, the radicalization of society abated and RSMH became more like a user-only group again. However, the group continued to receive substantial funding from the Swedish government, including subsidized salaries for workers. However, the biggest problem for RSMH today is that the national office is very strong with 20 to 25 paid workers, but they are all professionals. Nominally, there is a board of service users that directs this group of staff but, according to the reply we received to our internet questionnaire, this arrangement appears not to be working at all well.

Many groups in western Europe also contain family members. This can cause friction as the interests of users and relatives are not always the same. (Family-only groups have also emerged and are discussed in Chapter 16.) In mixed groups, relatives often dominate. In fact, this is clearest in the United States where user groups are very critical of the powerful relatives' organization, the National Alliance for the Mentally Ill (NAMI). This organization receives funding from the pharmaceutical industry and favours more coercive measures for users.

There are relatively few completely user-controlled groups in eastern Europe and in the new EU member states. Those that do exist in Bulgaria, Lithuania, Estonia, Ukraine, Georgia, Romania and Poland, for example, all have professional 'allies' who offer some kind of support, usually on request. There is no state support for user-led services or even for involving users in planning or managing services anywhere. On a more positive note, with some persuasion from organized user groups, there is now a growing acceptance of the need to listen to the voice of the user.

Looking at the experiences of the user-led groups in the Hamlet Trust's network, many remain fragile and depend on the strength of a few individuals and, as everywhere, are vulnerable to crises. In comparison to non-user led groups they find it hard to obtain funding as they have little access to formal structures and information, and have fewer resources. Many of the groups in the Hamlet network were, in fact, established by professionals willing to encourage users either to take part or move out and establish their own independent groups. These (mostly young) professionals recognized that the only way that they are going to generate change is to move outside the psychiatric system and be willing to share what little resources and power they have. However, there is still a lot of suspicion about the viability of user-led activities, which is only exacerbated by the crises that inevitably occur. These then tend to be seen as proof that such groups cannot work rather than being seen a part of the everyday life faced by all organizations.

So, is it important whether groups are user-controlled or not? Those who say it is make the argument from experience. Only users know what it is like to be on the receiving end of psychiatric services and to experience mental distress. Therefore, only users can understand the situation of their fellows and are thereby enabled to engage in collective action. However, others believe that there is a role for non-users, especially when an organization is developing. They argue that people who use mental health services, especially those confined to hospital or residential care for long periods of time, do not have much experience of creating and running organizations and therefore may need help, at least in the beginning.

User-led research

We have not attempted here to collect information on the role of user groups in research across Europe. Evaluation of all interventions, including user-led projects is crucial, and it is important to briefly highlight the contribution that can be made by user-researchers. Service users are beginning to play a role in the area of research, most notably in the United Kingdom, where policy guidance recommends user involvement in the research process. On the ground, however, there may be tension, power differentials and suspicion between clinicians and professional researchers (who may have a narrow medical focus and misgivings about user-researchers' skills), and the broader perspective of user researchers.

Evidence is beginning to emerge on the contribution of user involvement to research, which shows that it can positively influence the content of research projects. User-researchers may ask different questions and obtain different responses to research conducted by professionals. User-researchers are more likely, for instance, to be interested in how interventions are delivered and what their impact is on individual empowerment (Trivedi and Wykes 2002; Chamberlin 2005).

Important outcomes of an intervention may be more apparent to a service user than to professionals; for instance, one study looking at how the work of different professionals working with a service user is coordinated concluded that this did not lead to greater involvement or awareness among service users (Rose 2003). Outcomes regarding advocacy, being listened to and having an opportunity to contribute to meetings were things that were overlooked by professionals but were important to service users, and had important implications for the success of the intervention.

User-researchers' understanding of an issue may also lead to alternative explanations of why things do or do not work and their impact on quality of life (Faulkner and Thomas 2002). One example of how such important insights into quality of life may be identified comes from a recent user-researcher-led systematic review of patient perspectives on electroconvulsive therapy (ECT) (Rose *et al.* 2003). This review examined the differences between measures of effectiveness and efficacy reported in the clinical literature and user satisfaction with treatment. User-led studies reported significantly less benefit than clinician-led studies; this, it was argued, may be due to clinical studies obtaining information from those undergoing ECT too soon after treatment, using simplistic questionnaires that do not pick up complex patient views. The study highlighted the need for more qualitative research to identify outcomes of value to those who undergo treatment.

Credibility remains a crucial issue for user research. In an evidence-based culture, evidence from service users frequently fails to measure up to the 'scientific' standards of evidence-based medicine (Campbell 2005). One response to this has been the establishment of the Service User Research Enterprise (SURE). This is a partnership between service-user researchers and clinical academic staff that 'aims to involve service users in all aspects of research'. It is one of only two units within United Kingdom universities to employ people who have used mental health services and the only one where *most* employees are users or former users of mental health services as well as having research skills. The unit is funded through winning grants on a competitive basis from research funding bodies (SURE 2005). As part of their remit, SURE also provides training for service users to help give them the skills to undertake research. The National Institute for Mental Health in England has also funded SURGE (Service Users Research Group for England) through the Mental Health Research Network. This is a partnership between the Mental Health Foundation, Shaping Our Lives, the Centre for Citizen Participation at Brunel University, the NIMHE Experts by Experience group and the Survivor Researcher Network. Again, it was set up to support mental health service users and people from universities and National Health Service trusts to work together on mental health research. SURGE supports service user input to the MHRN through service user involvement in local hub committees, research project teams and at a national level (SURGE 2005).

In addition, Suresearch is a Midlands-based, user-led network of mental health service users and their allies based in the Institute of Applied Social Studies, University of Birmingham (Suresearch-SURGE 2005). Members undertake mental health research and education on a paid basis. Suresearch also provides research training for members and users from other local service user organizations (Davis 2005; SURGE 2005).

The Hamlet Trust has also run some user research training for groups in Estonia and Georgia, and as a consequence has supported some user evaluation of programmes in those countries.

Influences on policy-making

Finally, we look at what impact, if any, the user movement has had on policy across Europe, turning first to recent developments at the European level. The mental health *Declaration* for Europe and the mental health *Action Plan* for Europe, endorsed by ministers from all 52 European countries in January 2005, were developed through a process of consultation with many different stakeholders, including user groups over a number of years. The *Declaration* recognizes the need to empower and support people with mental health problems, importantly acknowledges 'the experience and knowledge of service users and carers as an important basis for planning and developing mental health services', and supports the creation of service user organizations (WHO 2005a). The detailed *Action Plan* invites member states to consider setting standards on the representation of users on committees and groups responsible for planning, delivery, review and inspection of mental health activities, empowering service users to take responsibility for their care and increase the level of social inclusion (WHO 2005b). Only time will tell if these words are translated into effective action.

Turning to policy at the national level, and starting this time with the countries of the ex-Soviet bloc, there is still little evidence of users having any influence whatsoever on state policy. Indeed, this lack of link with policy-making led the Hamlet Trust to develop an initiative called Pathways to Policy in five countries, establishing local policy forums and arranging a number of stakeholder meetings (Hamlet Trust 2003, 2004). The forums can help to establish communication channels between groups and are beginning to have some kind of impact in making people think in new ways about the importance of listening to the experience of users. In Estonia, where some of this thinking had already begun, the Policy Forum is taking off with active support from the Ministry of Social Welfare. There is, however, little interest from the Ministry of Health or mainstream psychiatry.

It is also worth noting that there is little well-developed mental health policy in this region. This could be seen as a positive thing in that by the time governments become willing to develop and implement good policy, the user movement might be well developed enough to take a natural part in that process. In fact, this appears to be happening in Hungary already, with the national user organization involved in many activities and campaigns.

In western Europe, large groups with national, regional and local structures and networks usually have a direct influence on government policy on mental health. This is true, for example, in France, Sweden, Denmark and the Netherlands. Southern European countries whose health and social welfare systems are decentralized have few national organizations and the limited influence on policy-making must take place at a regional level. In Catalonia, for instance, a region-wide group can directly lobby the Catalan government.

In the United Kingdom, policy-making related to mental health is an issue for the devolved administrations in Wales, Scotland and Northern Ireland (when devolution is restored). Thus, there is no over-arching user empowerment group and most organization is at the local level. Since most funding is at local level, most influence is inevitably confined to that level. There are several national groups but they tend to be specific to issues (Hearing Voices Network) or part of other organizations (MINDlink). However, very recently there have been attempts to establish a 'network of networks' in an effort to develop a national user/survivor organization.

In England there is currently a strong emphasis on consumer involvement in all aspects of health policy, and certainly groups of individual users were involved in the process of developing the National Service Framework (NSF) for mental health. However, these users were not elected by national groups and most found it a very unhappy experience (Wallcraft *et al.* 2003). Moreover, although the final version of the NSF states that there should be arrangements in place for user involvement, there are few additional references to users in the seven standards in the NSF or in the recent *Five Years On Review* (Tait and Lester 2005).

This brings us back to the issue of consultation and 'user involvement'. Funding for groups may be contingent on them providing representatives to sit on committees that have some influence on policy-making. Some are happy to do this. However, others see 'user involvement' as, at best, tokenism. One or two users sit round a table with 10 or 20 professionals, with a huge agenda and a discussion couched mainly in jargon and acronyms. It is felt by many, especially those from more developed user organizations, that users cannot possibly have a voice or an influence under such circumstances.

This can be illustrated by studies looking at the involvement of service users at the local level in England. One study which looked at the involvement of all types of service users (including non-mental health service users) in the clinical governance of 12 primary care trusts (PCTs) found that user members on the boards of these trusts had very little role in setting priorities, and beyond participating on these boards, any other participation of service users in the planning of mental health services only occurred in 2 of the 12 Trusts (Pickard *et al.* 2002). Another study looked at how service users are involved in the planning and delivery of psychiatric services across Greater London. Of 29 (48 per cent) user groups responding to a questionnaire, only 6 (21 per cent) were satisfied with their local PCT's commitment to user involvement. None of the PCTs had systems for user involvement in place that met national standards, although both Trusts and user groups were able to identify areas where users had contributed to service development and change (Crawford *et al.* 2003).

A further issue concerns the way users are involved. Many feel that they are involved only to 'rubber-stamp' decisions already made by the authorities. It is argued very strongly that users need to be there at the start of policy changes and be meaningfully involved throughout. Some have argued that consultation with stakeholders, including service users, in health policy-making in general has moved towards a 'stakeholder' model in which it is accepted that there are inequalities in power between different stakeholders. In this model, elected politicians are likely to have the final say on policy issues (Rush 2004). This approach is clearly not going to satisfy those who believe in all stakeholders having an equal say in the decision-making process. Research in two London PCTs reported that service managers tightly controlled the level of involvement of users in Trust business, and excluded them from some aspects of this (Rutter *et al.* 2004).

These criticisms have led some activists to expend their energies elsewhere. Creative groups, discussed above, are one option that many favour. There is also the beginning of a new form of anti-psychiatry in some countries. Both the United Kingdom and Denmark have organizations of people who prize their experience of madness and wish to celebrate it. The United Kingdom organization is called 'Mad Pride'. In the Netherlands there are philosophical differences between the Patients' Councils' members and the users movement known as the Clientenbond, with the latter being 'abolitionists' (Van Hoorn 1992). For such organizations, user involvement is a waste of time as it can only lead to minor changes within a system that structurally stays the same. Both the

United Kingdom and the Dutch organizations prefer street demonstrations, pop concerts and attempts to 'reclaim madness'.

Conclusion

The level and nature of the user movement in Europe is contingent on the social, economic and political conditions that pertain in a country, as well as its mental health policy and the way it provides services. In this chapter we have tried to map the terrain of user and survivor activity in Europe and draw out some of the issues that are important in most countries, even though they may be embryonic concerns in some regions. We live in a time of tension. Certainly, the user and survivor movement is claiming increasing authority in many countries but, at the same time, mental health legislation is mooted in some countries that will erode the few rights that users had previously come to expect.

At a European level, the recent mental health *Declaration* for Europe and the mental health *Action Plan* for Europe, endorsed by ministers from all 52 European countries, are a positive development, with a welcome, if overdue, recognition of the importance of service users in the development and planning of services, and encouragement for the use of legislation on disability rights on an equal basis for people with physical and mental disabilities. Little attention, however, has been paid to how user groups might be funded and sustained, but yet retain their autonomy (Thornicroft and Rose 2005). Thus, at both national and pan-European level the user/survivor movement remains a site of struggle.

Acknowledgement

Thanks to Mary Nettle for sparing the time to be interviewed and for her comments on an earlier draft of this chapter. Thanks also to all colleagues and friends in the Hamlet Trust network whose energy and experience created the work that is described here.

Note

1 The countries of central and eastern Europe, including those which have recently acceded to the EU (in the spring of 2005), can no longer be seen as a cohesive region. While they all experienced Soviet domination in some way, the transitions they have experienced since the fall of the Berlin wall and the Soviet Union has been unique and significantly different in each case.

References

Allam, S., Blyth, S., Fraser, A., Hodgson, S. *et al.* (2004) Our experience of collaborative research: service users, carers and researchers work together to evaluate an assertive outreach service, *Journal of Psychiatric and Mental Health Nursing*, 11(3): 368–73.

Brown, G. and Fleischmann, P. (1999) *Luxury Hotels for the Mentally Ill! What the UK Can Learn from Swedish User-run Mental Health Services*. London: Brent Lund Alternatives.

Campbell, P. (1996) The history of the user movement in the UK, in T. Heller, J. Reynolds, R. Gomm, R. Muston and S. Pattison (eds) *Mental Health Matters*. Basingstoke: Macmillan.

Campbell, P. (2005) From little acorns. The mental health service user movement, in Sainsbury Centre for Mental Health (ed.) *Beyond the Water Towers. The Unfinished Revolution in Mental Health Services 1985–2005*. London: Sainsbury Centre for Mental Health.

Chamberlin, J. (2005) User/consumer involvement in mental health service delivery, *Epidemiologica e Psichiatria Sociale*, 14(1): 10–14.

Crawford, M. J., Aldridge, T., Bhui, K., Rutter, D. *et al.* (2003) User involvement in the planning and delivery of mental health services: a cross-sectional survey of service users and providers, *Acta Psychiatrica Scandinavica*, 107(6): 410–14.

Davis, A. (2005) User involvement in mental health research and development, in D. Sallah and M. Clarke (eds) *Research and Development in Mental Health: Theory, Frameworks and Models*. Amsterdam: Elsevier Science.

ENUSP (2005) European Network of (Ex-) Users and Survivors of Psychiatry website, www.enusp.org/.

Faulkner, A. and Thomas, P. (2002) User led research and evidence-based medicine, *British Journal of Psychiatry*, 180: 1–3.

Hamlet Trust (2003) *Annual Report 2003*, www.hamlet-trust.org.

Hamlet Trust (2004) *Annual Report 2004*, www.hamlet-trust.org.

Henderson, C., Flood, C., Leese, M., Thornicroft, G. *et al.* (2004) Effects of joint crisis plans on use of compulsory treatment in psychiatry: single blind randomised controlled trial, *British Journal of Psychiatry*, 329: 136–41.

Hölling, I. (1999) The Berlin runaway house – three years of antipsychiatric practice, *Changes – An International Journal of Psychology and Psychotherapy*, 17(4): 278–88.

Hölling, I. (2001) About the impossibility of a single (ex-) user and survivor of psychiatry position, *Acta Psychiatrica Scandinavica*, 104(Suppl. 410): 102–6.

Laing, R. (1959) *The Divided Self*. London: Tavistock.

MDAC (2003) *Caged Beds Report*. Budapest: Mental Disability Advocacy Centre, www.mdac.info.

Pickard, S., Marshall, M., Rogers, A., Sheaff, R. *et al.* (2002) User involvement in clinical governance, *Health Expectations*, 5(3): 187–98.

Rose, D. (2003) Partnership, co-ordination of care and the place of user involvement, *Journal of Mental Health*, 12(1): 59–70.

Rose, D., Wykes, T., Leese, M., Bindman, J. and Fleischman, P. (2003) Patients' perspectives on electroconvulsive therapy: systematic review, *British Medical Journal*, 326: 1363–8.

Rush, B. (2004) Mental health service user involvement in England: lessons from history, *Journal of Psychiatric and Mental Health Nursing*, 11(3): 313–18.

Rutter, D., Manley, C., Weaver, T., Crawford, M. J. and Fulop, N. (2004) Patients or partners? Case studies of user involvement in the planning and delivery of adult mental health services in London, *Social Science and Medicine*, 58(10): 1973–84.

Simpson, E. L. and House, A. O. (2002) Involving users in the delivery and evaluation of mental health services: systematic review, *British Medical Journal*, 325: 1265–70.

SURGE (2005) Service User Research Group for England website, www.mhrn.info/surge.html.

SURE (2005) Service User Research Enterprise website, http://web1.iop.kcl.ac.uk/iop/Departments/HSR/sure/index.shtml.

Suresearch-SURGE (2005) *Guidance for Good Practice: Service User Involvement in the UK.*

Mental Health Research Network, accessible from the SURGE website: www.mhrn. info/surge.html.

Szasz, T. (1972) *The Myth of Mental Illness*. London: Granada.

Tait, L. and Lester, H. (2005) Encouraging user involvement in mental health services, *Advances in Psychiatric Treatment*, 11(3): 168–75.

Thornicroft, G. and Rose, D. (2005) Mental health in Europe, *British Medical Journal*, 330: 613–14.

Thornicroft, G. and Tansella, M. (2005) Growing recognition of the importance of service user involvement in mental health service planning and evaluation, *Epidemiolgia e Psichiatria Sociale*, 14(1): 1–3.

Trivedi, P. and Wykes, T. (2002) From passive subjects to equal partners: qualitative review of user involvement in research, *British Journal of Psychiatry*, 181: 468–72.

Van Hoorn, E. (1992) Changes? What changes? The views of the European patients' movement, *International Journal of Social Psychiatry*, 38(1): 30–5.

Wallcraft, J., Read, J. and Sweeney, A. (2003) *On Our Own Terms*. London: The Sainsbury Centre for Mental Health.

World Health Organization (2005a) *Mental Health Declaration for Europe*. Copenhagen: World Health Organization Regional Office for Europe.

World Health Organization (2005b) *Mental Health Action Plan for Europe*. Copenhagen: World Health Organization Regional Office for Europe.

Websites

European Disability Forum: www.edf-feph.org

European Network of (Ex-) Users and Survivors of Psychiatry (ENUSP): www.enusp.org

Hamlet Trust: www.hamlet-trust.org

Mental Disability Advocacy Centre (MDAC): www.mdac.info

Mental Health Initiative of the Open Society Institute: www.soros.org/initiatives/mhi

Service User Research Enterprise (SURE): http://web1.iop.kcl.ac.uk/iop/Departments/HSR/sure

Service User Research Group for England Website (SURGE): www.mhrn.info/surge.html

chapter fifteen

The mental health care of asylum seekers and refugees

Charles Watters

The mental health care of asylum seekers and refugees in Europe is a highly specific and complex area of investigation. To do justice to the field, it is essential to adopt a multi-disciplinary approach that embraces the study of political processes and social policies relating to migrants and refugees, and the impact these may have on the contexts in which refugees receive mental health care. These political and social factors should not be examined solely at the level of nation states but include significant developments at an international level led by bodies such as the European Commission (EC). The Treaty of Amsterdam (1997) raised the issue of asylum and immigration to the 'first pillar' of policy-making within the European Union (EU). The implication of this is that all member states should work to achieve common minimum standards in the area of immigration and asylum, including standards relating to health and welfare provision for asylum seekers.

At the time of writing there is a growing convergence in procedures for processing asylum applications and the nature of the support received by asylum seekers once they enter an EU country. Under a 2003 EC Council Directive all member countries of the EU are required to adhere to explicit minimum standards for the reception of asylum seekers. National governments within the EU were required to have incorporated the Directive into national laws by February 2005 (EC 2003).

Analysis at the social and political levels informs us of the contexts in which mental health care is offered. To form a complete picture it is also important to examine the micro level at which individuals and families experience mental health problems and may have direct contact with service providers. Here consideration must be given to the impact of stressors in the pre-migration, flight and post-migration contexts as these may have a significant effect on the mental well-being of refugees (Ager 1993, 2000). It is also important to focus on the service providers themselves and examine the institutional contexts in which services are provided (Watters 2002).

This chapter will proceed with an overview of migrants and refugees in the European context. Refugees will initially be identified as a particular type of migrant and attention will be given to the relationship between refugees and undocumented migrants. As part of this background, statistical information on refugees in Europe will be presented and discussed, drawing attention to the significant differences that exist between refugee numbers in southern and northern Europe. The second section of the chapter will focus on the mental health needs of refugees, drawing on evidence of the mental health problems experienced by this group and debates concerning diagnosis. This section will include an examination of refugees' mental health in the post-migration context and evidence linking post-migration experiences with mental illness. The third section will focus on the provision of mental health services for refugees within Europe. This section will draw on work on good practices in the mental health of refugees and will comment in particular on developments in four European countries – the United Kingdom, the Netherlands, Spain and Portugal – before drawing more general conclusions regarding the position in Europe as a whole and the potential for disseminating good practice in this area.

Migrants and refugees in a European context

The period between the middle of the twentieth century and the present time has been referred to as the 'age of migration'. Commentators have noted that while historically people have crossed borders and settled in other lands since time immemorial, the scale, global scope and social and economic consequences of migration in the present age is unprecedented (Castles and Miller 2003). Of course, migration may occur for a variety of reasons. Historically, millions of people have left their countries of origin or moved to different regions to pursue a better life in other lands. The driving force behind this may have been religious or political persecution or economic deprivation, or it may have been a perception that a better standard of living was achievable elsewhere. The interrelationship between factors that drive people from their home countries and those that attract them to new ones is typically referred to as 'push/pull', and the analysis of migration frequently focuses on this interrelationship (Hollingfield 2000).

Castles and Miller (2003) have identified five 'tendencies' that characterize migration in the early twenty-first century. The first is the 'globalization of migration' in that migration affects a wide diversity of 'receiving' countries at the same time. It is also globalized in the sense that countries of immigration may receive a very wide diversity of migrants from different economic, social and cultural backgrounds. Secondly, there is an acceleration of migration in that migration has grown in volume in all the regions of the world. This is not to say that certain *types* of migration cannot reduce from time to time. For example, at the time of writing, there has been a notable decrease in the number of asylum seekers entering the industrialized world (UNHCR 2004). However, as will be noted below, there may be a direct relationship between a reduction in one type of migration and an increase in another and, arguably, there are increases in undocumented migrants that accompany decreases in those seeking asylum (Crisp 2003).

A third factor or tendency is the differentiation of migration in that most countries do not have one type of immigration but a large variety of types including labour migration, those migrating temporarily to study, those attached to multinational corporations that spend circumscribed periods of time in a range of countries, and refugees and asylum seekers. The policies of governments may be both actively encouraging one type of migration while discouraging others and, as Zolberg (1989) has demonstrated, the formulation and implementation of policies has a direct impact on the movement of migrants into and between countries. Thus, for example, in many European countries at the present time there is both a strong tendency to restrict access by asylum seekers while, simultaneously, actively encouraging well skilled or educated migrants to fill gaps in certain sectors, for example in health care. The encouragement of migration is also driven by demographic changes in Europe resulting in steep declines in the adult working population that threaten standards of living.

A fourth tendency identified by Castles and Miller relates to the notable increase in the number of women migrants in all categories. This includes labour migration, incorporating potentially exploited roles as domestic servants or, more perniciously, as undocumented migrants recruited for the sex industries. It also includes women travelling abroad to study or work in international corporations. The increasing numbers of women in these categories challenges the established model of 'chain migration' that is initiated by a male family member migrating for work who is then followed by his wife and other family members. By contrast, women migrants may form the majority in groups 'as diverse as those of Cape Verdians to Italy, Filipinos to the Middle East and Thais to Japan' (Castles and Miller 2003: 9). In identifying persons 'of concern' to the United Nations High Commissioner for Refugees (UNHCR) in 2002, 51 per cent were women. A report to the UNHCR suggests that while women and men may face the same kind of harm, 'women are often subject to specific forms of gender-related abuse and violence such as rape, abduction or an offer of protection documents or assistance in exchange for sex' (UNHCR 2002).

The final tendency identified is the politicization of migration in which migration has an increasingly significant role in both domestic and international politics. As noted above, migration, in recent years, has moved to the top of the EU policy-making agenda. It is also a critical element in bilateral and regional relations. Examples include the diplomatic strains between Britain and France over the Red Cross Sangatte refugee camp situated close to the ferry and rail crossings between France and England, and disputes regarding the influx of migrants between Albania and Greece, Morocco and Spain and Germany and a number of its central and eastern European neighbours.

Refugees in Europe

Refugees are thus a particular category of migrants, one occupying a specific political and legal position. A refugee is defined in Article 1 of the 1951 UN convention as any person who:

> owing to a well founded fear of being persecuted for reasons of race, religion, nationality, membership of a particular social group or political opinion, is outside the country of his nationality and is unable, or owing to such fear, is unwilling to avail himself of the protection of that country . . .

The immediate concern of those who drafted the Convention was the situation in Europe following the end of the Second World War and the Convention originally only referred to those who became refugees 'as a result of events occurring before 1 January 1951'. However, this time limitation was removed in 1967 and the 1951 Convention and the 1967 Protocol are still the most important, and the only universal, instruments of international refugee law. The fundamental challenge for those seeking refugee status is to demonstrate that they have a well-founded fear of persecution while receiving countries have their own systems of deciding whether a person fits the UN definition, and national courts may interpret the Convention differently. Some countries, for example, interpret the Convention as referring only to state persecution and do not accord refugee status to those suffering from persecution from non-state agencies. Other countries include both state and non-state persecution when considering the granting of refugee status (Justice 2002).

The term 'refugee' is often used in a generic sense to include both asylum seekers and those who have achieved refugee status. It is also, on occasion, used to refer to 'undocumented migrants' who enter countries clandestinely and do not actively seek asylum. Here the term will be used to include asylum seekers and refugees except where specific issues relating to one or other category are addressed, in which case the more precise terminology will be used. Undocumented migrants occupy a quite different legal, political and social position. Their rights to welfare benefits, health and education may be significantly different to those of refugees and asylum seekers and they may be largely 'invisible' to service providers. In short, with respect to mental health care, being an asylum seeker or refugee will affect the context and content of the care provided and this may be significantly different in content and availability to that which undocumented migrants may have access to (PICUM 2001).

Despite this, there are important reasons for considering the position of undocumented migrants in an examination of the mental health care of refugees. Firstly, there is an interrelationship between asylum-seeking and undocumented migration. In many European countries with low numbers seeking asylum (for example, most of the countries in southern Europe), there is evidence of very high numbers of undocumented migrants. Bernal (2003: 85), for example, cites evidence of between 200,000 and 300,000 undocumented migrants in Spain while the number of asylum applications annually since 1995 never exceeded 10,000. In the years 2001 and 2002 Spain received 9200 and

6200 applications respectively. Greece received 5600 and 5700, and Portugal records 200 applications in each of the two years. This compares with northern European countries such as Germany (88,300 and 71,100 in 2001 and 2002) and the United Kingdom (92,000 and 110,700 in 2001 and 2002).

There is a range of potential reasons for this variation. It may be linked to low rates of acceptance in some countries. The recognition rates in southern European countries have tended to be low, rarely exceeding 10 per cent of applicants while in some northern European countries the rate is significantly higher. For example, the United Kingdom recorded a 34.9 per cent recognition rate for those granted refugee or humanitarian status between 1990 and 1999, and the Netherlands recorded 27.3 per cent in the same period (UNHCR 2000). In countries with low acceptance rates but high numbers of applicants (e.g. Germany and Austria) this may be accounted for by the proximity of borders to refugee 'exporting' countries. There are concerns that, as access to asylum becomes more restrictive, potential claimants will not put their cases before the relevant authorities and will join swelling numbers of undocumented migrants either through not registering a claim in the first place, or absconding when a negative decision is reached (Crisp 2003).

Table 15.1 provides evidence of asylum claims submitted in the EU between 1990 and 2003. It is notable that over this period Germany had over 40 per cent of asylum claims with the United Kingdom in second position with 16 per cent. This order was reversed in 2003, when the United Kingdom had a total of 103,080 applications as compared with Germany's 71,130. In 2003, there was a significant decrease in asylum applications across the EU-15 countries (down by 22 per cent) and in Europe overall (down 20 per cent). Governments claim that this downward trend was the result of stricter border controls and asylum procedures although it is frequently argued that the flow of asylum seekers may have been stemmed by a degree of stability returning to major 'sending' countries such as Somalia and Iraq. In the United Kingdom a Home Office minister hailed figures produced in August 2004 as showing the impact of successful government policies adding, 'This has been achieved by bringing in tough new legislation to tackle abuse and cut delays, securing our borders, rolling out detection technology and UK immigration controls to foreign soil, closing Sangatte, introducing fast-track processing, ending in-country appeals for nationals of safe countries and bringing in new visa regimes'.

This downward trend was not uniform, however, as some of the countries joining the EU in 2004 recorded an increase in applications. UNHCR reports 34 per cent increases in the Czech Republic and Poland and a 364 per cent increase in Cyprus. It is too early to draw any firm conclusions as to the reasons behind this difference, although one possible contributory factor is that asylum seekers whose intended destination is the EU are now lodging their applications in countries they may have previously passed through *en route* to their intended destination. A further possible contributory factor may lie in improvements in reception and recording procedures in the accession countries. A notable feature in asylum applications in Poland and the Czech Republic is the significant number of asylum seekers from eastern Europe. In Poland the highest number of asylum seekers in 2003 were from the Russian Federation, and for the

Table 15.1 Asylum claims submitted in the EU-15, 1990–2003

Country	Total	Share (%)	Per 1,000 population
Sweden	349,700	6.60	39.4
Austria	249,800	4.70	30.8
Belgium	283,400	5.30	27.5
Netherlands	433,500	8.10	27.0
Germany	2,168,000	40.70	26.3
Denmark	117,900	2.20	22.0
Luxembourg	9,700	0.20	22.0
Ireland	59,300	1.10	15.2
UK	851,930	16.00	14.4
France	485,700	9.10	8.1
Finland	29,600	0.60	5.7
Greece	47,000	0.90	4.3
Spain	113,100	2.10	2.8
Italy	118,800	2.20	2.1
Portugal	6,400	0.10	0.60
Total	5,323,830	100.00	14.0

Czech Republic the Ukraine was the leading country of origin (UNHCR 2004). Table 15.2 shows the top five European asylum seeker nationalities between 2001 and 2003.

An examination of asylum figures is important in indicating the challenge facing mental health and other service providers. Firstly, there is the unpredictability of asylum and undocumented migrant flows. Services developed to address the needs of specific migrant groups may have to adapt quite dramatically in response to new flows from different regions, involving different languages and cultural knowledge. Secondly, there is the shifting political and policy contexts requiring swift adaptation from service providers in trying to ensure a degree of continuity and appropriateness of care. Thirdly, there are specific issues in responding to the needs of individuals whose claims are rejected and who may be placed in holding or detention centres pending removal from the country. As indicated below, this group may face particularly acute mental health problems.

Refugees and mental health

Research on refugees and mental health may be classified as being of four types: epidemiological studies of mental illness within refugee populations; studies of aetiological factors in mental illness, including the impact of the post-migration

Table 15.2 The top five European asylum seeker nationalities in Europe between 2001 and 2003

Country/region of asylum	2001	2002	2003	Total Absolute	Total Share	Total Rank	Annual change 2001–2	Annual change 2002–3	Per 1,000 population Total	Per 1,000 population Rank
Germany	88,290	71,130	50,450	209,870	12.60%	3	–19%	–29%	2.55	17
Greece	5,500	5,660	8,180	19,340	1.20%	18	3%	45%	1.76	20
Portugal	230	250	110	590	0.00%	35	9%	–56%	0.06	38
Spain	9,490	6,310	5,770	21,570	1.30%	17	–34%	–9%	0.53	30
United Kingdom	91,600	103,080	61,050	255,730	15.40%	1	13%	–41%	4.33	11

environment; research into mental health service provision; and research on the socio-legal context of mental health care.

Much of the debate on refugees and mental health has, in recent years, focused on post-traumatic stress disorder (PTSD) (Silove *et al.* 2000b). PTSD is widely regarded as one of the major mental health problems experienced by refugees. Most frequently it refers to the impact of a traumatic event in the refugee's country of origin, for example the direct or indirect experiencing of torture, beatings, killings or rape. These distressing experiences are then relived with intrusive flashbacks or vivid memories and the afflicted person may seek to avoid circumstances and locations that they associate with the original trauma (Goldberg *et al.* 1994). PTSD is a relatively recent addition to the psychiatric canon, having only been recognized as a distinct psychiatric category in 1980 and entered into the *Diagnostic and Statistical Manual* of the American Psychiatric Association. Vietnam War veterans and those who lobbied the health insurance industries on their behalf crucially influenced the recognition of PTSD (Young 1995). Since then there has been considerable clinical and academic interest in the extent to which refugee populations suffer from PTSD. A range of epidemiological studies has been undertaken on diverse refugee populations to seek to determine the prevalence of the illness. For example, Mollica *et al.* (1999) found that 15 per cent of Cambodian residents in a refugee camp on the Thai border suffered from PTSD while a study of Bosnian refugees in treatment indicated that between 18 per cent and 53 per cent suffer from PTSD. Silove *et al.* (2000b) have argued that, in general, only a minority of those exposed to mass violence suffer from PTSD, with numbers normally varying between 4 and 20 per cent. Silove has drawn attention to the context of research and pointed to the significant sampling bias that may exist between the findings of community studies and those focused on clinic populations, with the former studies recording consistently lower rates of PTSD (Silove 1999).

The past decade has seen significant challenges to the application of the PTSD diagnosis to refugee populations. There has been a sociological critique of the way in which the numbers of 'victims' of PTSD may be inflated to support the programmes of humanitarian aid organizations. Drawing on work in the former Yugoslavia, Stubbs (2004), for example, has challenged the epidemiological underpinnings for a process he describes as 'talking up the numbers' in which rash statements such as that 'more than 700,000 people in Bosnia Herzegovina . . . suffer from severe psychic trauma' are made. Summerfield (1999) provides a wide-ranging and sustained critique of the widespread application of the PTSD diagnosis. Drawing on the work of Allan Young, he points to the relatively recent 'discovery' of PTSD and contrasts its historical contingency with its widespread association with the problems of various refugee and non-western populations. A central concern of Summerfield's is what he sees as a form of psychiatric imperialism whereby large numbers of those suffering from the effects of war are categorized as mentally ill and as needing mental health interventions regardless of the sufferers' own views of their condition or what would alleviate it. While acknowledging that, on occasions, exaggerated statements have been made regarding the incidence of PTSD in post-conflict and refugee populations, authors have argued that an unforeseen consequence of this critique may be to undermine much-needed mental health programmes for refugees (Silove *et al.* 2000a, 2001). Furthermore, there is evidence that even small-scale mental health programmes for refugees can have a significant impact. Drawing on an evaluation of the impact of the introduction of a community psychiatric nurse in a large refugee camp, Kamau and colleagues have argued that even a small amount of mental health care can have a dramatic impact on the mental well-being of refugees (Kamau 2004).

Further research on the mental health of refugees focuses on the impact of 'stressors' arising from external events such as displacement and resettlement and 'stresses', the latter referring to subjective reactions to these events (Ahearn 2000). The effect of stressors can be ameliorated through coping strategies and external support. The impact of these has been the subject of extensive research activity focusing, for example, on work on the impact of religious faith, on social networks and material support. These factors have been mapped onto a chronological sequencing of the refugee's experience in which the stressors relating to the pre-flight, flight, post-migration and resettlement environments are identified (Ager 1993). The pre-flight environment is associated with a combination of stressful factors that commonly include economic hardship, social disruption, political oppression and physical violence. A common feature of 'social disruption' is the loss of family and friends either through them having been killed or through becoming separated in the chaotic circumstances of refugee migration. McCallin (1992), for example, observed that out of a sample of 109 Mozambican women who fled to Zambia, 24 per cent had been separated from their children. According to Beiser (1999), the loss of family members frequently results in long-term emotional problems that make the process of readjustment and integration into a new society more difficult.

The impact of the process of flight on the mental health of refugees has been given relatively little attention in the literature. According to one authority, this is regrettable because 'flight from one's homeland represents a major life event which – even if accomplished swiftly and in safety – is likely to prompt major emotional and cognitive turmoil, with concomitant risk to mental health' (Ager 1993: 9). Refugees may be particularly vulnerable, during the process of flight, to violence and sexual and economic exploitation. Besides these external factors they may experience subjective stresses arising from the recent loss of family, friends and homelands. Eisenbruch (1991) has argued that the profound sense of loss should be more clearly recognized in the mental health field and has proposed the establishment of a specific psychiatric category of 'cultural bereavement' that, he argues, may more accurately encapsulate refugees' experience than current western psychiatric categories. He cites, for example, the case of a Cambodian patient who is possessed by spirits, 'troubled by visitations of ghosts from the homeland, hears voices commanding him to make merit on behalf of his ancestors, and feels that he is being punished for having survived' (p. 675). In these instances the person is suffering from culturally normal signs of bereavement that may be misinterpreted as PTSD in a western psychiatric context.

While the emphasis on mental health research on refugees has been, until recently, on the impact of 'stressors' arising in the pre-migration environment on mental health, over the past decade there has been a considerable growth in literature on the impact of post-migration factors. This emphasis has reflected the emergence of increasingly restrictive policies towards asylum seekers and illegal immigrants in America, Europe and Australasia. Measures have included confinement in detention centres, enforced dispersal in the community, the implementation of more stringent refugee determination procedures, increasingly severe restrictions on access to work, education and housing and restrictions in access to health care (Silove *et al.* 2000b). Researchers have examined the relationship between factors relating to bureaucratic procedures, living conditions, low social support and discrimination in the post-migration environment and concluded that these can have a significant impact on the increased risk of PTSD symptoms among traumatized asylum seekers (Silove *et al.* 1993). Increased levels of depression have been shown to be associated with low levels of social support and financial difficulties. On the basis of a study of 84 Iraqi refugees, Gorst-Unsworth and Goldenberg conclude that, 'Social factors in exile, particularly the level of "affective" social support, proved important in determining the severity of both post-traumatic stress disorder and depressive reactions, particularly when combined with a severe level of trauma/torture. Poor social support is a stronger predictor of depressive morbidity than trauma factors' (1998: 90). According to Silove *et al.*, 'salient ongoing stressors identified across several studies included delays in the processing of refugee applications, conflict with immigration officials, being denied a work permit, unemployment, separation from family, and loneliness and boredom' (2000b: 606).

Internationally there has been a significant increase over the past decade in the detention of asylum seekers. A number of studies have been undertaken to examine the mental health implications of detention. Research in the United Kingdom indicated that psychological distress is evidenced through the high incidence of attempted suicide and hunger strikes (Pourgourides *et al.* 1996). As reported in research undertaken on 25 detained asylum seekers in Australia, there were higher rates of depression, suicidal ideation, post-traumatic stress, anxiety, panic and physical symptoms among the detained asylum seekers as compared to compatriot asylum seekers, refugees and immigrants living in the community (Thompson *et al.* 1988).

What these studies indicate is the interrelationship between specific policies towards asylum seekers and refugees and the mental health problems experienced by this group. Increasing restrictions on the facilities and support offered to refugees and the tightening of bureaucratic procedures may be significant 'stressors' that are detrimental to mental health. A recently developing area of study has shifted the emphasis from a clinical focus on the impact of policies of deterrence on mental health status to a more sociological approach that examines the impact of ill health, including mental ill health, on the socio-legal contexts in which asylum applications are generated and status is determined (Fassin 2001; Watters 2001a). This research is influenced by Zolberg's seminal paper in which he directs attention to the impact of state immigration policies on patterns of migration and away from early neo-classical push/pull theories (Zolberg 1989).

The routes taken by asylum applicants have been described as 'avenues of access' that are influenced by the prevailing immigration laws and policies (Watters 2001b). The 'avenues' followed by asylum seekers may be influenced by the extent to which they are experiencing health and mental health problems but also by the opportunities offered within the prevailing policies on asylum and immigration. Commenting on the situation in France, Fassin has pointed to a significant decrease over the past ten years in the number of claims for refugee status being accepted while, at the same time, there has been a sevenfold increase in the number of people receiving leave to remain on the basis of humanitarian concerns relating to ill health (Fassin 2001). One of the few routes to legitimacy available is through ill health. Fassin concludes from this that 'Thus greater importance is ascribed to the suffering body than to the threatened body, and the right to life is being displaced from the political to the humanitarian arena' (p. 4). Elsewhere, this argument has been extended to refer to a process of 'strategic categorization' wherein medical professionals may highlight refugees' health problems as they provide one of a limited range of 'avenues of access' to health and social care benefits (Watters 2001b). This is not to imply that professionals are wilfully exaggerating the mental health problems faced by some refugees. It is rather to suggest that, in a context where a refugee may have a range of problems relating to health, mental health and social care, some of these may enhance the refugee's case and may be duly emphasized. It is thus important that researchers examining the mental health of refugees in Europe are aware of the social and legal context of diagnosis and treatment.

Mental health services for refugees in Europe

In undertaking an examination of the mental health care of refugees in Europe one is immediately struck by the difficulties in mapping the field. In some countries with large, or relatively large, numbers of asylum seekers and refugees, mental health services are closely integrated into the systems established for processing asylum claimants. In others, there is very little planning or management and considerable variation in the quantity and quality of care from city to city, region to region. Many of the problems in mental health care provision are common to those experienced by migrant and settled minority ethnic communities across Europe. Six characteristics of these services are: a lack of monitoring and evaluation; a 'bottom up' unplanned approach resulting in considerable variability in service availability and quality; an absence of consultation with service users; poor access to appropriate counselling services; presence of racial discrimination in some services; and poor quality and quantity of staff training (Watters 2002).

It is useful to consider these features in the light of international recommendations for service provision in this area. The 2001 *World Health Report* highlights the specific needs of refugees and internally displaced persons. They are identified as a vulnerable group with 'special mental health needs'. The report identifies the importance of a holistic approach in stipulating that mental health policy 'must deal with housing, employment, shelter, clothing and food, as well as the psychological and emotional effects of experiencing war, dislocation and the loss of loved ones'. The report adds that in this area, 'community intervention should be the basis for policy action' (WHO 2001: 83). An earlier manual produced by the World Health Organization (WHO), and which drew on the experiences of a range of international experts, stressed the key features of an appropriate response to the mental health needs of refugees. These included integrating mental health care with traditional forms of healing, the empowerment of refugees through active consultation and participation in mental health programmes, and the interrelationship between mental health and physical health (WHO 1996). The manual stressed the importance of integrating mental health work with other forms of supportive activity and repeatedly emphasizes the importance of ensuring that refugees have a maximum level of autonomy in work and leisure activities. This approach is underpinned by a view of refugees as resourceful individuals who 'should not be seen as helpless people who totally depend on help that they are given' (WHO 1996: 1). In the manual the emphasis on empowerment is not merely ideological but it is seen as having practical consequences in the care of refugees: 'Broad participation and giving a say to refugees or other displaced persons prevents the harmful sense of helplessness and enforced dependence which can drain their energy' (1996: 133).

A further report by the WHO, in collaboration with the Red Cross and Red Crescent organizations, identifies a 'rapid assessment tool' for assessing the mental health needs of refugees and the resources that may be available in designated areas. In presenting the tool the authors stress the importance of adopting an approach to mental health care that moves away from psychiatric care only. They argue that 'any traumatic event will result in distress and suffering that will have a powerful effect on individuals and communities. However, distress and suffering are not psychiatric illnesses' (WHO 2001: 1). Consequently, 'generalized psychiatric care is inappropriate and thus must be prevented'. The above documents stress the importance of an integrated approach to mental health and social care, both in the sense of providing a service to clients that crosses traditional boundaries between mental health and social care and in the sense of providing a multi-disciplinary professional approach. The integration also crucially incorporates the role of 'service users' and the provision of traditional therapeutic approaches.

In 2002 and 2003 a detailed examination of mental health services for refugees in four European countries was undertaken. Specifically, researchers undertook an examination of services for refugees in the United Kingdom, the Netherlands, Spain and Portugal (Watters and Ingleby 2003). The remainder of this chapter draws on the findings of this study. The study concluded that across the four countries there were significant problems in relation to the provision of basic information on the use of mental health services by refugees. Monitoring was virtually non-existent, as in Portugal and Spain, or undertaken using very broad ethnic categorizations, as in the Netherlands and the United Kingdom. These were of limited utility in such a diversified group. The problems here were twofold: general service monitoring did not capture the wide range of national and ethnic origins and, being ethnically based, it did not expose important legal distinctions between refugees, asylum seekers, those granted forms of humanitarian status and undocumented migrants. As noted in the report, disarmingly simple questions such as 'how many refugees use your service?' led to consternation among mainstream service providers who attempted to guess or explained that monitoring systems did not accommodate this knowledge.

The evidence presented in the report confirmed the vital role of specialist NGOs in service provision to this group. As a consequence of their day-to-day interaction, these groups often held specialist knowledge about asylum seekers' and refugees' needs. The fact that these organizations are not structurally embedded in distinct health and social care services allows them to play a crucial coordinating role in meeting a wide range of practical, social care and mental health needs. While providing important services, however, these agencies typically existed in a marginal position in relation to mainstream health, mental health and social care. Mainstream services were routinely oriented almost exclusively to the majority population, and were severely limited in terms of the education and training of staff and in the availability of interpreting services (Watters 2002). In general terms, in Europe there is a significant polarization between specialist services for refugees existing in a marginal position, and mainstream health and social care agencies lacking knowledge and awareness of the needs of refugees. Consequently, there were severe challenges for specialist refugee services in attempting to offer mental health and social care services. In practical terms the establishment of such services relied on identifying mental health professionals and general practitioners within localities who were sympathetic to, and knowledgeable of, the needs of refugees and had the requisite skills and resources to address these needs. Thus, mental health initiatives for refugees normally involved partnerships between at least two agencies with a commitment to the field.

At the time of writing, examples of initiatives include Breathing Space in the United Kingdom, a partnership between the Refugee Council and the Medical Foundation for the Care of Victims of Torture, Pharos in the Netherlands, that evolved through a merger between the Social Psychiatric Service for Refugees and the Refugee Health Care Centre set up in the Dutch Ministry of Health, and SAPPIR in Spain, that grew out of a multi-disciplinary grouping of health professionals – the Health Assistant Service for Immigrants and Refugees. However, while their unique development was inextricably linked to their ability to offer distinctive services that crossed traditional boundaries in service provision, this aspect was also a source of potential weakness. With the possible exception of the Dutch example, mental health and social care services for refugees are rarely structurally embedded in mainstream mental health and social care services. The funding base for such services is rarely long term and secure. Initiatives normally take the form of 'special projects', or in larger organizations, emerge from forums in which a number of special projects may be developed. They are established for a finite period during which they are normally subject to an evaluation initiated by the funding body. The long-term survival of special projects thus is often in doubt.

As concluded in the report, a further feature was that services for refugees were typically the product of an initiative taken by an individual or group of individuals with an interest in the mental health and social care of refugees. The group had specialist interest in the field but had to balance this with employment within mainstream services. After formulating a plan for a service, typically the group then sought funding from a government department, an international body or charitable foundation. Time was often divided between refugee and mainstream services; for example, a psychiatrist who has commitments to a generic local team or psychiatric hospital. Projects directed at mental health and social care thus were rarely the result of top-down policy development supported by appropriate resources.

This had implications for the distribution of services in that some areas had dedicated professionals who secured resources for projects in their localities. However, this geographical distribution may not be based on demographic and epidemiological realities. For example, the study in Spain indicated that the majority of asylum seekers and refugees were based in Madrid while the most significant service developments in the field were recorded in Barcelona. In the United Kingdom, some areas to which asylum seekers had been dispersed had good service infrastructures while others, with similar numbers of asylum seekers, had minimal facilities. A top-down approach is necessary to ensure that there is an equitable distribution of services to areas of greatest need.

The political and legal contexts of migration may have a significant impact on access to mental health and social care services. However, the studies also recorded the impact of a secondary level of access, through professional gatekeepers within the localities in which refugees are based. Examples highlighted in the Netherlands suggest problems that may be faced by asylum seekers who only access the support of a specialist after going through two professional gatekeepers in the form of the *Medische Opvang Asielzoekers* (Medical care for asylum seekers) in the accommodation centre and, subsequently, the general practitioner in the community. The study points to barriers that may exist in gaining access to services through these gatekeepers arising from the latter's lack of knowledge and cultural competence in dealing with refugee clients. This may be compounded by the refugees' own lack of knowledge of the health care system resulting in their feeling of being 'fobbed off' by the service. In the United Kingdom, dispersed refugees may be faced with a situation in which they have little knowledge of the health care system in their locality and where general practitioners may feel they have neither the time, expertise or resources necessary to treat refugees. This has, on occasions, resulted in explicit decisions being made by individual practices not to treat refugees. Thus, while entitlement to services may be present, actual access to services may not.

The question of access may be addressed by agencies that act as brokers or advocates for refugees. In Portugal, the Portuguese Refugee Council is a fundamental mediator between users and health care services. In the United Kingdom, Breathing Space acts as an advocate in ensuring that refugees receive an appropriate range of mental health and social care services. In each of the countries studied, and in the broader international report, advocacy was widely viewed as a vital component of good practice in the mental health and social care of refugees.

Research into the mental health care of refugees in Europe is at an early stage. However, even at this point it is possible to suggest some elements of mental health care that may constitute good practice in this field. The elements identified in the research project included the following:

- cultural sensitivity;
- an integrated approach;

- political awareness;
- accessible services.

Those services that were identified as offering good practice have combined, to a greater or lesser degree, these four components.

Cultural sensitivity here refers to the development of mental health and social care services that are knowledge-based and reflect the cultures of the refugee groups with whom the service seeks to engage. It directly challenges mono-cultural models of service provision and seeks to develop systems of classification and treatment that reflect the problems identified by refugees themselves. The work of such services may result in the revision of categories to include 'cultural bereavement' and, on the basis of the work of the SAPPIR service in Barcelona, the 'Ulysses Syndrome' resulting from the experience of migrating across the Mediterranean Sea. Cultural sensitivity also implies recognition of the dynamic nature of cultures and awareness of cultural heterogeneity and the development of new cultural forms over time. Thus, the approach seeks to avoid the stereotyping and reification of refugee cultures that has dogged the development of mental health services to refugees and minority ethnic groups.

An integrated approach implies the integration of mental health and social care services. It involves recognition that the problems experienced by refugees are rarely appropriately differentiated into the categories of mental health *or* social care. As noted, within the post-migration context there is a crucial interrelationship between social circumstances and mental health with factors such as detention, bureaucratic processes, homelessness, poverty, loss of culture, loss of family and friends, and social isolation having a discernible impact on mental health status (Silove *et al.* 2000). If services are to be effective they must seek to identify the interplay of factors and function to ameliorate them at different levels. Services identified in the good practice study recognized this interplay and often operated on an implicit 'hierarchy of needs' model in which emphasis was placed on ensuring that basic needs such as food and shelter were addressed prior to offering what may be more clearly identified as mental health care. An integrated approach typically required the crossing of institutional boundaries and the creation of partnerships between statutory services, intergovernmental bodies and NGOs.

A further feature of good practice identified in the report concerned the development of *political awareness* among service providers and this may be seen to have functioned at both a macro and a micro level. At a macro level it involved awareness of the situations refugees were fleeing from and developing as up-to-date knowledge as possible of the volatile situations within the countries of origin. It also included knowledge of the political situations in the countries refugees passed through *en route* to western Europe. This included changes in laws and policies within countries developed at a national or supra-national level (e.g. through new EU policies). These macro changes were viewed by astute service providers not as mere background knowledge, but as having a direct and substantial impact on the lives of the refugees they were supporting. Changing conditions in one country, for example, Afghanistan or Iraq, had a considerable impact on relatives and friends living there and on refugees' perceptions of their future lives. On some occasions a host country's perception of improving conditions led to anxieties about being forced to return to a situation in which refugees may continue to feel very unsafe. Consequently, macro level changes may have very direct impact on the lives and mental health of refugees. Political awareness was also of vital importance in relation to the changing laws and policies of the host societies and the pressures that arise from public perceptions of refugees. Public hostility in particular localities greatly increased anxiety, isolation and depression.

A fourth component identified in the study was *accessibility*, and this too is also appropriately viewed as operating at different levels. Each of the services identified in the research project were innovative in seeking to improve the access of refugees to services. At the most obvious level, they sought to create 'user friendly' environments where there was, for example, evident celebration of multiculturalism through the use of images in posters and ceramics and, on occasions, the promoting of multicultural events aimed towards generating or nurturing harmonious relations between refugees and the host communities. Access was also improved by organizational developments aimed at ensuring that services relevant to refugees were located in places where they congregated. It involved both a geographical analysis of refugee dispersal and settlement and an awareness of the contexts where refugees were most likely to be stressed, for example at ports of entry, and to encounter stressful reception conditions. Thus, the Breathing Space team, for example, located its service in one of the United Kingdom's major support centres for refugees. Access involved the development of relationships and pathways between principal 'gatekeepers' to health, mental health and social care. For example, it could mean forging close relationships with local doctors and undertaking outreach work into accommodation centres or places where refugees receive emergency accommodation. A further dimension to access was the employment of staff who would speak appropriate community languages and who would be aware of refugees' cultures, including subdivisions within cultural groups.

The above elements were shown in the study to be fundamental building blocks in appropriate refugee mental health services. Increasing emphasis on the standardization of reception arrangements across Europe provides unprecedented opportunities for sharing models of good practice across countries. The utilization and standardization of evaluation models and techniques provides new opportunities for assessing achievement in this field and ensuring that good practice is implemented as widely as possible.

References

Ager, A. (1993) *Mental Health Issues in Refugee Populations: A Review*. Working paper of the Harvard Center for the Study of Culture and Medicine. Project on International Mental and Behavioral Health. Cambridge, MA: Harvard Medical School, Department of Social Medicine.

Ager, A. (2000) Psychosocial programmes: principles and practice for research and evaluation, in F. Ahearn (ed.) *Psychosocial Wellness of Refugees*. New York: Berghahn Books.

Ahearn, F. (ed.) (2000) *Psychosocial Wellness of Refugees*. New York: Berghahn Books.

Beiser, M. (1999) *Strangers at the Gate: The 'Boat People's' First Ten Years in Canada*. Toronto: University of Toronto Press.

Bernal, M. (2003) Identification study: Spain, in C. Watters and D. Ingleby, *Good Practice in Mental Health and Social Care for Refugees and Asylum Seekers*. Canterbury: University of Kent.

Castles, S. and Miller, M. (2003) *The Age of Migration: International Population Movements in the Modern World*. Basingstoke: Palgrave Macmillan.

Crisp, J. (2003) *A New Asylum Paradigm? Globalization, Migration and the Uncertain Future of the International Refugee Regime*. Working paper no. 100. Geneva: Evaluation and Policy Analysis Unit, UNHCR.

Eisenbruch, M. (1991) From post-traumatic stress disorder to cultural bereavement: diagnosis of Southeast Asian refugees, *Social Science and Medicine*, 33(6): 673–80.

European Commission (2003) *Council Directive 2003/9/EC of 27th January 2003*. Brussels: European Commission.

Fassin, D. (2001) The biopolitics of otherness: undocumented foreigners and racial discrimination in French public debate, *Anthropology Today*, 17(1): 3–7.

Goldberg, D., Benjamin, S. and Creed, F. (1994) *Psychiatry in Medical Practice*. London: Routledge.

Gorst-Unsworth, C. and Goldenberg, E. (1998) Psychological sequelae of torture and organized violence suffered by refugees from Iraq: trauma-related factors compared with social factors in exile, *British Journal of Psychiatry*, 172(Jan): 90–4.

Hollingfield, J. (2000) The politics of international migration, in C. Brettell and J. Hollingfield (eds) *Migration Theory*. New York: Routledge.

Justice (2002) *Asylum: Changing Policy and Practice in the UK, EU and Selected Countries*. London: Justice.

Kamau, M., Silove, D., Steel, Z., Catanzaro, R., Bateman, C. and Ekblad, S. (2004) Psychiatric disorders in an African refugee camp, *International Journal of Mental Health, Psychosocial Work and Counselling in Areas of Armed Conflict*, 2(2): 84–9.

McCallin, M. (1992) The impact of current and traumatic stressors on the psychological well-being of refugee communities, in M. McCallin (ed.) *The Psychological Well-Being of Refugee Children: Research, Practice and Policy Issues*. Geneva: International Catholic Child Bureau.

Mollica, R.F., McInnes, K., Sarajli, N., Lavelle, J., Sarajli, I. and Massagli, M. (1999) Disability associated with psychiatric comorbidity and health status in Bosnian refugees living in Croatia, *Journal of the American Medical Association*, 282(5): 433–9.

PICUM (Platform for International Cooperation on Undocumented Migrants) (2001) *Health Care for Undocumented Migrants*. Antwerp: PICUM.

Pourgourides, C.K., Bracken, P.J. and Sashidharan, S.P. (1996) *A Second Exile: The Mental Health Implications of Detention of Asylum Seekers in the United Kingdom*. Birmingham: Academic Unit, Northern Birmingham Mental Health Trust.

Silove, D. (1999) The psychosocial effects of torture, mass human rights violations, and refugee trauma, *Journal of Nervous and Mental Disease*, 187(4): 200–7.

Silove, D., McIntosh, P. and Becker, R. (1993) Risk of retraumatization of asylum-seekers in Australia, *Australian and New Zealand Journal of Psychiatry*, 27(4): 606–12.

Silove, D., Ekblad, S. and Mollica, R. (2000a) The rights of the severely mentally ill in post-conflict societies, *Lancet*, 355(9214): 1548–9.

Silove, D., Steel, Z. and Watters, C. (2000b) Policies of deterrence and the mental health of asylum seekers, *Journal of the American Medical Association*, 284(5): 604–11.

Stubbs, P. (2004) Transforming local and global discourses: reassessing the PTSD movement in Bosnia and Croatia, in D. Ingleby (ed.) *Forced Migration and Mental Health: Rethinking the Care of Refugees and Displaced Persons*. Amsterdam: Kluwer.

Summerfield, D. (1999) A critique of seven assumptions behind psychological trauma programmes in war-affected areas, *Social Science and Medicine*, 48(10): 1449–62.

Thompson, M., McGorry, P., Silove, D. and Steel, Z. (1988) Marlbymong Detention Centre Tamil Survey, in D. Silove and Z. Steel (eds) *Mental Health and Well-Being of On-Shore Asylum Seekers in Australia*. Sydney: Psychiatry Research and Teaching Unit, University of New South Wales.

UNHCR (2000) *The State of the World's Refugees: Fifty Years of Humanitarian Action*. Geneva: UNHCR.

UNHCR (2002) *Global Consultations on International Protection: Refugee Women*. Geneva: UNHCR.

UNHCR (2004) *Asylum Levels and Trends: Europe and non-European Industrialized Countries, 2003*. Geneva: Population Data Unit, UNHCR.

Watters, C. (2001a) Emerging paradigms in the mental health care of refugees, *Social Science and Medicine*, 52(11): 1709–18.

Watters, C. (2001b) Avenues of access and the moral economy of legitimacy, *Anthropology Today*, 17(2): 24.

Watters, C. (2002) Migration and mental health care in Europe: report of a preliminary mapping exercise, *Journal of Ethnic and Migration Studies*, 28(1): 153–72.

Watters, C. and Ingleby, D. (2003) *Good Practice in the Mental Health and Social Care of Refugees and Asylum Seekers: Report to the European Refugee Fund*. Brussels: European Commission.

World Health Organization (1996) *The Mental Health of Refugees*. Geneva: WHO.

World Health Organization (2001) *Mental Health: New Understanding, New Hope*. Geneva: WHO.

Young, A. (1995) *The Harmony of Illusions: Invention of Post-traumatic Stress Disorder*. Princeton, NJ: Princeton University Press.

Zolberg, A. (1989) The next waves: migration theory for a changing world, *International Migration Review*, 23(3): 403–30.

sixteen

Carers and families of people with mental health problems

Lorenza Magliano, David McDaid,
Susan Kirkwood and Kathryn Berzins

During the past two decades the responsibility falling on families to help in providing care and assistance to people with mental health problems has increased in most European countries. There has been a trend both towards shorter hospital stays and a reduction of inpatient beds, coupled with a more general shift towards providing community-based mental health care services wherever possible (see Chapter 10). It is now estimated that between 40 and 90 per cent of people with mental health problems remain in close contact or live with relatives who often provide them with long-term physical and emotional support (Hogman and de Vleesschauwer 1996; Rose 1996; Ostman and Hansson 2001; World Health Organization 2001; Ostman and Hansson 2002b; Lauber *et al.* 2003). These family members may have to undertake additional responsibilities and tasks, especially where insufficient resources have been transferred to community-based mental health systems (Kuipers 1993; Brand 2001).

These additional tasks and responsibilities, provided unpaid and informally, are therefore often referred to as the 'carer burden'. Although widely used, this term can sometimes be perceived to be unduly negative, and while we concentrate here on the challenges faced by caregivers and the support mechanisms they require, it is very important at the outset to recognize that there are both rewards and difficulties associated with the caregiving experience. A sense of satisfaction may be derived by carers from knowing that they are able to help and improve the quality of life of a loved one. 'Carer burden', however, does convey a sense of the great demands and strains that carers often report, and it can help to indicate a need to focus on integrated measures of physical and mental well-being and socioeconomic status that can reduce the negative aspects, and help reinforce the positive features of the caregiving experience. Negative experiences for carers that go unchecked can also have an impact on long-term outcomes for individuals with mental health problems.

In this chapter we begin by distinguishing between two distinct impacts of caregiving: subjective and objective burdens. We then go on to review briefly aspects of both and to highlight the health and socioeconomic consequences for all. Risk factors which can help identify a potential burden are discussed. We then look at the role that access to services, backed up by legislation, can have in supporting family carers. Voluntary family associations also play a vital role in empowering and supporting family carers. We end by looking at how they have evolved across Europe and consider the policy challenges to be faced.

The objective and subjective impact of care

Since the early 1960s, family 'burden' has been divided into objective and subjective dimensions (Hoenig and Hamilton 1966). The former relates to the practical problems experienced by an individual's family, such as the disruption of family relationships, constraints in social, leisure and work activities, financial difficulties and a negative impact on physical health. The latter describes the psychological reactions that family members experience; for example, a feeling of loss, depression, anxiety and embarrassment in social situations, the stress of coping with disturbing behaviours and the frustration caused by changing relationships (Lanzara *et al.* 1999; Pereira and de Almeida 1999; Ostman and Hansson 2000; Jungbauer and Angermeyer 2002; Magliano *et al.* 2002; Mory *et al.* 2002; Ohaeri 2003; Ostman and Hansson 2004; Magliano *et al.* 2005a, 2006b; Moller-Leimkuhler 2005). While objective burden is predominantly related to the close contact between families and people with mental health problems, subjective burden is determined by many factors, including the resilience and different coping mechanisms used by carers, the strength of relationships prior to the onset of illness, the level of support from social networks and the availability of, and access to, formal services.

The impact of caregiving

We begin by concentrating on some of the subjective burdens faced by carers of people with different types of mental health problems and then go on to consider some of the objective impacts on health and socioeconomic status that are common to all. To date, most research on the impact of caregiving has focused on cognitive disorders such as dementia and Alzheimer's disease. However, the number of published studies on caregiving burden, in general, has increased in recent years, with more attention being paid to other mental health problems, most notably psychoses (Ohaeri 2003; Schulze and Rossler 2005).

Psychoses

Following a first admission for treatment a substantial proportion of individuals with psychoses will return to live with their relatives. This can be a long-term commitment: in one study looking at 179 people with schizophrenia initially living with other family members, more than half were still residing with them 15 years later (Brown and Birtwistle 1998). The impact, of course, is not just restricted to those households where a person with psychosis lives with other family members. In the UK700 study, for instance, half of all people with schizophrenia had frequent contacts with at least one relative, and two-thirds met their families more than once a week (Harvey *et al.* 2001a, 2001b).

The EPSILON study looked at the impact of schizophrenia in five different cities across Europe – Amsterdam, Copenhagen, London, Santander and Verona. This demonstrated that the most common consequences for families were worries about their loved one's health and future, as well as their own personal safety and financial situation (Thornicroft *et al.* 2004). The impact was higher when the person with schizophrenia lived with and/or had more contact with their family. Other studies have also emphasized concerns about the behaviour of people with psychoses – for instance, their restlessness, hypochondria, sleep disturbances or aggressiveness (Grad and Sainsbury 1968; Bury *et al.* 1998; Schene *et al.* 1998). Suicide attempts and depressive moods are also frequently reported by relatives as contributing to subjective burden. The lack of independence and social skills, low levels of interest in leisure activities and a poor state of self-care are other aspects of the disorder with which relatives can have difficulty coping (McCarthy *et al.* 1989).

All of these factors can contribute to reduced quality of life for caregivers. One recent, albeit relatively small, study in Sweden which compared the parents of people with schizophrenia to a random sample of the population reported that these parents were significantly less satisfied with their quality of life; moreover, there was a correlation between lower overall quality of life and higher perceived burden (Foldemo *et al.* 2005). This impact on quality of life can be long-standing. In one study, around one half of all relatives initially experienced moderate or severe distress at the onset of caregiving, with little change found 15 years later (Brown and Birtwistle 1998).

Affective disorders

Much less attention has focused on affective disorders, but like psychoses they can also cause great distress for individuals and their families (Sartorius 2001). The partners of people with persistent depression, in particular, have marked difficulties in maintaining social and leisure activities, complain about a decrease in total family income and may have considerable strains placed on their marital relationships (Jungbauer *et al.* 2004; van Wijngaarden *et al.* 2004).

Substantial subjective distress has also been reported in relatives of individuals with bi-polar disorders. Again, burden is significantly related to symptoms and changes in family roles. Burden has been found to be greatest among family members who believe that their relative is able to control symptoms, and among those who were aware of the prognosis of the illness. Moderate or great distress in at least one of the domains of burden has been reported by as many as 93 per cent of caregivers (Perlick *et al.* 1999, 2001). The cyclical nature of bi-polar disorders requires even more emphasis on the long-term assessment of the impact they have has on families. It is likely that families are greatly involved in care only during critical periods of the disorder (Perlick *et al.* 2005).

Cognitive disorders

There has been more focus on the burden of care faced by the family members of people with dementia or Alzheimer's disease than any other mental health problem. Looking after someone with dementia can sometimes be, literally, a 24-hour-a-day activity. People may become isolated from their social network of family and friends as the disease progresses and caregiving becomes a full-time occupation (Leinonen *et al.* 2001). Evidence of high levels of distress and depression among carers of people with dementia can be seen in many studies of service users and in community surveys (Clipp and George 1993; Livingston *et al.* 1996; Murray *et al.* 1999; Coen *et al.* 2002; Thomas *et al.* 2005).

Other disorders

Although only limited data are available on the difficulties experienced by the families of people with obsessive-compulsive disorder (Steketee 1997; Amir *et al.* 2002), again, it seems that this disorder has a considerable impact on families and can lead to a reduction in social activities, leading to isolation over time. People with obsessive-compulsive symptoms frequently involve their relatives in rituals, sometimes attracting anger and criticism towards them, which consequently has a negative impact on treatment outcomes (Calvocoressi *et al.* 1995).

Eating disorders have received little attention, although here, again, some research suggests that the impact on family members of anorexia nervosa may be even higher than for psychoses (Treasure *et al.* 2001). Recent, albeit small-scale, qualitative research on bulimia nervosa also indicates that carers have significant emotional and practical needs for support and information. However, there is some evidence of the positive rewards associated with caregiving, with 16 out of 20 carers reporting some positive experiences (Perkins *et al.* 2004; Winn *et al.* 2004).

The health impact of caring

Regardless of the mental health problem of a loved one, family carers are themselves vulnerable to physical and mental health problems, and as a consequence they may make greater use of medical resources (Jungbauer *et al.* 2002; Wittmund *et al.* 2002; Hirst 2005). A higher prevalence of depressive disorders also has been reported among caregivers of people with mental health problems than in the general population, especially when the level of disability is high (Jungbauer *et al.* 2002; Wittmund *et al.* 2002). Two studies found that over half of the family members in their study group believed that their own mental health had been affected and they experienced symptoms such as insomnia, headaches, excessive irritability and depression (Grad and Sainsbury 1968; McCarthy *et al.* 1989). Another reported that, among the negative consequences of caregiving cited by parents, the health impact was greatest. Among the symptoms cited, brooding, inner unrest, irritability, insomnia, fatigue, as well as neck and shoulder pains were most frequently mentioned (Angermeyer *et al.* 2001). The severity of these symptoms was a significant predictor of psycho-somatic complaints in carers, and compared with the general population they were found to visit physicians more frequently, particularly general practitioners, as well as psychiatrists and psychotherapists. One study in Finland, which looked at members of a local family association, found that 38 per cent were vulnerable to clinical depression. Mothers and wives, and respondents with low incomes or who were enduring economic hardship, in particular, were found to be at a high risk of depression (Nyman and Stengård 2001).

The impact on health and the need for health care resources may vary depending on the nature of the mental disorder. One recent study that looked retrospectively at the experiences of primary family caregivers in the United States over a seven-month period prior to the admission of a relative to a psychiatric outpatient unit or inpatient admission for bi-polar disorder reported much higher rates of mental health and primary care service utilization than those found in the general population (Perlick *et al.* 2005). Another study of 90 families of people with schizophrenia found that relatives were stressed by the individuals' disturbing behaviours at a 'pathological level in 38 per cent of cases' (Birchwood and Cochrane 1990). The health impacts on carers of people with cognitive disorders can also be substantial. As dementia and Alzheimer's disease are most prevalent in older age groups, their carers, the majority of whom are spouses, may be frail themselves and can suffer a deterioration in their own health as a result of the mental and physical strains of caring, such as lifting, washing and dressing (Meinland *et al.* 2001; Thomas *et al.* 2005).

Positive aspects of caring

As we noted at the beginning of this chapter, it is important to recognize that there are both rewards and difficulties associated with caregiving; yet often, the positive aspects may be overlooked. Appreciation of the positive aspects of caring can be significantly associated with low family burden (Nyman and Stengård 2001). Caregivers may, for instance, report that they benefit from feelings of gratification, love and pride. Moreover, although many relatives experience considerable distress, research evidence does not suggest that they avoid frequent contact with the patient as a consequence (Grella and Grusky 1989; Veltman *et al.* 2002). One Verona study reported that when adequately supported by professionals, 92 per cent of relatives continued to maintain contact with friends and relatives, 72 per cent did not see their family income decrease because of caregiving responsibilities, and 52 per cent could manage household disruptions during a crisis (Samele and Manning 2000).

Similar findings have been reported when looking at carers of older people with cognitive problems. One Canadian study of 211 caregivers reported that 73 per cent could identify at least one positive aspect of caregiving (Cohen *et al.*

2002). In another study of carers of people with dementia in England, Italy and Sweden, few informal carers were found to be willing to give up caring for their relatives even when the level of objective burden was great (McDaid and Sassi 2001). Similarly, studies looking at depressive disorders report that, despite problems, the majority of spouses are committed to remaining with their partner (Fadden *et al.* 1987; Keitner and Miller 1990; Ellring 1999). More generally, in a survey of nearly 1000 informal carers of people with a range of health conditions, nearly half reported positive aspects of caring and felt that their happiness would be reduced if they were to transfer their responsibilities to someone else (Brouwer *et al.* 2005).

The economic consequences of caregiving

The desire and willingness of family members to provide care can sometimes mean that policy-makers and other stakeholders treat informal care as a 'free resource'. However, it can entail significant economic costs for individuals and society. Economic analysis is primarily concerned with the opportunity costs of caring; i.e. what would have been done had an individual not been caring. While the availability of family carers may reduce the need for professional support, carers will incur a loss of time (and hence a cost) which they could have used for work, or to pursue leisure activities. They may also incur additional out-of-pocket expenses to support a relative financially and, as we have seen, may suffer from both physical and mental health problems which again can entail significant costs to the health system.

Inclusion of the full costs of caring can thus be very important in a comprehensive economic analysis and could make a difference when decision-makers have to determine whether it is cost-effective to introduce specific services or programmes to support family caregivers or provide other interventions. It also provides an indication of the costs that may fall on statutory services in future if there is a shortage of such carers due to the ageing of the population in most European countries. However, because of methodological difficulties in estimating informal care costs, and often too narrow a focus solely on the health care system alone, the cost to family carers has often been ignored within economic analyses. In particular, identifying the best alternative use of time is not always easy, particularly if a family carer already has been responsible, to some extent, for an individual – for example, the parents of a child. This has led to a considerable variation in estimates of the cost of caring (McDaid 2001).

Nonetheless, there is a growing number of studies that place a value on family care, particularly in two areas: psychoses and dementia. One American study estimated that the costs of lost employment to carers of people with schizophrenia alone was approximately 17.5 per cent of the total costs of the illness (Rice and Miller 1996). In one Italian study of the costs associated with schizophrenia it was estimated that approximately 29 per cent were due to lost employment, employment opportunities foregone and the leisure time costs of family carers (Tarricone *et al.* 2000). Estimates from Australia suggest that the annual costs to the 2379 carers of people with schizophrenia who had given up the opportunity to work ranged from $AUS 51.5 million (Carr *et al.* 2003) to

$AUS 88 million, or just over 6 per cent of the total costs of the illness (Access Economics 2002). The authors of this latter study considered this estimate to be conservative as it did not include the costs for part-time carers or those not designated as 'home carers'. Family and other informal carers can also account for a very high proportion of the total costs associated with Alzheimer's disease and other forms of dementia – ranging from 36 to 85 per cent of total costs in one review (McDaid 2001). For instance, another study looking at carers in London over a two-year period estimated that informal care accounted for at least 40 per cent of total costs (Schneider *et al.* 2003).

There is remarkably little discussion in the literature of carer costs related to depressive disorders. Studies sometimes recognize the important contribution of caring but find it impossible to place a value on this contribution (Evers and Ament 1995). Others have excluded costs on the grounds that there was no impact on paid employment, as in the case of one review for bi-polar disorders (Das Gupta and Guest 2002). Yet the costs go far beyond lost opportunities for paid employment. One approximation from Australia estimated that 9 per cent of people with bi-polar disorders have carers who have had to give up work to provide care full-time. The costs of lost wages to these 9000-plus carers was estimated in 2003 to be almost $AUS 200 million (Access Economics and SANE Australia 2003). There are also significant costs incurred by those carers who are beyond retirement age. The additional costs of caring for people over the age of 70 who have depression have been estimated in the United States. Most of these carers are themselves retired and provide an additional three to six hours per week of informal care, depending on the number of depressive symptoms shown, at a cost of some $US 9 billion per annum (Langa *et al.* 2004).

Risk factors associated with family burden

We have highlighted the subjective, objective and economic impacts of caregiving, but this is of little use unless we have some understanding of what contributes to and/or protects against the negative aspects of caring. Research in this area continues to grow (Schulze and Rossler 2005). A key predictive factor is expressed emotion. This is a measure of family involvement with a relative based on how they spontaneously talk about their loved one. It can be defined as notable attitudes of criticism and/or emotional over-involvement towards the individual (Foldemo *et al.* 2005). Several studies have examined the reciprocal influence of burden and expressed emotions as aspects of the relationship between people with mental disorders and their families (Wearden *et al.* 2002). High-expressed-emotion (HEE) relatives can have twice the level of burden of low-expressed-emotion (LEE) relatives, and may feel that they do not cope as effectively (Smith *et al.* 1993).

Other studies have suggested that coping styles such as coercion and negative criticism are associated with higher levels of burden (Jackson *et al.* 1990; Budd *et al.* 1998), while Perlick *et al.* (2004), looking at bi-polar disorder, reported an association between emotional over-involvement and higher levels of caregiver burden. A recent five-year follow up of the burden and predictors of burden for 83 caregivers of individuals hospitalized for schizophrenia or depression conducted in Germany found that relatives with HEE had significantly more objective and subjective burden, as well as lower satisfaction with life (Moller-Leimkuhler 2005). Scazufca and Kuipers (1996) found that relatives of people with schizophrenia were less burdened at a nine-month follow up than at the time of the initial episode. The largest improvement in burden was found among relatives who changed from HEE to LEE, while a significant increment in burden was observed among those who shifted from LEE to HEE.

Some studies suggest that relatives' coping strategies are influenced by the symptoms and level of disability seen in people with mental health disorders. Coercion is more frequently adopted by relatives of people with formal thought disorders and delusions (Magliano *et al.* 1995; Harvey *et al.* 2001a), or if they have high levels of social disability and experience frequent relapses. Acceptance of an individual's behaviours is higher among relatives of those with greater social functioning (Birchwood and Cochrane 1990). Emotion-focused coping strategies, such as avoidance, resignation and seeking spiritual help, as well as a low sense of mastery or control over the situation, have been found to be closely related to high family burden (Magliano *et al.* 1995; Bibou-Nakou *et al.* 1997). Also, it has been found that carers of chronic patients more frequently adopt a passive style of coping than those caring for individuals in the early phase, suggesting a change in coping style over time.

Burden has also been studied in relation to caregivers' social networks (Magliano *et al.* 1998; Ostman and Hansson 2001). High practical social support, as well as participation in self-help groups and psycho-educational programmes have been associated with effective coping strategies and lower family distress (Johnson 1990, 1995). Social networks of families and friends, for instance, are particularly vital for older carers; without access to such social support networks they have been found to be much more vulnerable to having a crisis in caring (Wenger and Burholt 2004). More generally, when family members have a supportive social network, they have greater protection against stress (Gore and Colten 1991; Olstad *et al.* 2001) and are better able to manage their relative's critical periods, with a consequent decrease in rates of hospitalization (Brugha *et al.* 1993).

A national study on family burden in routine clinical settings was carried out in Italy, where mental health care is strongly community-oriented. More than 700 families of service users with schizophrenia were consecutively recruited in 30 mental health departments randomly selected from across the country (Magliano *et al.* 2002). Ninety-seven per cent of relatives reported feelings of loss, and 83 per cent stated that they cried or felt depressed. In addition, 73 per cent of relatives had neglected their hobbies and 68 per cent had had difficulties going on holiday. Thirty-four per cent of the relatives reported that they felt confident enough to seek professional help in a crisis situation, and 43 per cent received adequate information from service staff on how to cope with an individual's disturbing behaviours. The practical and psychological burden was significantly higher in families of those with high disability and manic/hostility symptoms when relatives received poor support from professionals and from their social networks in emergencies, and when there was less practical social support. Moreover, practical burden was found to be lower in more affluent northern Italy, where professional resources were more frequently available and patients were more frequently involved in rehabilitative pro-grammes. However, social networks were stronger in the south where traditional community-orientated values remain strong.

The experience of these caregivers was also compared with a sample of 646 family carers of people with a long-term physical illness (brain disorder, heart disease, diabetes, kidney or lung diseases). While the impact of caring was substantial for all, subjective burden was greatest for those supporting someone with schizophrenia or a brain disorder. Moreover, access to social support and emergency help was much lower for the carers of people with schizophrenia; those with less access to social networks and support had higher levels of both subjective and objective burden (Magliano *et al.* 2005a). These groups of carers were also compared with 714 members of the general population. Sixty-one per cent of the general population had been contacted by family or friends during a two-month period compared to just 38 per cent of carers of people with schizophrenia (Magliano *et al.* 2006b).

At a European level, the availability of cross-cultural research in this area is poor; most studies have been carried out in just a single country. Findings are not necessarily applicable in other contexts, as burden is likely to be influenced by factors such as public attitudes toward mental illness and the level of service provision, which significantly vary both within and across countries. One European study, conducted between 1994 and 1997, that specifically explored family burden and coping strategies in schizophrenia, looked at 236 relatives of people with schizophrenia recruited in Italy, the United Kingdom, Greece, Germany and Portugal (Magliano *et al.* 1998, 1999). In all locations, relatives reported that caring for someone with schizophrenia resulted in restrictions in their own social activities, had negative effects on family life and engendered a sense of loss. A higher level of burden and a more frequent adoption of ineffective coping strategies such as resignation, reduction of social interests and avoidance of the person with schizophrenia were found among relatives who had poorer social network support. In contrast, relatives were better placed to use problem-solving strategies, such as involving their relative in their social activities, positive communication, seeking information and talking with friends to help them adapt to caring when they had access to a large and supportive social network.

While there were common findings across the five centres, there were also differences, some apparently reflecting a divide between the Mediterranean centres and the north-European centres. For example, relatives in the Mediter-ranean centres were more resigned and frequently used spiritual help as a cop-ing strategy, unlike those in northern centres. Similarly, the former group report a greater level of reduction in social interests, and lower levels of support from their social network. One-year follow-up data (Magliano *et al.* 1999) showed that burden was stable over time in the absence of significant changes in the pattern of care. However, when burden decreased, a related improvement over time was found in: a) relatives' tolerance of an individual's behaviours; b) practical support provided to families by their social network; c) course of illness; and d) the person with schizophrenia's social functioning.

Interventions and support for caregivers

Caring is not a free resource. If family carers cannot manage they may have to be replaced or supplemented by paid professional caregivers. Moreover, a high level of burden on caregivers not only impacts on their own health and eco- nomic productivity but also adversely affects the outcomes for the person with mental health problems (Falloon 1985; Perlick *et al.* 2004). From a policy perspective therefore, a key issue must be to ensure that there is an appropriate assessment of carers' needs, followed by access to appropriate support to help families enjoy the rewards of caregiving while minimizing the challenges that they face. These experiences are very much influenced by access to information, as well as professional support. Psychoeducational interventions targeted at family members may also be helpful in reducing family burden.

Improved access to advice and information

Despite the vital contribution made by family carers, their relationship with local mental health services has often been described as problematic and tense (Grella and Grusky 1989; Schene and van Wijngaarden 1995; Jungbauer and Angermeyer 2002). Relatives may feel hostility, resentment and dissatisfaction towards professionals who fail to understand their needs. Moreover, families report that they lack information about mental illness, are ignored by mental health professionals and are not consulted about treatment. One survey in five European countries of the help given during the first episode of psychosis (de Haan *et al.* 2002) reported that families expressed most dissatisfaction with the advice received on how to handle specific problems. Another study in Rome reported that satisfaction with services expressed by outpatients and their families was fairly good, except with respect to information on the condition and the level of family-member involvement in therapeutic programmes. In particular, dissatisfaction was associated with a lack of information during periods of inpatient care (Gigantesco *et al.* 2002).

Families are often in need of practical advice, information and education on psychiatric symptoms, use of medications, and management of disturbing behaviour and disabilities (Kuipers 1993; Reid *et al.* 1993; Angermeyer *et al.* 2000). Although information by itself has only a limited impact on families and does not change long-term outcomes, it improves relatives' hopes and con- fidence in professionals, and can have great value in facilitating coping with the emotional impact of mental disorders. Emotional support is particularly important in the first episodes of illness (Tennakoon *et al.* 2000; Lenior *et al.* 2002; Wolthaus *et al.* 2002). At this time, relatives must simultaneously cope with their own emotional reactions while providing support to their loved one.

Psychoeducational interventions

Effective family support interventions have been developed in the last 25 years (Falloon 1985; Leff *et al.* 1990). These psychoeducational interventions share a number of objectives: a) to provide the family with information on the disorder and treatment; b) to improve communication patterns within the family; c) to enhance family problem-solving skills; d) to improve family coping strategies; and e) to encourage their involvement in social activities.

Here we look at the use of such interventions for the families of people with psychoses. Since the 1980s, a growing body of evidence on the efficacy of psychological interventions for schizophrenia has been produced. Family therapy has clear preventive effects on the outcomes of psychiatric relapse and readmission, in addition to benefits of medication compliance and cost containment (Tarrier et al. 1988; Mueser et al. 2001; Pilling et al. 2002). Compared with routine case management, psychoeducational interventions have been shown to reduce fourfold the relapse rate in psychosis after a year, and twofold after two years. Moreover, they improve compliance with drug therapy, reduce the overall economic costs of care and may have a positive influence on the family situation (Canive et al. 1996; Szmukler et al. 1996; Stam and Cuijpers 2001). One study also reported that relatives' groups are more effective than behavioural family intervention groups in reducing the rate of relapse for individuals in a stable phase of schizophrenia (Montero et al. 2001).

Despite their proven efficacy, these interventions are not always available routinely across Europe. In western Europe, one study in the late 1990s suggested that less than 15 per cent of families of patients with schizophrenia received structured supportive interventions in routine settings (Magliano et al. 1998). In order to deal with their poor availability, the European Union (EU), within its Fifth Framework Programme for Research and Technological Development, promoted a study aimed at assessing, across six European countries, the impact of two alternative staff training programmes on the implementation and effectiveness of a well-known psychoeducational intervention for relatives of patients with schizophrenia. The study was carried out in 24 mental health services and involved 48 professionals who provided the intervention for one year to 55 families of people with schizophrenia. At one-year follow-up assessment, statistically significant improvements were found in these patients' symptoms and social functioning as well as in relatives' burden, coping strategies and social supports (Magliano et al. 2005b).

Initiatives to implement these psychoeducational interventions on a large scale were initiated in the United Kingdom and Italy. In the former, the provision of family supportive interventions has been included among the key actions for the management of schizophrenia. In the latter, the assessment of family burden and the provision of family support interventions were priority actions in the National Health Plan 2002–4. Furthermore, a national project on schizophrenia, commissioned by a national family association and the National Institute of Health, was funded in Italy to implement family supportive interventions in routine clinical settings. Recent evaluation suggests that it is indeed possible to introduce such interventions into the mental health system after a relatively brief period of training. Moreover, they have a significant impact both on functional outcomes and family burden when provided to service users and carers in ordinary service settings (Magliano et al. 2006a, 2006c).

Child caregivers

This chapter has until now concentrated solely on issues affecting adult family members, but it is important to remember that children can also be affected by the mental health problems of family members. In contrast with the large amount of data on the burden on adult relatives, information on children is sparse. One study reported that 28 per cent of people, especially mothers, admitted to an in-hospital psychiatric unit were most responsible for raising their children (Ostman and Hansson 2002a). Older children can sometimes find themselves providing care for a parent. They can experience a consistent level of practical and psychological difficulties including guilt over their parent's emotional disturbances and embarrassment about his or her behaviour. Such children may find it difficult to communicate with their parent or to discuss their delusions and hallucinatory behaviours. While few studies have attempted to look at the socioeconomic costs to these child caregivers, we can hypothesize that long-term costs may be substantial, arising, in particular, from the difficulty that child carers may have in keeping up with their education.

Aldridge and Becker (2003) reveal that both parents and their child carers experience fear and prejudice from local and professional communities. This study also reported that the exclusion of children from care plans and medical, health and social care interventions helps to perpetuate these adverse consequences. Family associations may be a major source of support and information. In Sweden, the National Family Association has successfully begun to hold support meetings for children of all ages. Other European family associations have also instigated, published and distributed books and other materials to support children within a family where a parent has a severe mental illness. The experience of young siblings of a person with a mental health problem has also been reviewed, again with an emphasis on the need for access to information, and in particular, on information which can provide reassurance as a child reaches the age at which their brother or sister developed their illness (Davtian 2003).

The role of European and national legislation

Legislation can play an important role. Not only can it be used to protect the rights of a person with mental health problems (see Chapter 13), but it also has an important role to play in setting out the extent to which families can receive information on their relative's mental health state and be involved in treatment decisions. Legislation can also ensure that families are involved in the development of mental health policy and practice. One recent review looked at European and national legislation, and in addition, conducted a survey by email questionnaire of family associations across 25 countries that were members of the European Association for Families of People with Mental Illness (EUFAMI). This was backed up by a review of previous research and, where possible, information from law and statute-making bodies (Berzins 2003). The survey addressed four key questions:

Do countries consult with carers and family members when they review/develop mental health legislation or policy?

Seven of ten EUFAMI country members responding to this question (Belgium, England, Ireland, Italy, the Netherlands, Norway and Scotland) stated that they had been, or were going to be involved in the formulation of new legislation. Two of these country members, including Italy, expressly said it had been a positive experience, while the only other association to express a view was a family association in England who felt that consultation was only tokenistic and not properly valued. The countries where family members had not been involved in consultation were Cyprus, Greece and Slovenia, although in Greece there had been consultation within a committee examining the rights of people with mental health problems, and while this process was not intended to develop legislation it does show an acknowledgement by legislators of the benefits of consultation.

How are family members affected by legislation that allows people with mental illness to be detained and treated?

Again, the involvement of families in treatment decisions is complex and sensitive. Families in some situations may feel that it is essential that they make the decision on whether a loved one should or should not receive professional treatment and/or services. This may go against the wishes of the individual with a mental health disorder, and hence in other situations families may wish not to be involved in such decisions, fearing that they later may be blamed by their relative for committing them (World Health Organization 2005c). Family members can also have an important right to appeal against involuntary detention or treatment decisions on behalf of their relative, if this individual is unable to do so.

In the survey (Berzins 2003), information was obtained from 12 countries on the involvement of families on these issues. Half of these, including Cyprus, England, Greece and Ireland, have legal involvement in authorizing a family member to be subject to compulsory admission. Countries that did not legally involve family members in this decision included Belgium, Portugal, Sweden and the Netherlands. In a review of Scotland's mental health legislation the involvement of family members in compulsory admittance was seen as having the potential to cause conflict between the person with mental health problems and the relative, and as such this role was subsequently removed in legislation passed by the Scottish Parliament in March 2003. Legislation in Norway has adopted a different approach, making this an optional responsibility for families.

Are there any legal family responsibilities to the individual with mental illness?

Eleven country associations responded to this third question and all but two stated that they had no legal obligations unless the relative was a legal minor or subject to general legislation concerning the neglect of a vulnerable adult. The exceptions were Cyprus and Spain. In Cyprus, the family could be held legally responsible for a relative on discharge or leave of absence from hospital. In Spain, whoever was living with a person with a mental illness could be held liable for that individual's actions, whether or not they were the person's official guardian. Families were not always aware of this responsibility.

How does legislation allow information about the individual with mental illness to be shared with families and carers?

Professionals may be reluctant to disclose confidential medical information to relatives of an individual with a mental health problem, even though they may be the primary caregiver(s). This is a complex issue as, on the one hand, there is a need to uphold an individual's rights to confidentiality, but at the same time families may require a certain level of information to be able to provide effective support. The extent to which information is shared will also be dependent on local culture and custom. Ten countries responded to this survey question, the majority raising legal issues surrounding confidentiality and many stating that the law would only permit information to be shared with the consent of the patient. However, the opposite situation exists in Greece where information is routinely shared with families unless the patient expressly forbids it. In Italy, in contrast, legislation made disclosure to family members more difficult, while it was felt in Cyprus that information was largely shared with families when medical staff wanted them to take on more responsibility. This was viewed negatively as it often left families feeling guilty. Other responses noted that this information might be shared 'informally' depending on the relationship between the professional and the family, particularly in Belgium. English respondents noted that medical personnel did not take account of the severity of symptoms and how they may affect the individual when deciding whether to share information with family members.

Empowerment of families – the role of family associations

The importance of empowering people with mental health problems to make their own decisions about what services best meet their needs has already been highlighted (see Chapter 3). Equally, the empowerment of family members is essential. In addition to formal services, a critical role can be played by family associations in empowering family caregivers by providing mutual support and information both on the illness and on the availability of formal services, as well as acting as advocates to protect the rights of both people with mental health problems and family members. Family associations have now been established in most European countries. While some associations have been in existence for 30 years, others have only been set up very recently. They have developed in different ways. In the United Kingdom, for example, the family associations Rethink, NSF (Scotland) and HAFAL (Wales) provide services for those with mental illness in addition to providing support to families. In several countries, including France, the focus of the family association is not on providing services, but instead on working with families to provide information, training and support.

In June 1990, EUFAMI was established at a congress in De Haan, Belgium, when family representatives from 16 European countries expressed a strong desire to collaborate to guarantee the rights and welfare of mentally ill people and their relatives throughout Europe. The levels of commitment were high. As one participant noted 'we even learned that a Romanian couple, a doctor and his wife, had sold their car in order to pay for the journey to De Haan'. The priorities for EUFAMI and its member associations are to fight stigma, to support families and to campaign for good practice. By the end of 2005, 41 family associations in 26 European countries, as well as neighbouring Morocco, were members of EUFAMI.[1]

The success of family associations has been the subject of review (Brand 2001). The principal achievement has been to obtain the active recognition by professionals that family members are partners in the care process. This process has been led by the World Psychiatric Association, which has actively sought to involve family members in developing policy statements. Human rights have been high on the policy agenda both at the Council of Europe, as well as in the European Commission and the World Health Organization (WHO). EUFAMI, in particular, was active in pressing for a 'seat at the table' for relatives. This has started to show results with family members being involved in high-level discussions and consultation with these organizations. One notable example has been the recent WHO *Action Plan* and *Declaration* on mental health (World Health Organization 2005a, 2005b), endorsed by all 52 countries of the European region in Helsinki in January 2005, where non-governmental organizations (NGOs) representing both service users and families, including EUFAMI, had been able to play an important role in preparatory discussions and consultations leading up to the event. As well as welcoming the final *Declaration* and *Action Plan*, which recognized the importance of supporting the needs of family carers, EUFAMI also noted that a number of countries for the first time had included family members and service users within their official delegations (EUFAMI 2005). Recently, EUFAMI has played an active role in stakeholder consultations on the European Commission's Green Paper outlining a strategy for mental health (Commission of the European Communities 2005).

As well as gaining recognition and having a greater say in the development of policy, both Europe-wide organizations such as EUFAMI and national organizations can help to share best practice – for instance, in respect of legislation and codes of practice. Good practice in one country might be used as an example for those elsewhere as part of their lobbying and campaigning activities. The availability of services and treatments across Europe can also be used to help make the case for improved services within any one country. During 2003, for example, family associations in Hungary and Poland were actively involved, with support from EUFAMI, in lobbying their governments on the case for access to newer but more expensive antipsychotic medications. Family associations also can play an important role in supporting research that looks not only at the care needs of people with mental health problems, but also at the needs of other family members such as siblings.

Conclusion

There is a substantial body of literature on the profound impacts, both positive and negative, on family carers of people with mental health problems. There is also evidence that family support for mental health service users can be important to their long-term quality of life. Some positive benefits for people with mental disorders of community-based care can be enhanced by access to everyday family support; for instance, it may reduce the chances of crisis events or rehospitalization.

The economic value of caring is substantial, yet too often this is perceived as a free resource. Without the support provided by family carers, additional professional support may be required in order to maintain the same level of help and support for people with mental health problems. Providing additional support for family carers can help enhance the positive aspects of caring while reducing some of the negative consequences in terms of the impact on carers' physical and psychological health, employment status and opportunities to enjoy leisure.

The balance of services in any mental health system, of course, will be dependent on the availability of human and capital resources. Strategies to promote the rewards of caring and reduce the burden on families ideally should be set within the context of a balanced package of mental health services. This might include a range of community mental health support providing community-based living arrangements, access to rehabilitation services and interventions for families.

The development of European, national and regional policies on mental health should encourage active contributions from all stakeholders including service users and family members. It is important not only to put in place, but also to enforce, national laws and international conventions aimed at protecting people with mental health problems and facilitating greater access to information and support. One key area where legislation can play a vital role is in ensuring that people with mental health problems and families have some assessment of their needs for support and also have access to information on what supports may be available.

Family associations can also play a vital role in providing information, support and a social network for family members who, in some circumstances, can become very isolated; they might also feature significantly in the mixed economy of mental health service provision (see Chapter 4). As we have seen, stigma and discrimination are major problems and awareness campaigns to debunk some of the myths that surround mental health may be helpful. Clearly, it is vital to look at ways to further empower people with mental health problems to make decisions about the services and support they wish to receive (see Chapter 14). Equally, carers can also benefit from greater empowerment over services and support that best meet their particular needs.

Note

1   See www.eufami.org for a detailed list of member organizations.

References

Access Economics (2002) *Schizophrenia: Costs. An Analysis of the Burden of Schizophrenia and Related Suicide in Australia*. Melbourne: SANE Australia.

Access Economics and SANE Australia (2003) *Bipolar Disorder: Costs. An Analysis of the Burden of Bipolar Disorder and Related Suicide in Australia*. Melbourne: SANE Australia.

Aldridge, J. and Becker, S. (2003) *Children Caring for Parents with Mental Illness*. Bristol: Policy Press.

Amir, N., Freshman, B.A. and Foa, E. (2002) Family distress and involvement in relatives of obsessive-compulsive disorder patients, *Journal of Anxiety Disorders*, 14(3): 209–17.

Angermeyer, M.C., Diaz Ruiz de Zarate, J. and Matschinger, H. (2000) Information and support needs of the family of psychiatric patients, *Gesundheitswesen*, 62(10): 483–6.

Angermeyer, M.C., Liebelt, P. and Matschinger, H. (2001) Distress in parents of patients suffering from schizophrenia or affective disorders, *Psychotherapy, Psychosomatik, Midizinische Psychologie*, 51(6): 255–60.

Berzins, K. (2003) *Legislation Affecting Carers of People with Mental Health Problems*. Brussels: EUFAMI.

Bibou-Nakou, I., Dikaiou, M. and Bairactaris, C. (1997) Psychosocial dimensions of family burden among two groups of carers looking after psychiatric patients, *Social Psychiatry and Psychiatric Epidemiology*, 32: 104–8.

Birchwood, M. and Cochrane, R. (1990) Families coping with schizophrenia: coping styles, their origins and correlates, *Psychological Medicine*, 20(4): 857–65.

Brand, U. (2001) European perspectives: a carer's view, *Acta Psychiatrica Scandinavica Supplementum*, 104(Suppl. 410): 96–101.

Brouwer, W.B., van Exel, N.J., van den Berg, B., van den Bos, G.A. and Koopmanschap, M.A. (2005) Process utility from providing informal care: the benefit of caring, *Health Policy*, 74(1): 85–99.

Brown, S. and Birtwistle, J. (1998) People with schizophrenia and their families, *British Journal of Psychiatry*, 173: 139–44.

Brugha, T.S., Wing, J.K., Brewin, C.R., MacCarthy, B. and Lesage, A. (1993) The relationship of social network deficits with deficits in social functioning in long-term psychiatric disorders, *Social Psychiatry and Psychiatric Epidemiology*, 28(5): 218–24.

Budd, R.J., Oles, G. and Hughes, I.C. (1998) The relationship between coping style and burden in the carers of relatives with schizophrenia, *Acta Psychiatrica Scandinavica*, 98(4): 304–9.

Bury, L., Zaborowski, B., Konieczynska, Z., Jarema, M., Cicowska, G., Kunicka, A., Bartoszewicz, J. and Muraszkiewicz, L. (1998) Family burden of schizophrenia patients with various forms of psychiatric care, *Psychiatria Polska*, 32(3): 275–85.

Calvocoressi, L., Mazure, C.M., Kasl, S.V., Skolnick, J., Fisk, D., Vesgo, S.J., Van Noppen, B.L. and Price, L.H. (1995) Family accommodation in obsessive-compulsive disorder, *American Journal of Psychiatry*, 152(3): 441–3.

Canive, J.M., Sanz-Fuentenebro, J., Vasquez, C., Qualls, C., Fuentenebro, F., Perez, I.G. and Tuason, V.B. (1996) Family psychoeducational support groups in Spain: parents' distress and burden at nine-month follow-up, *Annals of Clinical Psychiatry*, 8(2): 71–9.

Carr, V.J., Neil, A.L., Halpin, S.A., Holmes, S. and Lewin, T.J. (2003) Costs of schizophrenia and other psychoses in urban Australia: findings from the Low Prevalence (Psychotic) Disorders Study, *Australian and New Zealand Journal of Psychiatry*, 37: 31–40.

Clipp, E.C. and George, L.K. (1993) Dementia and cancer; a comparison of spouse caregivers, *Gerontologist*, 33: 534–41.

Coen, R.F., O'Boyle, C.A., Coakley, D. and Lawlor, B.A. (2002) Individual quality of life factors distinguishing low-burden and high-burden caregivers of dementia patients, *Dementia and Geriatric Cognitive Disorders*, 13(3): 164–70.

Cohen, C.A., Colantonio, A. and Vernich, L. (2002) Positive aspects of caregiving: round-ing out the caregiver experience, *International Journal of Geriatric Psychiatry*, 17(2): 184–8.

Commission of the European Communities (2005) *Improving the Mental Health of the Population: Towards a Strategy on Mental Health for the European Union*. Brussels: Health and Consumer Protection Directorate, European Commission.

Das Gupta, R. and Guest, J. (2002) Annual cost of bi-polar disorder to UK society, *British Journal of Psychiatry*, 180: 227–33.

Davtian, H. (2003) *Les Frères et Sœurs de Malades Psychique*. Paris: UNAFAM.

de Haan, L., Kramer, L., van Ray, B., Weir, M., Gardner, J.SA., Ladinser, E., McDaid, S., Hernandez-Dols, S. and Wouters, L. (2002) Priorities and satisfaction on the help needed and provided in a first episode of psychosis. A survey in five European Family Associations, *European Psychiatry*, 17: 425–33.

Ellring, J.H. (1999) Depression, psychosis and dementia, *Neurology*, 52(Suppl. 3): S17–20.

EUFAMI (2005) Caring families must be treated as equal stakeholders in the mental health team. Press release. Brussels: EUFAMI.

Evers, S. and Ament, A. (1995) Costs of schizophrenia in the Netherlands, *Schizophrenia Bulletin*, 21: 141–53.

Fadden, G., Bebbington, P. and Kuipers, L. (1987) Caring and its burden. A study of the spouses of depressed patients, *British Journal of Psychiatry*, 151: 660–7.

Falloon, I.R.H. (1985) *Family Management of Schizophrenia: A Controlled Study of Clinical, Social, Family and Economic Benefits*. Baltimore, MD: Johns Hopkins University Press.

Foldemo, A., Gullberg, M., Ek, A.-C. and Bogren, L. (2005) Quality of life and burden in parents of outpatients with schizophrenia, *Social Psychiatry and Psychiatric Epidemiology*, 40: 133–8.

Gigantesco, A., Picardi, A., Chiaia, E., Balbi, A. and Morosini, P. (2002) Patients' and relatives' satisfaction with psychiatric services in a large catchment area in Rome, *European Psychiatry*, 17: 139–47.

Gore, S. and Colten, M.E. (1991) Gender, stress, and distress: socialrelational influences, in J. Eckenrode (ed.) *The Social Context of Coping*. New York: Plenum.

Grad, J. and Sainsbury, P. (1968) The effects that patients have on their families in a community care and a control psychiatric service – a two year follow up, *British Journal of Psychiatry*, 114: 265–78.

Grella, C.E. and Grusky, O. (1989) Families of the seriously mentally ill and their satisfac-tion with services, *Hospital and Community Psychiatry*, 40(8): 831–5.

Harvey, K., Burns, T., Fahy, T., Manley, C. and Tattan, T. (2001a) Relatives of patients with severe psychotic illness: factors that influence appraisal of caregiving and psycho-logical distress, *Social Psychiatry and Psychiatric Epidemiology*, 36: 456–61.

Harvey, K., Burns, T., Sedgwick, P., Higgitt, A., Creed, F. and Fahy, T. (2001b) Relatives of patients with severe psychotic disorders: factors that influence frequency: report from the UK700 trial, *British Journal of Psychiatry*, 178: 248–54.

Hirst, M. (2005) Carer distress: a prospective, population-based study, *Social Science and Medicine*, 61: 697–708.

Hoenig, J. and Hamilton, M. (1966) The schizophrenic patient and his effect on the household, *International Journal of Social Psychiatry*, 12: 165–76.

Hogman, G. and de Vleesschauwer, R. (1996) *The Silent Partners: The Needs of the Caring Family of People with a Severe Mental Illness*. Brussels: EUFAMI.

Jackson, H.J., Smith, N. and McGorry, P. (1990) Relationship between expressed emotion and family burden in psychotic disorders: an exploratory study, *Acta Psychiatrica Scandinavica*, 82: 243–9.

Johnson, D.L. (1990) The family's experience of living with mental illness, in H. Lefley and D.L. Johnson (eds) *Families as Allies in Treatment of the Mentally Ill*. Arlington, VA: American Psychiatric Press.

Johnson, D.L. (1995) Current issues in family research: can the burden of mental illness be relieved? in H. Lefley and M. Wasow (eds) *Helping Families Cope with Serious Mental Illness*. New York: Breach and Gordon Publishers.

Jungbauer, J. and Angermeyer, M.C. (2002) Living with a schizophrenic patient: a comparative study of burden as it affects parents and spouses, *Psychiatry*, 65(2): 110–23.

Jungbauer, J., Mory, C. and Angermeyer, M.C. (2002) Does caring for a schizophrenic family member increase the risk of becoming ill? Psychological and psychosomatic troubles in caregivers of Schizophrenia patients, *Fortschritte der Neurologie-Psychiatrie*, 70: 548–54.

Jungbauer, J., Wittmund, B., Dietrich, S. and Angermeyer, M.C. (2004) The disregarded caregivers: subjective burden in spouses of schizophrenia patients, *Schizophrenia Bulletin*, 30(3): 665–75.

Keitner, G.I. and Miller, I.W. (1990) Family functioning and major depression: an overview, *American Journal of Psychiatry*, 147: 1128–37.

Kuipers, L. (1993) Family burden in schizophrenia: implications for services, *Social Psychiatry and Psychiatric Epidemiology*, 28: 207–10.

Langa, K.M., Valenstein, M.A., Fendrick, A.M., Kabeto, M.U. and Vijan, S. (2004) Extent and cost of informal caregiving for older Americans with symptoms of depression, *American Journal of Psychiatry*, 161: 857–63.

Lanzara, D., Cosentino, U., Lo Maglio, A.M., Lora, A., Nicolo, A. and Rossigni, M.S. (1999) Problems of patients with schizophrenic disorders and of their families, *Epidemiologia e Psichiatria Sociale*, 8(2): 117–30.

Lauber, C., Eichenberger, A. and Luginbuhl, P. (2003) Determinants of burden in caregivers of patients with exacerbating schizophrenia, *European Psychiatry*, 18: 285–9.

Leff, J.P., Berkowitz, R., Shavit, N., Strachan, A., Glass, I. and Vaughn, C. (1990) A trial of family therapy vs. relatives' group for schizophrenia, two-year follow up, *British Journal of Psychiatry*, 153: 571–7.

Leinonen, E., Korpisammal, L., Pulkkinen, L.M. and Pukuri, T. (2001) The comparison of burden between caregiving spouses of depressive and demented patients, *International Journal of Geriatric Psychiatry*, 16: 387–93.

Lenior, M.E., Dingemans, P.M., Schene, A.H., Hart, A.A. and Linszen, D.H. (2002) The course of parental expressed emotion and psychotic episodes after family intervention in recent-onset schizophrenia, a longitudinal study, *Schizophrenia Research*, 57(2–3): 183–90.

Livingston, G., Katona, C. and Manela, M. (1996) Depression and other psychiatric morbidity in carers of elderly people living at home, *British Medical Journal*, 312: 153–6.

Magliano, L., Veltro, F., Guarneri, M. and Marasco, C. (1995) Clinical and sociodemographic correlates of coping strategies in relatives of schizophrenic patients, *European Psychiatry*, 10(3): 155–8.

Magliano, L., Fadden, G., Madianos, M., de Almeida, J.M., Held, T., Guarneri, M., Marasco, C., Tosini, P. and Maj, M. (1998) Burden on the families of patients with schizophrenia: results of the BIOMED I study, *Social Psychiatry and Psychiatric Epidemiology*, 33(9): 405–12.

Magliano, L., Fadden, G., Fiorillo, A., Malangone, C., Sorrentino, D., Robinson, A. and Maj, M. (1999) Family burden and coping strategies in schizophrenia: are key relatives really different to other relatives? *Acta Psychiatrica Scandinavica*, 99(1): 10–15.

Magliano, L., Marasco, C., Fiorillo, A.C.M., Guarneri, M. and Maj, M. (2002) The impact of professional and social network support on the burden of families of patients with schizophrenia in Italy, *Acta Psychiatrica Scandinavica*, 106(4): 291–8.

Magliano, L., Fiorillo, A., De Rosa, C., Malangone, C. and Maj, M. (2005a) Family burden in long-term diseases: a comparative study in schizophrenia vs. physical disorders, *Social Science and Medicine*, 61(2): 313–22.

Magliano, L., Fiorillo, A., Fadden, G., Gair, F., Economou, M., Kallert, T., Schellong, J., Xavier, M., Pereira, M.G., Torres-Gonzales, F., Palma-Crespo, A. and Maj, M. (2005b) Effectiveness of a psychoeducational intervention for families of patients with schizophrenia: preliminary results of a study funded by the European Commission, *World Psychiatry*, 4(1): 45–9.

Magliano, L., Fiorillo, A., Malangone, C., De Rosa, C. and Maj, M. (2006a) Implementing psychoeducational interventions in Italy for patients with schizophrenia and their families, *Psychiatric Services*, 57(2): 266–9.

Magliano, L., Fiorillo, A., Malangone, C., De Rosa, C. and Maj, M. (2006b) Social network in long-term diseases: a comparative study in relatives of persons with schizophrenia and physical illnesses versus a sample from the general population, *Social Science and Medicine*, 62: 1392–402.

Magliano, L., Fiorillo, A., Malangone, C., De Rosa, C., Maj, M. and Family Intervention Working Group (2006c) A pragmatic randomised controlled trial on the impact of a psychoeducational family intervention for schizophrenia on patients' personal/social functioning and relatives' burden and perceived support, *Psychiatric Services*, in press.

McCarthy, B., Lesage, A., Brewin, C.R., Brugha, T.S., Mangen, S. and Wing, J.K. (1989) Needs for care among relatives of long-term users of day care: a report from the Camberwell High Contact Survey, *Psychological Medicine*, 19: 725–36.

McDaid, D. (2001) Estimating the costs of informal care for people with Alzheimer's disease: methodological and practical challenges, *International Journal of Geriatric Psychiatry*, 16(4): 400–5.

McDaid, D. and Sassi, F. (2001) The burden of informal care for Alzheimer's disease: carer perceptions from an empirical study in England, Italy and Sweden, *Mental Health Research Review*, 8: 34–6.

Meinland, F.J., Danse, J.A., Wendte, J.F., Klazinga, N.S. and Gunning-Schepers, L.J. (2001) Caring for relatives with dementia-caregiver experiences of relatives of patients on the waiting list for admission to a psychogeriatric nursing home in the Netherlands, *Scandinavian Journal of Public Health*, 29: 113–21.

Moller-Leimkuhler, A.M. (2005) Burden of relatives and predictors of burden: baseline results from the Munich 5-year-follow-up study on relatives of first hospitalised patients with schizophrenia or depression, *European Archives of Psychiatry and Clinical Neuroscience*, 255: 223–31.

Montero, I., Asencio, A., Hernandez, I., Masanet, M.J., Lacruz, M., Bellver, F., Iborra, M. and Ruiz, I. (2001) Two strategies for family intervention in schizophrenia: a randomized trial in a Mediterranean environment, *Schizophrenia Bulletin*, 27(4): 661–70.

Mory, C., Jungbauer, J., Bischkopf, J. and Angermeyer, M.C. (2002) Financial burden on spouses of patients suffering from schizophrenia, depression or anxiety disorder, *Fortschritte der Neurologie-Psychiatrie*, 70(2): 71–7.

Mueser, K.T., Sengupta, A., Schooler, N.R., Bellack, A.S., Xie, H., Glick, I.D. and Keith, S.J. (2001) Family treatment and medication dosage reduction in schizophrenia: affects on patient social functioning, family attitudes, and burden, *Journal of Consultation and Clinical Psychology*, 69(1): 3–12.

Murray, J., Schneider, J., Banerjee, S. and Mann, A. (1999) EUROCARE: a cross-national study of co-resident spouse carers for people with Alzheimer's disease II: a qualitative analysis of the experience of caregiving, *International Journal of Geriatric Psychiatry*, 14(8): 662–7.

Nyman, M. and Stengård, E. (2001) *Mielenterveyspotilaiden omaisten hyvinvointi (Well-being of caregivers of the mentally ill)*. Saarijärvi: Omaiset mielenterveystyön tukena keskusliitto ry.

Ohaeri, J. (2003) The burden of caregiving in families with a mental illness: a review of 2002, *Current Opinions in Psychiatry*, 16: 457–65.

Olstad, R., Sexton, H. and Sogaard, A.J. (2001) The Finnmark Study. A prospective population study of the social support buffer hypothesis, specific stressors and mental distress, *Social Psychiatry and Psychiatric Epidemiology*, 36(12): 582–9.

Ostman, M. and Hansson, L. (2000) The burden of relatives of psychiatric patients. Comparisons between parents, spouses, and grown-up children of voluntarily and compulsorily admitted psychiatric patients, *Nordic Journal of Psychiatry*, 54: 31–6.

Ostman, M. and Hansson, L. (2001) The relationship between coping strategies and family burden among relatives of admitted psychiatric patients, *Scandinavian Journal of Caring Science*, 15: 159–64.

Ostman, M. and Hansson, L. (2002a) Children in families with a severely mentally ill member: prevalence and needs for support, *Social Psychiatry and Psychiatric Epidemiology*, 37: 243–8.

Ostman, M. and Hansson, L. (2002b) Stigma by association, *British Journal of Psychiatry*, 181: 494–8.

Ostman, M. and Hansson, L. (2004) Appraisal of caregiving, burden and psychological distress in relatives of psychiatric inpatients, *European Psychiatry*, 19: 402–7.

Pereira, M.G. and de Almeida, J.M. (1999) The repercussion of mental disease in the family: a study of the family members of psychotic patients, *Acta Medica Portuguesa*, 12(4–6): 161–8.

Perkins, S., Winn, S., Murray, J., Murphy, R. and Schmidt, U. (2004) A qualitative study of the experience of caring for a person with bulimia nervosa. Part 1: the emotional impact of caring, *International Journal of Eating Disorders*, 36(3): 256–68.

Perlick, D., Clarkin, J.F., Sirey, J., Raue, P., Greenfield, S., Struening, E. and Rosenheck, R. (1999) Burden experienced by care-givers of persons with bipolar affective disorder, *British Journal of Psychiatry*, 175: 56–62.

Perlick, D.A., Rosenheck, R.R., Clarkin, J.F., Raue, P. and Sirey, J. (2001) Impact of family burden and patient symptom status on clinical outcome in bipolar affective disorder, *Journal of Nervous Mental Disorders*, 189: 31–7.

Perlick, D.A., Rosenheck, R.A., Clarkin, J.F., Maciejewski, P.K., Sirey, J., Struening, E. and Link, B.G. (2004) Impact of family burden and affective response on clinical outcome among patients with bipolar disorder, *Psychiatric Services*, 55(9): 1029–35.

Perlick, D.A., Hohenstein, J.M., Clarkin, J.F., Kaczynski, R. and Rosenheck, R.A. (2005) Use of mental health and primary care services by caregivers of patients with bipolar disorder: a preliminary study, *Bipolar Disorders*, 7(2): 126–35.

Pilling, S., Bebbington, P., Kuipers, E., Garety, P., Geddes, J., Orbach, G. and Morgan, C. (2002) Psychological treatments in schizophrenia: meta-analysis of family intervention and cognitive behaviour therapy, *Psychological Medicine*, 32(5): 763–82.

Reid, A., Mancy Lang, C. and O'Neil, T. (1993) Services for schizophrenic patients and their families: what they say they need, *Behavioural Psychiatry*, 21: 107–13.

Rice, D.P. and Miller, L.S. (1996) The economic burden of schizophrenia: conceptual and methodological issues and cost estimates, in M. Moscarelli, A. Rupp and N. Sartorius (eds) *Handbook of Mental Health Economics and Health Policy, Volume 1, Schizophrenia*. London: Wiley.

Rose, L.E. (1996) Families of psychiatric patients: a critical review and future research directions, *Archives of Psychiatric Nursing*, 10(2): 67–76.

Samele, C. and Manning, N. (2000) Level of caregiver burden among relatives of the mentally ill in South Verona, *European Psychiatry*, 15(3): 196–204.

Sartorius, N. (2001) The economic and social burden of depression, *Journal of Clinical Psychiatry*, 15(Suppl.): 8–11.

Scazufca, M. and Kuipers, E. (1996) Link between expressed emotion and burden of care in relatives of patients with schizophrenia, *British Journal of Psychiatry*, 168(5): 580–7.

Schene, A.H. and van Wijngaarden, M.A. (1995) A survey of an organisation for families of patients with serious mental illness in the Netherlands, *Psychiatric Services*, 46(8): 807–13.

Schene, A.H., van Wijngaarden, B. and Koeter, M.W. (1998) Family caregiving in schizophrenia: domains and distress, *Schizophrenia Bulletin*, 24(4): 609–18.

Schneider, J., Hallam, A., Kamrul Islam, M., Murray, J., Foley, B., Atkins, L., Banerjee, S. and Mann, A. (2003) Formal and informal care for people with dementia: variations in costs over time, *Ageing and Society*, 23(3): 303–26.

Schulze, B. and Rossler, W. (2005) Caregiver burden in mental illness: review of measurement, findings and intervention in 2004–2005, *Current Opinion in Psychiatry*, 18: 684–91.

Smith, J., Birchwood, M., Cochrane, R. and George, S. (1993) The needs of high and low expressed emotion families: a normative approach, *Social Psychiatry and Psychiatric Epidemiology*, 28: 11–16.

Stam, H. and Cuijpers, P. (2001) Effects of family interventions on burden of relatives of psychiatric patients in the Netherlands: a pilot study, *Community Mental Health Journal*, 37(2): 179–87.

Steketee, G. (1997) Disability and family burden in obsessive-compulsive disorder, *Canadian Journal of Psychiatry*, 42: 919–28.

Szmukler, G.I., Herrman, H., Colusa, S., Benson, A. and Bloch, S. (1996) A controlled trial of a counselling intervention for caregivers of relatives with schizophrenia, *Social Psychiatry and Psychiatric Epidemiology*, 31(3–4): 149–55.

Tarricone, R., Gerzeli, S., Montanelli, R., Frattura, L., Percudani, M. and Racagni, G. (2000) Direct and indirect costs of schizophrenia in community psychiatric services in Italy. The GISIES study. Interdisciplinary Study Group on the Economic Impact of Schizophrenia, *Health Policy*, 51(1): 1–18.

Tarrier, N., Barrowclough, C., Vaughn, C., Bamrah, J.S., Porceddu, K., Watts, S. and Freeman, H. (1988) The community management of schizophrenia: a controlled trial of a behavioural intervention with families to reduce relapse, *British Journal of Psychiatry*, 153: 532–42.

Tennakoon, L., Fannon, D., Doku, V., O'Ceallaigh, S., Soni, W., Santamaria, M., Kuipers, E. and Sharma, T. (2000) Experience of caregiving: relatives of people experiencing a first episode of psychosis, *British Journal of Psychiatry*, 177: 529–33.

Thomas, P., Hazif-Thomas, C., Delagnes, V., Bonduelle, P. and Clement, J.P. (2005) La vulnérabilité de l'aidant principal des malades déments à domicile. L'étude Pixel, *Psychologie et Neuropsychiatre Vieilissement*, 3(3): 207–20.

Thornicroft, G., Tansella, M., Becker, T., Knapp, M., Leese, M., Schene, A. and Vazquez-Barquero, J.L. (2004) The personal impact of schizophrenia in Europe, *Schizophrenia Research*, 69(2–3): 125–32.

Treasure, J., Murphy, T., Todd, G., Gavan, K., Schmidt, U., Joyce, J. and Szmukler, G. (2001) The experience of caregiving for severe mental illness: a comparison between anorexia nervosa and psychosis, *Social Psychiatry and Psychiatric Epidemiology*, 36: 343–7.

van Wijngaarden, B., Schene, A.H. and Koeter, M.W. (2004) Family caregiving in depression: impact on caregivers' daily life, distress, and help-seeking, *Journal of Affective Disorders*, 81(3): 211–22.

Veltman, A., Cameron, J. and Stewart, D.E. (2002) The experience of providing care to relatives with chronic mental illness, *Journal of Nervous Mental Disorders*, 190: 108–14.

Wearden, A.J., Tarrier, N., Barrowclough, C., Zastowny, T. and Armstrong, A. (2002) A review of expressed emotion research in health care, *Clinical Psychology Review*, 20(5): 633–66.

Wenger, G.C. and Burholt, V. (2004) Changes in levels of social isolation and loneliness among older people in a rural area: a twenty-year longitudinal study, *Canadian Journal of Aging*, 23(2): 115–27.

Winn, S., Perkins, S., Murray, J., Murphy, R. and Schmidt, U. (2004) A qualitative study of the experience of caring for a person with bulimia nervosa. Part 2: carers' needs and experiences of services and other support, *International Journal of Eating Disorders*, 36: 269–79.

Wittmund, B., Wilms, H.U., Mory, C. and Angermeyer, M.C. (2002) Depressive disorders in spouses of mentally ill patients, *Social Psychiatry and Psychiatric Epidemiology*, 37: 177–82.

Wolthaus, J.E., Dingemans, P.M., Schene, A.H., Linszen, D.H., Wiersma, D., van den Bosch, R.J., Cahn, W. and Hijman, R. (2002) Caregiver burden in recent onset schizophrenia and spectrum disorders: the influence of symptoms and personality traits, *Journal of Nervous Mental Disorders*, 190(4): 241–7.

World Health Organization (2001) *The World Health Report 2001 – Mental Health: New Understanding, New Hope.* Geneva: World Health Organization.

World Health Organization (2005a) *Mental Health Action Plan for Europe: Facing the Challenges, Building Solutions.* Copenhagen: World Health Organization.

World Health Organization (2005b) *Mental Health Declaration for Europe: Facing the Challenges, Building Solutions.* Copenhagen: World Health Organization.

World Health Organization (2005c) Rights of families and carers of persons with mental health disorders, in *WHO Resource Book on Mental Health, Human Rights and Legislation.* Geneva: World Health Organization.

seventeen

Mental health policy in former eastern bloc countries

Toma Tomov, Robert Van Voren,
Rob Keukens and Dainius Puras

Introduction

This chapter attempts to provide an evidence-based contribution to mental health policy in some of the former eastern bloc[1] countries. The difficulties associated with such a task are formidable and first need to be stated.

General health versus mental health reforms

The medical literature in health policy focuses on policy content rather than policy processes and power structures, and employs methods developed within public health disciplines (Walt 1994). From this perspective, the current health policy concern in former eastern bloc countries is general health care reform or the replacement of free health care by paid services. To that end, most 'transition countries' attempt, firstly, to improve the availability of care by enhancing the gatekeeping role of primary care services, and secondly, to sustain quality of care by introducing structured clinical practices – thus enabling evaluation.

Mental health poses problems for both these priorities – for the first, there is the issue of treatment adherence, while the therapeutic alliance requirement poses problems for the second. Neither adherence nor alliance yields to impartial analysis. Both make technological solutions somewhat misleading because such solutions necessarily disavow individual uniqueness when handling relationships. Not surprisingly therefore, these pertinent problems are often left out of the public agenda of mental health reforms.

However, when a real problem is prevented from entering the agenda at the content level of policy it still penetrates at the level of process and power

(Walt *et al.* 1999). This chapter will touch on these issues in an attempt to demonstrate the importance of hidden agendas in the interpretation of mental health service data obtained through positivist research in societies in flux. The hope is to attract attention to the key role of governance. In this we are guided by the concern that dictatorial cultures, with their blatant disregard for human decency, humane approaches and individual dignity, seem to survive long after the dictators are formally removed.

The spurious similarity

The downfall of the Berlin wall revealed that the assumed similarity between eastern bloc countries was more fictional than real, resulting from a suppression of differences. What appeared to be similar was, in fact, a misleading impression created by biased data, obstructed access to information and the manipulation of findings.

On the other hand, observers of the sociopolitical scene in the former eastern bloc began to identify the lasting impacts of totalitarian rule on individuals and communities, such as a poor ability to manage change and a failure by human services and the economy to respond to the challenges of transition (Dahrendorf 1990). In particular, the huge public health crisis was attributed to an inability to cope with unexpected and prolonged psychosocial stress, resulting from the failure of coping strategies built on social passivity and a dependence on the state to guide countries in their transformations into open societies (Cornia and Paniccia 2000).

In distancing themselves from the imposed image of 'Second World' nations, these countries took different routes. Those from central Europe snugly settled into the mould of western democracies, and established mental health care of a kind that is accountable in terms of comparative quantitative analysis, with all its strengths and weaknesses. The relatively high degree of structuring of their services, and the considerable uniformity in their handling of the constructs involved, have contributed to this accountability. These countries are outside the focus of this chapter.

In the rest of the eastern bloc, mental health systems had been reconciled with the excessive control of the previous regimes to a much larger degree. The more pronounced the role of traditional values in regulating communal, family and professional life prior to dictatorial times, the easier it was for health systems to yield to authoritarian pressure. In the case of the former Soviet Union, psychiatry had deliberately been used for the pursuit of the political goal of controlling minds. This brought about an institutional culture in the psychiatric domain which is difficult and painful to leave behind, even to this day.

Although little research has been done, it is important to bear in mind how this practice has left an imprint on the culture of psychiatry in the countries of the former Soviet Union and how pervasive this imprint is. It is evident in hospitals and nursing homes, but also in the infamous dispensaries which became outposts of institutionalism in the community. Azerbaijan, Georgia, Ukraine and the Russian Federation are used here to illustrate this analysis.

What they all share, despite economic and cultural differences, is the common legacy of their mental health systems. Unlike Russia, after 1989 it has been much easier for sizeable groups of the psychiatric profession in the other three countries to draw a distinction between propaganda and reality. Much of this debate, however, has not yet involved official decision-makers, including health administrators in particular.

In a third group of eastern bloc countries, after 1989 the need for progress in psychiatry was not contested but innovation was met with prejudice and stigma. Discrimination against psychiatry was structural and manifested itself not only as the prevailing layperson's attitude to mental illness, but also as legal restrictions in many domains of life. Although political abuse of psychiatry had not occurred in these countries, respect for pluralism and human rights was regarded as political clutter rather than as a realistic opportunity for new mental health policy. For example, the authorities in these countries could afford to tolerate the unduly dismal quality of life experienced in psychiatric institutions without fear of public condemnation at home. Bulgaria and Lithuania are two countries from this third group, which first saw reformist developments in the non-governmental sector. Unlike Russia, which passed an impeccable mental health law as early as 1992, even to this day Bulgaria has not reformed its mental health legislation despite constant debate. The impression is, however, that in reality the culture of psychiatric institutions in Russia has changed far less than the culture of those in Bulgaria. Unfortunately, this finding can be substantiated with 'soft' data only – a fact that pinpoints the limitations in shedding light on social change exclusively with the help of quantitative analyses.

Sources of information

This chapter draws on a variety of different sources of information which are often difficult to compare. Official country statistics were used for six countries: Azerbaijan, Bulgaria, Georgia, Lithuania, Russia and Ukraine. Instrumental in complementing this information with 'insider' interpretations were national teams established for collaborative projects sponsored by international donors and which constituted a regional network. Two projects in particular need to be mentioned here. The first, 'Attitudes and Needs Assessment in Psychiatry' (Tomov 2001) examined the attitudes to mental illness and psychiatry, and the expectations for reform, that prevailed in these six countries. This study was conducted against a background of mounting criticism of health policy in eastern Europe, which had seen a move away from universal access and tax-funded health systems to more pluralist systems with a greater reliance on health insurance. The principal criticism levelled against this move was that during times of economic recession it would lead to a widening of inequity in access to health care (Domenighetti 2003). This attitudinal study suggested that the introduction of psychiatric reforms in such circumstances might not be wise if there was little participation in the reform process by the community (as is the case in all post-totalitarian countries), particularly if this fact is not acknowledged by political and health governance institutions.

The second project, 'Analytic Studies of Mental Health Policies and Services' produced descriptions (called 'mental health profiles') of countries from all World Health Organization (WHO) regions, including eastern Europe. The Country Profile instrument (Jenkins *et al.* 2004) attempted to bring together all the evidence that conceivably bore upon the explicit or implicit mental health policies of a country. The objective was to explore whether a generic mental health policy template (Townsend *et al.* 2004) could be developed and offered for decision-makers to use across the globe. However, one finding from the region was that after life under political dependence, the art of hypocrisy that this life had instilled within state administrations had remained – and actually became their hallmark. The conclusion was that reforms orchestrated by those in office in the region would often be compromised by corruption (Mladenova *et al.* 2002).

It is important to see the findings from the two studies as part of a whole. The abstention of regular citizens from involvement with issues of change dumps authority and power on administrations, which usually exceed their proper competences, inciting them to perform hypocritically and fraudulently. This inevitably becomes public knowledge and further reinforces abstention from citizens' participation in public matters. This explanatory pattern is very familiar in organizational research, pointing to flawed leadership, and suggests a particular type of intervention which has very little to do with expertise in mental health (Chisholm and Elden 1993; Elden and Chisholm 1993). In the case of most former eastern bloc countries flawed leadership is a problem on a nationwide scale, penetrating all domains and thus not allowing leverage for intervention. The sheer magnitude of flawed leadership is unprecedented. This is the single most salient contextual factor that any mental health policy in the region needs to take into account (Tomov *et al.* 2003).

Information on the history of the political abuse of psychiatry in the former Soviet Union is drawn from work documented by the Global (formerly Geneva) Initiative on Psychiatry (GIP). This non-governmental foundation has forged extensive links with both dissident psychiatry in the former eastern bloc and the reformist movement in the region since 1989.[2] GIP helped to invoke the human rights argument within mental health policy and to demonstrate that respect for ethical principles is a universal requirement across the globe, independent of ethnic, cultural or political traditions. Currently, GIP engages in many attempts to precipitate critical self-assessment among stakeholders in mental health by initiating projects that bring home the concept of community psychiatry. As an initiative developed to engage with those with severe mental illness, while respecting individual differences and free choice, community psychiatry often poses problems of meaning and comprehension that require careful consideration of differences in experience and culture. GIP is developing a special sensitivity to the quagmire of civil law that affects mental health in the region.

Objectives

There is a paradox that this chapter hopes to disentangle, or at least bring to greater awareness. Policy development is a governance task; yet poor governance repeatedly comes up as the component of mental health policy that causes the most difficulties in the region's mental health care systems. The crux of this problem is that state administration employees appear to hate their work, which in democratic countries would normally involve mental health policy-making and implementation. This alienation from work is a most salient (albeit unacknowledged) feature of the workplace ethos of the region's state adminis-trations. It has been referred to many times in focus group discussions, inter-views and other events that were part of the action research methodology adopted by some studies. It is therefore the action research paradigm that those authors see not just as a key method that helps to reveal the problem, but also as a method for generating solutions.

The discussion below has been guided by this concern. It begins with a con-sideration of the broad picture of life under dictatorship, followed by a descrip-tion of the changes brought about by the political events in Europe after 1989. A special emphasis is placed on the political abuse of psychiatry in the former Soviet Union, seen from the perspective of human relations. This helps to cap-ture more clearly the legacy that individuals and governance institutions need to cope with. The chapter then proceeds to briefly sketch the sociodemographic features of the populations in the region and outline mental health resources, service provision and utilization. Governance in mental health is described, followed by an attempt to align this vast quantity of information into a comprehensible account of mental health policy.

The sociopolitical context in former eastern bloc countries

In order to understand why mental health policy and practice in former eastern bloc countries have so critically lagged behind developments in the rest of Europe, the sociopolitical context is crucial. Meriting special attention is the unprecedented scope of political change that took place almost overnight in 1989 and affected the lives of hundreds of millions. The impact on the health and well-being of individuals and communities caused by the upheaval in values, status, social cohesion and the like since then has been enormous. Yet psychiatry in the region has only risen to the task in a stuttering fashion, if at all. This hesitation to embrace social engagement has its roots in history.

The political context: the abuse of psychiatry

The last decades of the Soviet Union were marked by a relative thaw that started after the death of Josef Stalin in March 1953. In his secret speech to the Twentieth Party Congress in 1956 the new leader Nikita Khrushchev criticized his pre-decessor who, after years of mass terror, had left a paralysed nation soaked with 'the inertia of fear and passivity' (Sakharov 1975). When Brezhnev took over, repression and stagnation increased once again and criticism of the regime was considered to be a 'destructive activity' that had to be contained. Control by deportation to the gulag or exile was less appropriate after de-Stalinization, however, and particularly after Nikita Khrushchev claimed that the USSR no longer had political prisoners (Tomov 1999). Critics of the regime were accused of 'anti-Soviet agitation and propaganda' or of 'slandering the Soviet state'; thus, they qualified as 'parasites' and 'antisocial elements' and were interned in 'corrective' labour camps and prisons or sent into exile (Sjalamov 1995). Political psychiatry came to complement this practice. The mental health care system, unthinkable as this may seem, was turned into an instrument of repression and those who wanted to reform the existing political and social order were labelled psychiatric cases.

The conception of political psychiatry

Commenting on the initiation of the political abuse of psychiatry, Bukovsky (1974) wrote:

> Khrushchev figured that it was impossible for people in a socialist society to have antisocialist consciousness . . . Wherever manifestations of dissidence couldn't be explained away as a legacy of the past or as a provocation of world imperialism, they were simply the product of mental illness.

Khrushchev had said this in a speech published in the state newspaper *Pravda* on 24 May 1959:

> A crime is a deviation from generally recognized standards of behaviour frequently caused by mental disorder. Can there be diseases, nervous disorders among certain people in a Communist society? Evidently yes. If that is so, then there will also be offences, which are characteristic of people with abnormal minds. Of those who might start calling for opposition to Communism on this basis, we can say that clearly their mental state is not normal.

The campaign to declare political opponents mentally ill and to incarcerate dissidents in psychiatric hospitals started in the late 1950s and early 1960s. The Soviet secret service became interested in this branch of medicine as early as 1948. Dissident poet Naum Korzhavin reported that the atmosphere at the Serbsky Institute for Forensic and General Psychiatry in Moscow changed almost overnight when a Dr Daniil Lunts was appointed head of the Fourth Department, known as the Political Department. Previously, psychiatric departments had been considered a 'refuge' against being sent to the gulag, but from that moment onwards this policy changed. The first reports of dissidents being hospitalized for non-medical reasons date from the early 1960s, not long after Dr Georgi Morozov became director of the Serbsky Institute. Both Lunts and Morozov were notorious abusers of psychiatry for political purposes and were personally involved in many well-known cases.

Why the Soviet authorities decided to use psychiatry as a means of repression still has not been clearly answered. While Khrushchev publicly claimed that the Soviet Union no longer kept political prisoners, he continued to have dissidents sent to the camps. It does not appear likely, therefore, that he tried to use psychiatry to cover up the practice of political imprisonment. By the same token, the psychiatric professionals involved in this practice could not have possibly believed that dissidence was a mental disorder. Most Russian doctors were indeed unfamiliar with world psychiatry and were exposed to the Soviet school of thought only. But the *nomenclature* cadre had full access to the *spets-khran* (special closed departments) of the medical libraries, where 'bourgeois' psychiatric literature was kept. They travelled to international conferences, were aware of western criticism and knew that they were lying when stating that formerly hospitalized political prisoners were admitted for treatment as soon as they arrived in the West. Understanding political psychiatry requires a grasp of how Soviet culture misconstrued science and humane care.

The disgrace of science

In 1927, *Pravda* published an article claiming that a young researcher, Trofim Denisovitch Lysenko (1898–1976), had resolved the food shortages in the Soviet Republic of Azerbaijan by growing peas during the winter season. The food shortage was caused in the first place by the massive reallocation of labour from agriculture to industrial production and threatened to expose the party policy of rapid industrialization as shortsighted. Lysenko's solution came at an opportune time, providing a rationale that allowed his deceptive (and now discredited) but highly desirable version of genetics to rescue party authority. Unfortunately, the price was disastrous because Lysenko's solution concealed the ignorance of the party from itself and legitimated the abuse of science by precipitating a decision that placed the whole domain of research under party jurisdiction (Faria 1995; Soyfer *et al.* 1997).

In 1951, in a manner that was almost identical to the abandonment of Soviet genetics for Lisenko's quackery, Nobel-prize winner Ivan Pavlov's behaviourism was enforced as the only acceptable ideology of mental health practice and research at a joint meeting of the All-Union Neurological and Psychiatric Association and the Academy of Medical Sciences. This act legitimated yet another disastrous development – biological reductionism in Soviet psychiatry. It seems that in this case the originator of the ideas that were carried over from neurophysiology to mental health, in violation of all principles of science, was not even colluding with the 'partocracy': his thinking was just brutally misappropriated by others.

By far the most egregious among those who benefited from the imposed monopoly of neurophysiological ideas on the science of psychiatry was the academician Andrei Snezhnevsky. He acted as a man craving to make history and the totalitarian ethos colluded with him in declaring reformist thinking, obstinacy of character, religious faith and concern with truth all to be manifestations of mental illness. He coined the term 'sluggish schizophrenia', implying a clinical condition of disguised course that could present itself as a normal mental state on psychiatric examination. Renowned psychiatrists who questioned the evidence for his claims lost their jobs; some were even exiled to Siberia. This made it blatantly clear that it was unwise to observe the ways of science with people like Snezhnevsky, who cunningly made use of the terror that reigned in the Soviet Union during Stalin's last years. Thus, his views, unchallenged and glorified, were taught to many generations of Soviet psychiatrists and even today have not been openly exposed as political and scientific fraud. The instrument for such social practice – science as a paradigm based on evidence of an agreed type, and its interpretation within scientific discourse – had been effectively abolished and its recovery has not yet taken place.

The Soviet view on disability

With proper scientific discourse on mental health out of the way, an important instrument for testing the realities of political leadership had been eliminated, thus allowing notions of social policy to deviate from human decency beyond anything modern societies have faced or have been able to admit to being possible. The hallmark of this policy was to maintain and reinforce dependency, a strategy presumed to postpone indefinitely the removal from power of those who had usurped it forcefully. Aspects of human nature that were inconvenient to the cultivation of eternal dependency had to be eliminated without any respect for human rights whatsoever. The architects of 'Soviet Man' did not even spare the trust of children, as attested by the children's stories from the period. Books suggested that the party was by far a more enduring, reliable and trustworthy parent than a biological parent could ever be.

Loss, grief and sadness had no place in the newly-constructed human nature: hence, human decline, either physical or mental, was regarded as depravity. The combination of a 'scientific' interpretation of mental life as tantamount to the physiology of the higher nervous system, and the view that disability was base, could allow for the complete disavowal of the medical, social and vocational needs of people with disabilities.

The system of institutional care was predicated by this attitude. It did not provide for recovery and social integration: it was, by design, a way to eliminate those who had become a nuisance and who were dispensable. In 1980, when the Soviet Union organized the Olympic Games in Moscow, it was suggested that the Paralympics be held there as well. The Soviets answered curtly: 'We have no invalids'. Indeed, people with physical disabilities were hardly ever seen on the streets: understandably so, because only one factory (in Zaporozhe, now in the Ukraine) produced wheelchairs, and these were of very poor quality. Individuals who had lost their legs in wars or were paralysed could leave their homes only by using a board with wheels and wooden clogs to propel themselves forward. The 'Action Group to Defend the Rights of the Disabled', which was established in 1980 to set up a Disabled Union, met with repression from the secret police; within a year its members were jailed, forced into emigration or put under constant surveillance.

Care for the 'substandard'

Institutional care for children in need of parental care and for people with intellectual disabilities and mental illness is an old European tradition that was introduced to prevent abuse and even the violent death of these vulnerable people where communities were not reliably governed by the concerns of human rights and related ethics (Shorter 1997). With advances towards democracy and civil society, concern grew over the apparent abuse of the human rights of people in custody. The detrimental consequences of this practice on individual development and quality of life triggered the process of deinstitutionalization.

After 1989, concern for human rights penetrated the new democracies and entered public debate through the publications of human rights organizations like the Helsinki Committee. According to one World Bank study, at least 1.3 million children, people with disabilities and the elderly in the eastern bloc live in 7400 large, highly structured institutions. These institutions absorb much of the limited financial resources that could be used to create alternative, community-based support systems for people with mental health needs. In Lithuania, for example, 1.75 per cent of the national budget is used for the institutional care of vulnerable individuals (Tobis 2000).

Custodial care, which has remained in most former eastern bloc countries, appears to be inherent to the notion of 'governance' espoused by totalitarianism. Systems of institutional care had also been introduced in the social, health and education sectors as separate legal entities. In most countries, infant homes and psychiatric hospitals were governed under the auspices of ministries of health, special boarding schools for disabled and socially deprived children were the responsibility of ministries of education, while responsibility for special psychoneurological facilities for both the mentally ill and children and adults with intellectual difficulties rested with ministries of social welfare. The three systems had little in common in terms of coordination. However, they were identical in their mission to socially exclude 'substandard' individuals. Any moral doubts related to this practice must have been abated by the boundless trust in centrally-planned economies and the common belief that the evils of human nature had forever been relegated to the other side of the Iron Curtain.

Looking back, it can be seen how the failure of the economy to bring prosperity left totalitarian rule with no option but to eliminate the less fit. The ability to adjust production technologies and work roles to better suit the limited competencies of disabled people suggests prosperity rather than economies of survivalism. It can also be argued, on the basis of research, that raising children in institutions while both parents were alive and well has negatively affected the social capital of countries like Bulgaria (Markova 2004). The difficult question faced now is whether political change is enough to make a difference to this institutional legacy – particularly when the prospects for economic growth in the region are considered to be certain with the advent of democracy and free markets.

In answering this question it is essential to take into account the serious social defences that institutional systems develop. In practice this means that the process of deinstitutionalization will be slow and the reallocation of staff will be as difficult and time consuming (if not more so) as the reallocation of institutionalized mental health patients to alternative systems of care. Retraining staff into new professional roles and skills will be crucially important.

Another essential barrier that requires considerable attention is the peculiar type of 'patienthood' that develops under systems of care provision that are excessively paternalistic. Self-stigmatization, a most unfortunate product of this kind of care, severely limits the impact that consumers can have through organizations as key stakeholders in the deinstitutionalization movement. Other major stakeholders, including relatives, professionals, politicians, the general public and the mass media are heavily influenced in their views and expectations concerning mental illness by the kind of psychiatry practised in institutions. Unsurprisingly, since 1989 the common trend in the countries with growing economies (such as the Baltic countries) has been to increase government investment in improving standards of care in institutions. The move to care in the community is seriously impeded by the widely-held belief that the primary task of the mental health care system is the safety of 'regular' citizens.

Understanding political psychiatry

The silencing of science as a crucial reminder of reality, the attitude of aversion towards the disabled, and the party hierarchy serving as a social defence against the anxiety arising from enforced dependency (Jaques 1955; Menzies 1992) provided the breeding ground for political psychiatry. The perception of political dissent as a derangement of the mind was only a step away. It took a few aberrant personalities within the profession to launch a practice of abuse wrongly construed by the unassuming many, and culpably misrepresented by the malicious few, as humane care for the 'non-insightful mentally disordered'.

This practice burgeoned due to many additional aspects of the Soviet context: the political apparatus for central control, the downgrading of the professions, the political purges, the abolishment of democratic freedoms, the misinformation of the public, to mention just a few. By the late 1970s and early 1980s approximately a third of all dissident cases were processed through the 'politically insane' procedure. The usual diagnoses were schizophrenia and having paranoid personalities. The treatments were heavy, given without consent, and had severe side-effects and debilitating consequences. The duration of commitment matched that of the sentences given to political prisoners – three to seven years. A growing need for more institutions was recognized by the party Politburo under Yuri Andropov and dozens of new mental hospitals, identical in design, were built across the country. In 1989, at the World Congress of Psychiatry in Athens, after years of international pressure, the Soviet delegation publicly acknowledged that, indeed, systematic political abuse of psychiatry had taken place, admitting that setting up political hospitals had been a wrong move. Hospitals have since been closed but what has remained behind is a culture of passive compliance and corrupt state administration.

The change of 1989

In 1989 political change, which had been in the air for a decade, became a fact of history. This happened by and large peacefully, revealing a significant capacity to contain anxiety and anger across the whole of the former eastern bloc even during the collapse of hierarchical social organizations. This was good news because hierarchies were believed to be an indispensable instrument of social defence against anxiety in this part of the world, largely because of people's limited experience with democracy. This did not mean, however, that dependency needs, reinforced for many generations by mother parties, could be outgrown overnight.

As time went by, efforts to come to grips with democracy resulted in the establishment of processes and structures by virtually all the countries in the region, only to discover that these institutions were feckless (Carothers 2002). The long and painful process of substituting psychic structures of self-governance for external enforcement had started, but only sporadically, and in the minds of only a few individuals. Social exclusion, non-participation, stigmatization, abuse of rights and a host of other manifestations of dependency gradually began to be acknowledged. This happened at varying rates across countries and sectors of life. The education, health and social sectors lagged behind considerably in comparison to the economic, defence and legal systems. The further away historically, geographically and culturally a compact population had been from the values favouring individual over group interests, the slower was the pace of transformation.

While these broad tendencies reveal a direction of positive change there are enormous, only partially recognized, and poorly understood problems frustrating millions in the region that impinge directly on demographic processes and suggest huge health needs.

The demographic and economic context

Since 1989 most countries in the region have fallen behind the rest of Europe in terms of fertility, mortality and morbidity figures. The socioeconomic demise is clearly visible in the *UN Human Development Index* (HDI) *2002*, a report that considers factors such as per capita income, resource development, human freedom, dignity and the role of people in shaping development. The report calls attention to the pain of the economic transition which has taken its toll in many countries in the former Soviet Union, with countries ranked from 42 (Estonia) to 105 (Moldova, the lowest-ranking European country). The Russian Federation is listed sixtieth. Since the first *HDI* was published in 1990, Russia and Ukraine have moved down 20 places, with Moldova shifting at least 30 places towards the bottom (United Nations 2002).

The population of the Russian Federation peaked in 1992 at 148.3 million but it has been declining ever since at a rate of 400–500,000 annually. The most urgent socioeconomic, political, and medical-demographic problem is the high mortality rate. Annually, more than 2 million people die in Russia (Shkolnikov *et al.* 2001; World Bank 2005a). Diseases such as tuberculosis, anaemia and dysentery, previously curtailed through primary health care structures and vaccination programmes, are on the rise again (for tuberculosis there has been a 40 per cent increase since 1990). At the same time, new social and health problems rapidly add to the demise of social cohesion. Examples of such phenomena are HIV/AIDS, suicide, drug addiction, divorce (67 per cent of new marriages end with divorce), malnutrition and poor diet (2 million children do not get proper nourishment). At least 40 per cent of all deaths are potentially avoidable with adequate and timely prevention and treatment: in other words, with a proper health care system. Similar trends, though less pronounced, can be traced in most countries in the region.

Nine of the ten countries with the highest suicide rates in the world are in the former eastern bloc (Varnik 2000). The high levels of mortality and morbidity in the region are related to a cluster of stress and helplessness-related conditions, including suicide, violence, risk-taking behaviour and self-destructive lifestyles (Rutz 2001). The rate of youth homicide (10–29 years), which is around 1 per 100,000 in the countries of western Europe, reaches 1.2–1.6 in the countries of central Europe, 5.4–7.7 in the Baltic countries and around 18 in the Russian Federation (Krug *et al.* 2002). The growth of positive social capital in the region is slow (Paldam and Svendsen 2001). Trust in the relationships between individuals, groups and organizations, and a sense of citizenship, are missing. So are the values of civil society in health governance (Kickbusch 2002).

In terms of economic prosperity, some of the countries have done better than others since 1989 but in general the region falls well behind the rest of Europe. There appears to be disquiet, envy and shame among the public and politicians, even though these countries have generated genuine economic growth in recent years. An unhealthy preoccupation with the consumption of goods and services seems to underlie this intolerance for delay. Examples can be found in any domain, including health. Thus for instance, demands for the availability of, and access to, sophisticated health care (that is way out of proportion with economic potential) come from politicians, the media and the professions.

As deregulation of health care advances, bursts of entrepreneurship tend to deliver care on a fee-for-service basis – a development that is presumed to be driven by market demands but actually is a result of pre-emptive action by individuals in control of easy money. This illustrates the problem of redistribution of wealth that countries face, but their governments seldom seem intent on finding just solutions. Governments often use the excuse of having externally imposed restrictions on budgets to allay discontent over the failure to meet basic needs related to income, quality of life and health. Most people accept this with resignation, particularly when it is accompanied by the argument that free markets rather than central planning drive development, even in health. Those in office in the region come from the ranks of the new ruling elite who are considered to have become rich almost overnight by a combination of entrepreneurial zeal and callousness. These people have a genuine difficulty in comprehending the struggle of millions of others in coming to terms with the values of globalization. This is a continuous source of turmoil in the region that has failed to attract the attention of health research.

Assessment of the mental health needs of populations using epidemiological approaches has very little application in the region. When available, findings have usually failed to bring about any change in the provision of services. It had not been uncommon before 1989 for researchers themselves to tailor conclusions so as to reinforce established organizations and service structures. Epidemiological findings that did not support the balance of service provision would rarely be disclosed, presumably because a system that reduced administration to subservience made this pointless.

In adult psychiatry, two major areas of needs stand out as woefully under-estimated and unaccounted for in service design. These are the vocational, residential and psychosocial rehabilitation needs of people with severe mental illness on the one hand, and the needs of people with common mental illnesses on the other. Major areas of unacknowledged needs across the region include community care for patients with dementia (old-age psychiatry), educational needs and family support services (child and adolescent psychiatry) and prison services and risk management (forensic psychiatry). All these examples of gaps in services expose one of the direst consequences of institutional care in the former eastern bloc: the disastrous lack of collaboration across sector boundar-ies. Once again, this is essentially a failure of governance rather than a lack of proper mental health expertise.

Several conclusions can be drawn. Politically, a period of particularly mis-guided social practice came to an end around 1989. The economic and social consequences are numerous, have varying profiles and intensities across the countries, and have only recently been acknowledged. The transition to a free market economy by the former eastern bloc countries has come at a time of globalization, which adds further frustrations to those based on the need to drop passivity and accept social participation. The complications of globaliza-tion arise from the fact that the challenge is no longer to find a dependable employer or patron but to compensate for dependency needs by adopting an entrepreneurial stance, i.e. organizing psychiatric services in ways that enable interdependence (Daulaire 1999; Lee 2000). A huge proportion of the ageing population in the region appears to be completely deprived of the chance to ever make this transition. An awareness of being doomed filters into the minds of millions but has not been stated authoritatively or on the basis of strong evidence in any of the eastern bloc countries. However, it does manifest itself strongly in sociodemographic statistics.

The human toll of transition is huge, but so far no governance structure appears to have risen to the task of predicting a realistic future and the way ahead for health systems. The persistent failure of governance in the com-munities of the former eastern bloc is predicated on the deeply instilled culture of dependency and corruption in the workplace. The evil indifference of, and attack on, individuality was the hallmark of previous regimes, as the example of the political abuse of psychiatry illustrates. This painful issue is still disavowed by governance structures.

Health resources

Health policies adopted by most countries in the region since 1989 have been based on the belief that health markets can function well and improve health care without the need for much governance. The transition to systems funded through social health insurance stands out as a core component of health reforms and has driven changes in legislation, taxation, ownership and the management of health systems. The fragility of economies has meant that most countries depend on international loans and have to accept restrictions enforced on their health budgets. Central health administrations are still directly responsible for the financial viability of almost every hospital without having the resources to achieve this task. Health ministries have had to face the consequences of introducing private practice and emerging markets in health care without even having a local word for 'stakeholder', not to mention strategies for coalition-building with consumer organizations.

Little data is available on health care expenditure or on mental health in particular. State-owned insurance agencies have been set up. These have unhealthy links with health administrations and inherit their propensity for tight central control by way of bureaucratic pressure. The purchase of services suffers all the difficulties of unregulated markets: a lack of rules, monopolies, disrespect for the consumer, bribery, blackmail, corruption and a lack of accountability. The allocation of resources on policy priorities is not transparent and reflects widespread beliefs about what conditions are worthy of cure (e.g. heart disease) and what are not (e.g. mental illness).

Most countries have a long way to go before they are able to prioritize investment in health on the basis of outcome data and sound health economic analysis. An example from Bulgaria is revealing. In line with new legislation the government regulates service provision on a geographic principle with the help of a National Health Map. This instrument determined the number of psychiatrists with whom the National Insurance Fund could contract services for 2003 (273), 43 of them in the capital, Sofia. By June 2003 contracts had been signed with 485 psychiatrists (almost twice the number), 137 of them in Sofia (3.2 times the target). No explanations were given for this. There are many similar examples of flawed governance.

Most countries in the region have inherited a huge number of hospitals with poor equipment and staff with poor training. This constitutes a formidable obstacle to health reforms in general and to mental health reforms in particular. At the heart of the problem, once again, is a lack of competence to effectively handle the organizational components of their health care systems. Prerequisites for efficient management, such as clinical standards with criteria that allow evaluation and arrangements that produce valid data, are not an integral part of the image of health care organization cherished by decision-makers. For example, almost none of the countries in the region seem to have a strategic plan which goes beyond a vague statement that transition from institutional to community care is planned. Existing policy and strategy documents fail to discuss the implications of closing down large institutions for re-engineering professional roles, tasks and jobs, for the acquisition of requisite skills, and for the redesign of information linkages and interfaces (Puras *et al.* 2004; Sharashidze *et al.* 2004; Tomov *et al.* 2004).

There is much talk of the need to close down psychiatric hospitals and to reduce bed numbers. The usual arguments, however, seldom go beyond borrowing the human rights rhetoric from organizations such as the Helsinki Committee. High-level officers within the health administrations deem careful case-by-case planning and individual solutions for transition from institutional to community care to be unthinkable. Arguments that psychiatric stigma is culturally diverse and that self-stigmatization in particular is driven by the psychiatric tradition of primitive paternalism fall on deaf ears. On second thought, one should not find this surprising given that the idea of care through partnership and community participation has established very few roots in the cultures of post-totalitarianism.

The tradition of central planning for health makes it difficult for new governance structures to call for an enlightened citizen and employer partnership in establishing adequate health funds, but nevertheless many countries are making significant progress in terms of pooling financial resources. Where most countries stumble is in the management of available funds, largely due to a lack of expertise and fiscal instruments.

Physical resources for health care are in poor condition and often there are problematic issues of ownership. This impedes shifting to a needs-based practice governed by a service culture informed by consistent quality assurance of care. This is a huge barrier to good health management. Adopting a managerial as well as a clinical perspective appears to be a major task for staff retraining now that the economic viability of the health systems in the region needs to be demonstrated continuously with the help of evidence on outcomes.

Provision and utilization of mental health services

Data on the provision of services in the region traditionally has been limited to a few general categories, allowing few conclusions to be drawn. Service utilization, to the degree to which it can be studied, is much less than estimated need, comparing poorly to the rest of Europe. Data on provision are reported to the local and central administrations and pooled for annual health statistics reports. This practice is not guided by articulated managerial needs to gauge progress on policy because policy (to the extent that it exists) is seldom translated into operational plans or expected changes in outcomes.

Focus groups run during a study on the attitudes of front-line health managers (Schider *et al.* 2004) revealed that people felt they were left out of the cycle of decision-making. The participants, who were usually medical specialists by training, expected to enforce the authority of the ministry of health and to streamline and oversee the collection of statistics tailored to needs other than their own. There was consensus in the focus groups that they produced work of poor quality. This attitude was explained by the lack of ownership of their work, and a feeling of being divorced from the governance aspects of service provision. The groups also agreed that the methods employed by health administrations, and even more so by the health insurance operatives, had an alienating influence. Their attitude was described as dictatorial and subversive to progress, in terms of both the humane and technological aspects of care provision. Issues of effectiveness, quality of life or satisfaction with mental health services were not seen as relevant or of general concern for the current operation of clinical services in the region. This was due to technological backwardness and a lack of prospects for investment. These sentiments, however, could not find expression in official reports or policy documents: they were shared only off the record (Mladenova *et al.* 2002).

Process analysis of mental health care at either local or central level has not been informed by a tradition of managerial, evidence-based decision-making.

This has resulted in the view that data collection is a chore of little relevance to clinical practice. Thus, there has been a general neglect of process data.

As recording the cost and volume of services becomes more vital to staff income there has been some revival of interest in process data collection and analysis. Most countries, however, still lack both the conceptual framework and the tools of structured clinical practice, operational protocols, clinical standards and indicators, as well as the requisite agencies to operate data-based management.

Governance

Good governance is a combination of leadership and management, for which the state sets the tone in society. Governance (or stewardship) (WHO 2000) combines ethics, legitimacy and trust with accountability, efficiency and substantive outcomes. Good governance includes a capable, ordered and respected bureaucracy, checked by the judiciary and subject to legislation, with the capacity to impose democratically approved law and to provide a sense of direction and meaning to individuals and communities. This capacity is poorly developed in most former eastern bloc countries (Brown 2001).

One of the findings from a recent study on mental health profiles (Mladenova 2002) was particularly illuminating. The information concerned the split between what was officially claimed and written about health and what one saw to be the day-to-day situation in the field. On a number of occasions the research teams were faced with the fact that one of the central roles of the health administration was to ascertain whether the claims about the situation in health services should be accepted or refuted, not on the basis of evidence but on the basis of whether or not they are made by those in authority. The underlying assumption is that authority firmly belongs with those who hold office. For example, the director of the Sofia Office of the Health Insurance Fund dismissed the proposal that small group sessions with people with severe mental illness counted as proper vocational rehabilitation, and thus should not be considered for remuneration by his agency. His grounds for refusing the proposal were that it had been made by psychiatrists, who by virtue of this fact could not be considered impartial on issues of psychiatry. Hence, this official saw himself as having the authority to reject the request and reprimand the petitioners.

The views of experts from a particular field (such as mental health) on problems could be tolerated by the central administration only as long as they did not question the role of management as a contributing factor. Certainly this stance appears hypocritical to observers and definitely requires clarification. One obvious explanation could be to draw parallels between the current stifling and unsuitable managerial culture and the party *apparatchiks* arguing that it takes time for social systems to change.

Policy in times of transition

Summarizing the evidence

It has repeatedly been affirmed that clear policy is of key importance in promoting mental health care and that such policy should be based on evidence (WHO 2003). Summarizing the evidence that bears on mental health policy in former eastern bloc countries, it could be concluded that the situation is dominated by the amazing political developments that occurred in 1989, following several years of *perestroika* (political and economic restructuring). Independently of how countries chose to proceed with reforms thereafter, health statistics slumped, making it obvious that health crises attest not just to the unhealthy nature of totalitarian societies. They also suggest that the capacity of post-totalitarian societies to turn to a reality free of preconceived notions could be damaged, and there might be a failure to grab opportunities for change whenever they arise. What would a hypothesis about such damage look like?

During the past decade most of the mental health systems in the region have been operating outmoded facilities and exercising beliefs about treatment, therapy, rehabilitation and prevention that are outdated and certainly out of sync with the values of civil society and democracy. Research into mental health services in the region has been negligible and almost all the evidence that is available for decision-making has come from service activity data. However, the quality of these data is poor, largely because the lack of demand for technological innovation had failed to drive developments in information systems. The economic slumps and the obsolete managerial ethos within countries in the region may account for a delay in innovation in mental health policy but it certainly cannot explain the large-scale denial of the issue of mental health problems within governance structures that was reported in a number of these countries by human rights organizations and other international bodies (Bulgarian Helsinki Committee 2001).

Most importantly, the review of the evidence on mental health policy presented above attests to the failure of governance structures to engage with the realities within the mental health sector by entering into constructive dialogue with consumers, personnel, partners and other stakeholders. Governance in most countries has not been able to develop the capacity to abide by commitments made to mental health services and often resorts only to paying lip service to responsibilities – a practice that is reminiscent of the hypocrisy of the totalitarian paternalism of the past. As the years have gone by, this practice has reinforced a mistrust of authority. In most countries the capacity to develop coherence in stakeholder groups and mutual goals in response to deprivation has not been improved.

Translating the evidence into policy

How does a national mental health policy face this state of affairs effectively? Clearly, there is a compelling argument that any such policy should take full account of the social transition that is occurring; or in other words, change by far outweighs continuity. The management of change then becomes the problematic issue. This invariably invokes the function of leadership with the core elements being an adequate interpretation of reality (providing a vision attuned to the *zeitgeist*) and containment (providing certainty amidst the lack of evidence, since evidence to support visions is never adequate) (Alford 2001; Barker 2001).

We know of one attempt in the former eastern bloc countries to formulate a context-relevant vision for psychiatry in the region, the GIP-supported Association of Reformers in Psychiatry.[3] In line with the human rights spirit of the time and the quest for participatory involvement, this body developed a vision of community psychiatry built on personalized, lifelong case coordination with support from social care and rehabilitation programmes. It targeted individuals with social impairments that were considered to be too disturbing for local communities if such individuals were trusted to reside unassisted within them. One contribution of this group was to express this vision in a long list of statements about mental illness, psychiatry and psychiatric reforms and to test if these were shared by local stakeholders. It appeared that they were not; at least, not with any enthusiasm (Tomov and Butorin 1997; Geneva Initiative on Psychiatry 2000).

In hindsight, it should have been possible to predict this. The rapid decline of strong central authority since 1989 had frustrated the dependency needs of all citizens. In the minds of many the issue of how to develop self-sufficiency and interdependence, which was the order of the day, had been eclipsed by anxiety at the loss of a dependable state and by anger directed at the authorities for abdicating from their incontestable obligations to protect the weak. Under the circumstances it was easy to read into the community psychiatry project the further withdrawal of institutions from exercising control (in this case over madness).

It is now clear that there are many preoccupations related to the social transition of those who are 'well' in former eastern bloc countries and these push mental disorders to the bottom of the social agenda. It appears that the community mental health vision cannot call forth either champions or leadership. This suggests that it would be unwise, under the circumstances, for mental health policy reform to place too much emphasis on community care for the severely mentally impaired. By the same token however, if the heavy toll of transition on mental 'wellness' is recognized and if the priorities of reform policies are construed in terms of attending to those affected by the process of change, the chances of gaining public support may improve significantly.

Most analysts are beginning to recognize this, as the strain of transition on the emotional and group life of people becomes more apparent (Dahrendorf 1990). Previously, mental well-being, and its promotion, were non-issues in the region because the notion of a mental disorder was confined to severe disabling illness. Mental illnesses were seen as involving a dispensable minority, which should be left entirely to the public sector to manage. These days, however, the salience of mental health is invoked by growing awareness of the rates of violence, homelessness, crime, prostitution and drug addiction. Communities have been taken by surprise by this surge in irrationality, and the response, so far, has been confusion, disbelief, frustration and the search for someone to blame.

Framing the problem: the psychosocial dynamics of change

In established democracies the wider acceptance of civil society values has made it possible to put mental health reform onto the public policy agenda. The former eastern bloc countries, however, are still struggling to contextualize these values within the economic, political and social domains. Their leaders and the demands of globalization are pushing for reform, including reforms in mental health care. But for many, what is happening is experienced as a hostile intrusion into their environment. They cannot see opportunities for themselves in these developments, or they may view these changes as involving them in activities that are counterproductive to social progress. Basically, they respond as their ancestors did to crisis, by revitalizing kinship networks. As a result, clans re-emerge, familism (division into kin and alien) becomes a fundamental line of distinction, and meritocracy is hampered in finding its way into community affairs (Stability Pact for South Eastern Europe 2004). Paradoxically, the values that emerge and are reinforced in this process are exactly those that the architects of transition were intent on replacing with the values of democracy.

In order to comprehend this, it is important to acknowledge the role of psychological and social defences in resistance to change (Jaques 1955). The defensive mode of functioning in individuals and organizations is triggered by the anxiety stemming from the preoccupation with differences brought about by change. This manifests itself in many ways: refusing to accept difference at face value, attributing negative meaning to it, a selective perception of only its negative consequences, jumping to pessimistic conclusions, and so on. Caught in this mode of functioning, individuals may more readily experience emotional distress and social impairment, develop disorders of sub-threshold or clinical severity, or have their pre-existing conditions aggravated. Those who have been well are prone to such problems as well as those who have had a history of psychiatric illness.

At the level of service provision the massive effects of the stress of transition may call into question the established boundaries between primary health and specialist services (Thornicroft and Tansella 1999). This may raise the need to reconsider the very principles of service provision in a country in terms of assigning priority status not only to severe disorders but also to those mental health problems triggered by transition. Governance structures should respond by shifting policy and directives respectively. They may conduct surveys to assess the scope of the problem or engage in public and professional debates to elicit attitudes. Straightforward as this may seem, it misses the fact that when minds are in defensive mode people find it difficult to be constructive and may employ their organizations as a shield against change. The mental health system is certainly not immune to being used as a social defence against the anxiety of change by its employees. In this context, an additional task for management is to turn the minds of those in the system of care away from this defensive mode so that they can start responding rationally to new policies, directives and work tasks.

Demands on mental health policy in the region

Being defensive because of anxiety provoked by nascent change is part of human nature. Finding a way around it is a serious challenge for mental health policy-makers, particularly as the solution should respect the rights of individuals to be true to their nature. Good governance in mental health is exactly about this and is not readily available in times of transition, times that place huge demands on leadership (Tomov *et al.* 2003). To get an idea of such demands one needs to consider that at times of transition mental health policy should at least:

- provide for the expected new needs within the general population precipi-tated by the stress of transition, which may manifest themselves as an epidemic of common mental illnesses;
- plan additional services for major psychiatric disorders in anticipation of the fact that the turmoil of change will aggravate their clinical severity and course;
- proceed with the restructuring of general psychiatric services, to re-orient them towards community-based care in line with the demands of the political agenda;
- respond to the rising demands for specialist psychiatric service – child and adolescent, geriatric, forensic, substance abuse – demands that erupt when the lid of central control is lifted off a community.

But first, and above all, mental health policy during times of transition should take good care of the country's mental health system itself – the single most important tool needed to deliver all of the measures listed above. However, the system can also be a tool that employees predictably will use as a social defence against their own anxiety about change, rendering it a much less pliable health instrument than it is normally. This becomes the case particularly when a coun-try's political agenda prescribes reform of the health system itself. It should be clear by now that reform policy is linked with the social power implicit in posi-tions and roles, or rather with their loss, or the threat of loss. Such things are painful and many people will go to great lengths to avoid or postpone them. In this they follow identifiable patterns, including:

- *Reframing* is a strategy of resistance to change that boils down to stripping the proponents of reform of all positive human qualities, ascribing these to one-self, while assigning to reformers all the negatives, including those introduced to the situation by oneself. It is a particularly vicious way of going *ad hominem.*
- *Obstructing entrepreneurship.* At times of transition, entrepreneurship mani-fests itself as the capacity to act within the real world constructively and with an awareness of the risks involved. An example would be to ask consumers what they want and eventually integrate it into the service profile. The bar-riers to achieving this in the countries of the region are formidable and are rooted in the quagmire of centralized bureaucracy.
- *'Rubber fence' responses* are an organizational defence whereby no new devel-opment provokes curiosity but is played down by claims that it is already part of routine activities.

- *'Privatization'* is a maladaptive way of acquiring ownership over work tasks by replacing, in a subtle and unacknowledged way, the primary task of an organization (e.g. care for people with mental health problems) with a private task (e.g. attending to staff anxieties provoked by transition).
- *Anonymity* is a denial of the need to acknowledge the patient as an individual in order to build the trust upon which to base interventions. It exposes the thwarted capacity of staff to enter into personal relationships with patients and with each other.

This list of maladaptive patterns that plague the organizational culture of health services, and that governance structures have to take into consideration, can be extended (Geneva Initiative on Psychiatry 2000). The more pertinent issue, however, is what action can be taken regarding the aspects of human nature that threaten failure for health systems. Are there limits where governance can afford to play down the importance of attending to tasks with the genuine excuse that the well-being of the organization should not be jeopardized? Such limits certainly exist but they cannot be set in the culture of the region as the example of political psychiatry clearly attests. The reason why this is the case is pretty much the same now as it was then. It is the fact that the answers to questions of governance strategy are traditionally addressed behind the scenes and out of public view, which is exactly the setting that favours defensive-mode solutions, solutions which disavow large portions of reality.

Participatory action research

Cultures of non-participation can embark on the road of mental health reform if defensive responses to change are repeatedly challenged in open debates until behind-the-scene decision-making is banned. Complicated as this approach may seem, it is well established in developed democracies and much discussed in the literature on leadership and management in the area of action research. There are many attempts to make it intelligible for actors in all domains facing the challenges of innovating human systems. When devising the method, K. Lewin (in 1946) reportedly meant '. . . research that would solve practical problems and contribute to general scientific theory' (Elden and Chisholm 1993).

Introducing the practice of deliberating on mental health policy while it is being made, rather than just imposing it, is indeed a practical problem of huge social significance, not only within this region. Thus, in 1985 Korman and Glennerster wrote: 'the reason why some policies are not implemented is that no one ever expected them to be. Acts are passed or ministerial speeches made to satisfy some party pressure or some awkward interest group, but civil servants know that they need not strain themselves too hard to achieve results. The policy is symbolic'. The specific policy Korman and Glennerster were referring to was the closure of a psychiatric hospital in the United Kingdom. The community mental health policies developed by health administrations in many countries in eastern and central Europe are regarded by influential corporate groups precisely as documents that are not meant to be implemented. Gill Walt (1994), who quotes Korman and Glennerster in her book on health policy, asserts that the policy process works interactively. Indeed, limiting policy-making to the development of coherent documents is hardly worth the effort even when such policy is evidence-based, context-relevant and criterion-guided. The interactive nature of the policy process implies that those who will implement policy would not be empowered to do so unless they have participated in the decision-making process.

Organizational cultures that impede progress need to import expertise for innovative change from outside the organization. In the case of the former eastern bloc countries this can only be achieved through international aid. In the case of action research such importation always begins with obtaining a mandate from local administrative structures. A mandate codifies awareness of the problems and a commitment to searching for solutions by those with whom the power of decision-making lies. In this sense it represents a promise for success.

Under the action research paradigm 'social defence' entails an intrusion into the activity of the organization by the interests and motives coming from the private lives and histories of its members. This intrusion is attributed to anxiety, related to the task faced by the organization (e.g. mental health policy reform) and is experienced as a threat (see 'Privatization' above).

In order to handle such experiences governance practices informed by action research would draw a distinction between the technical system (e.g. psychiatric care and treatment), the social system (e.g. staff, administration, patients) and the relationship structures that bring the two systems together (e.g. management, leadership, group life) (Pasmore 1995). Action research argues that 'because organizations employ whole persons, it is important to pay attention to human needs beyond those required for the regular performance of tasks dictated by technology' (Emery and Trist 1971). Such practices would also ensure the closer involvement of the participants in observing how their organization functions and would encourage them to generate findings and interpretations. In the process they would acquire ownership over the organization, its tasks and future.

An example of good practice

Experience in coping with the complexity of transition in mental health systems in the former eastern bloc is being gradually accumulated. Social defence issues would usually be identified when reformist groups, supported by grants from international bodies, would attempt to set up services in response to needs that had been neglected for decades and could be brought into the open due to political change. The scope of this practice has been growing since the early 1990s. The moment has now come when the monolithic control of the psychiatric establishment over decisions in mental health policy is being challenged regularly by activist groups of patients, relatives and professionals. Politicians have begun to acknowledge the existence of diversity of opinion and conflict of interests in this area. The new policy documents that most countries have developed in mental health policy reflect this important development.

A good illustration of how the power and policy scene is changing is a deinstitutionalization initiative in the Lithuanian capital, Vilnius, launched in 2003, to restructure a municipal mental hospital on Vasaros Street. The Vasaros project became possible as a result of unusual circumstances. A young, energetic hospital director decided to invest time in upgrading the hospital and opened it up to reforms. A young mayor understood the need to improve the quality of health care services in his city. Vasaros Hospital, unlike most other mental institutions in this part of Europe, had the opportunity to be established within the city centre. Finally, the Dutch Ministry of Foreign Affairs agreed to finance the development plan.

The project's objective was to develop a network of coordinated services with a seamless transition between them as clients' needs might dictate. In addition, three new modules of specialist psychiatric care were designed for implementation: crisis intervention, assertive community treatment and specialized services for eating disorders. Financially, the project envisaged municipal investment to upgrade premises and add new buildings. In addition, the project provided for the systematic involvement, throughout all stages, of both relatives and service users in the hospital's management, and a patients' council was established to undertake this task. Finally, there were negotiations with health insurance companies to provide adequate reimbursement for new services not covered by existing regulations. This was the key issue in sustaining the quality of the costly new services in an organizational culture that fails to provide for quality assurance.

The project met with opposition from two sides. Firstly, the site on which Vasaros was built was considered to be a prime location and a target for urban redevelopment. Secondly, the project was considered a threat by a group of psychiatrists and officials who favoured institution-based psychiatry and who – with regard to psychiatric hospitals – adhered to the concept of 'the bigger the better'. They countered the proposals by suggesting instead that Vasaros close all inpatient wards and run only outpatient services. They did so while being fully aware that only inpatient psychiatric services could be adequately reimbursed under Lithuania's health insurance laws (outpatient services being funded only in primary care centres via a capitation system). In fact, the opponents of the Vasaros project were advocating that the Vilnius Republican Psychiatric Hospital in Naujoji Vilnia, a suburb of Vilnius, be given a monopoly in providing mental health services. This hospital, a classical example of a large national psychiatric hospital with special privileged status under the direct authority of the Ministry of Health, was facing its own institutional anxieties. To prevent potential closure in the event that Lithuania's new mental health policies should gain momentum in the future, pressure was placed on the Ministry of Health to give this hospital a monopoly over inpatient psychiatric services for the whole of the Vilnius region which has a catchment area of around 1 million inhabitants.

By the end of 2003 a stalemate had been reached: the Minister of Health decreed that Vasaros Hospital should be affiliated to Naujoji Vilnia, with the clear intention of closing the small hospital at Vasaros and concentrating all inpatient psychiatric services, without any possibility of having a choice in inpatient treatment, in Naujoji Vilnia. In response, the mayor of Vilnius publicly protested, emphasizing the need for a modern vision of mental health services in Vilnius and denied the minister the right to take a decision regarding a municipal hospital. In addition, other public protests were made by both Lithuanian and foreign organizations.

A fragile consensus was eventually reached allowing the Vasaros project to go ahead as long as the Dutch government continued to provide investment. Thus, two years' valuable time was secured for Vilnius to develop a long-term mental health policy that would guarantee a future for Vasaros hospital. Interestingly, after parliamentary elections at the end of 2004 a new coalition government was formed. The new health minister openly favoured the development of modern mental health services and officially cancelled the affiliation decree of his predecessor, thus giving an important political signal and supporting the need for the development of modern approaches to mental health services in Lithuania.

Moreover, the new minister supported the formulation of a new national mental health policy with a clear emphasis on the development of community-based services as an alternative to the highly centralized system of large psychiatric institutions, protection of human rights in the field of mental health and the development of an evidence-based public health approach in accordance with the recommendations of the WHO ministerial conference held in Helsinki in 2005.

At this point it is still too early to predict the future of mental health services in Lithuania and other countries in transition, and how successfully these changes will be managed in the light of continued resistance within their mental health systems and prevailing attitudes. Nevertheless, projects like Vasaros provide a unique chance to change the mental health scene in a European capital and to challenge outdated Soviet-style mental health care provision by offering an integrated chain of mental health services.

Conclusion

The political transition started in 1989 is the single most important factor in shaping the mental health political agenda in former eastern bloc countries. There are many priorities on this agenda but they share a common root – the culture-bound disregard of the importance of mental well-being for prosperity and happiness. For over 50 years totalitarian indifference to human dignity and freedom had colluded with prejudice to block mental illness and its consequences from entering public debate and receiving its due share of attention and resources. This resulted in a deterioration of mental health services and parochial solutions, the most hideous of which was the political abuse of psychiatry in the former Soviet Union. Health governance in the region by and large disregards these bitter lessons of recent history and denies any connection between poor health indicators and inadequate national mental health policy.

Mental health policy awareness in the countries of the region increased rapidly after 1989 due to the work of human rights movements – not by evidence-based assessment of needs or concerns for quality assurance or the cost-effectiveness of mental health care systems. Lack of national mental health policies and the absence of operational policy at local service level are a serious

Table 17.1 General information and service provision data by country

Indicator/country	Azerbaijan	Bulgaria	Georgia	Lithuania	Russian Federation	Ukraine
Population* (2004, millions)	8.3	7.8	4.4	3.4	143.8	47.3
Live births* (per 1000 population)	13.8 (2003)	9.0 (2004)	10.7 (2003)	8.9 (2004)	10.5 (2004)	9.0 (2004)
Deaths 0–64* (per 100,000)	379 (2002)	383 (2004)	294 (2001)	471 (2004)	783 (2004)	648 (2004)
Infant deaths* (per 1000 live births)	12.8 (2002)	11.7 (2004)	10.4 (2001)	7.9 (2004)	11.5 (2004)	9.4 (2004)
Literacy in population 15+ (%)* (2003)	99	98	100	100	99	98
Gross national product* (USD) per capita (2004)	950	2740	1040	5740	3410	1260
Unemployment rate (%)* (2004)	1.4	12.2	12.6	6.0	7.8	8.6
Health expenditure* (% of GDP)	1.6 (2004)	4.8 (2001)	3.6 (2004)	6.0 (2004)	5.4 (2001)	3.5 (2004)
Suicide rate* (per 100,000)	1.4 (2002)	11.0 (2004)	2.1 (2001)	38.9 (2004)	31.7 (2004)	22.0 (2004)
Population below $2 per day*** (%)	9.1 (2001)	16.2 (2001)	15.7 (2001)	6.9 (2000)	7.5 (2002)	45.7 (1999)
Schizophrenia reported prevalence**** (per 10,000)	48	42	42	45.6	–	33.6
Mental health policy document**	No	Yes	Yes	Yes	Yes	Yes
Mental health law**	Yes	No	Yes	Yes	Yes	Yes
Psychiatrists** (per 10,000)	0.5	0.9	0.6	1.5	1.4	0.9
Psychiatric beds* (per 100,000) (2004)	45.5 (2003)	57.9	28.3	106.8	113.6	94.8

Sources:
* WHO, Health For All Database (January 2006)
** WHO, *Atlas* of mental health (2005)
*** World Bank Group, World Development Indicators (2005b)
**** Country teams

barrier to the introduction of structured clinical practice in the mental health sector. As a consequence the whole idea of policy-driven and accountable mental health is not taking root in the rapidly transforming cultures in the region. While international bodies like the WHO and the European Union readily provide road maps for the reform of services, transformational leadership stands out as the scarcest commodity in terms of managerial and governance resources. The profound crisis of leadership and governance, which is striking to external observers, fails to register with or capture the minds of local citizens and politicians, largely because of the enforced discontinuation of the participatory tradition suffered by the region under totalitarian rule. Participatory action research, as a way of introducing sustainable and progressive transformation, so far appears to have evaded the attention of the architects of change inside and outside the region.

In addition to focused efforts aimed at enhancing governance, all countries struggle to implement reforms. This remains the case even though the development of community-based mental health services as a replacement for institutional care by and large lacks support from local communities and funding from budgetary and external sources. Nevertheless, most countries push ahead with such reforms without any real understanding of the mechanisms of social defence operating counterproductively within society. The real challenge all countries face is the retraining of middle-level staff employed within mental health services in the skills of psychosocial rehabilitation and in coping with the anxieties of clinical work in ways that are more productive than the use of repression and similar defences. Action research seems to hold some promise to accomplish this mammoth task but few advisers and donors see the mission of international aid as encompassing the transformation of organizational culture as well as upgrading clinical practices.

Unlike most established democracies, which closed hospital beds under policies of reform, the former eastern bloc countries face the need to invest significantly, though selectively, in upgrading hospital facilities because of the expected high share of severely ill people in need of continuous hospital rehabilitation before being considered for community care. Moreover, specialist psychiatric services for geriatric patients, adolescents and children, drug addiction and anorexia services are suddenly in big demand but in very short supply. Last but not least, the human toll of transition in many countries of the former eastern bloc has turned out to be very high, causing disproportionately high rates of early death in middle-aged males, which many believe has been precipitated by psychosocial stress. This finding poses a formidable problem for mental health policy in the region. The consequences of not handling this properly could be dire.

Acknowledgement

We are grateful to Fuad Ismailov, Lyudmila Scoropada and Nana Sharashidze for their assistance in compiling data from Azerbaijan, Georgia and Ukraine.

Notes

1 The (former) eastern bloc consists of the following countries: Albania, Bulgaria, the Czech Republic and Slovakia (formerly Czechoslovakia), former German Democratic Republic, Hungary, Poland, Romania and the countries of the former Soviet Union.

2 The Geneva Initiative on Psychiatry (now the Global Initiative on Psychiatry) is an international non-profit organization registered in Amsterdam, with its headquarters in Hilversum, the Netherlands. Since 2001, the Geneva Initiative also has had offices in Vilnius (Lithuania), Sofia (Bulgaria) and Tbilisi (Georgia). It is the only organization in the world that concentrates solely on the reform and humanization of all mental health care in central and eastern Europe. In the past, the organization's work has been awarded several prestigious prizes for its efforts, namely the Human Rights award from the American Psychiatric Association, and the 2000 Geneva Prize for Human Rights in Psychiatry.

3 The Association of Reformers in Psychiatry was an attempt by non-governmental organizations in former eastern bloc countries to build a coalition and thus support each other's efforts. It was established in 1998 and dissolved several years later due to lack of funds.

References

Alford, C.F. (2001) Leadership by interpretation and holding, *Organizational and Social Dynamics*, 2(2): 153–73.

Barker, R. (2001) The nature of leadership, *Human Relations*, 54(4): 468–94.

Brown, J.F. (2001) *The Grooves of Change: Eastern Europe at the Turn of The Millennium.* Durham, NC: Duke University Press.

Bukovsky, V. (1974) *To Build a Castle, My Life as a Dissenter.* Washington, DC: Ethics and Public Policy Center.

Bulgarian Helsinki Committee (2001) *Inpatient Psychiatric Care in Bulgaria and Human Rights.* Sofia: www.bghelsinki.org.

Carothers, T. (2002) The end of the transition paradigm, *Journal of Democracy*, January–April, 13(1): 5–2.

Chisholm, R. and Elden, M. (1993) Features of emerging action research, *Human Relations*, 40(2): 275–98.

Cornia, G.A. and Paniccia, R. (eds) (2000) *The Mortality Crisis in Transitional Economies.* Oxford: Oxford University Press.

Dahrendorf, R. (1990) *Reflections on the Revolution in Europe.* New York: Random House.

Daulaire, N. (1999) Globalization and health, *Development*, 42(4): 22–4.

Domenighetti, G. (2003) *Evolution of the Health Care Systems in the Countries of Central and Eastern Europe and Newly-independent States.* Report for the Swiss Embassy, Sofia.

Elden, M. and Chisholm, R. (1993) Emerging varieties of action research: introduction to the special issue, *Human Relations*, 40(2): 121–42.

Emery, F.E. and Trist, E.L. (1971) Analytical model for sociotechnical systems, in P. Hill (ed.) *Towards a New Philosophy of Management.* London: Gower.

Faria, M. (1995) *Vandals at the Gates of Medicine: Historic Perspectives on the Battle Over Health Care Reforms.* Macon, GA: Hacienda Publishing.

Geneva Initiative on Psychiatry (2000) *Attitudes and Needs Assessment in Psychiatry: Final Report on a Study.* Sofia: MATRA, New Bulgarian University.

Jaques, E. (1955) Social systems as a defence against persecutory and depressive anxiety, in M. Klein, P. Heimann and R. Money-Kyrle (eds) *New Directions in Psychoanalysis.* London: Tavistock Publications.

Jenkins, R., Gulbinat, W., Manderscheid, R., Baingana, F. *et al.* (2004) The mental health country profile: background, design and use of a systematic method of appraisal, *International Review of Psychiatry*, 16(1–2): 31–47.

Kickbusch, I. (2002) Mobilizing citizens and communities for better health: the civil society context in central and eastern Europe. A background paper for USAID Conference, 'Ten Years of Health Systems Transition in Central and Eastern Europe and Eurasia', Washington, DC, 29–31 July.

Korman, N. and Glennerster, H. (1985) Closing a hospital: the Darenth Park Project, *Occasional Papers in Social Administration*, 78. London: Bedford Square Press.

Krug, E.G., Dahlberg, L.L., Mercy, J.A., Zwi, A.B. and Lozano, R. (eds) (2002) *World Report on Violence and Health*. Geneva: WHO.

Lee, K. (2000) Globalization and health policy: a review of the literature and proposed research and policy agenda, in Pan American Health Organization (ed.) *Health Development in the New Global Economy*. Washington, DC: PAHO.

Markova, G. (2004) The relationship between parental mental representations and attachment style and institutionalization of children in Bulgaria. PhD Thesis, School for Social Work, Smith College, USA.

Menzies, I.E.P. (1992) *Containing Anxiety in Institutions. Selected Essays*. London: Free Association Books.

Mladenova, M., Tomov, T. Broshtilov, A. and Okoliyski, M. (2002) The agenda of reforms and the attitudes to it: a report from Bulgaria. Paper presented at 5th ENMESH Conference, 31 May–2 June, Sofia.

Paldam, M. and Svendsen, T. (2001) Missing social capital and the transition in eastern Europe, *Journal for Institutional Innovation, Development and Transition*, 5: 21–34.

Pasmore, W. (1995) Social science transformed: the socio-technical perspective, *Human Relations*, 48(1): 1–21.

Puras, D., Germanavicius, A., Povilaitis, R., Veniute, M. and Jasilionis, D. (2004) Lithuania mental health country profile, *International Review of Psychiatry*, 16(1–2): 117–25.

Rutz, W. (2001) Mental health in Europe: problems, advances and challenges, *Acta Psychiatrica Scandinavica*, 104 (Suppl. 410): 15–20.

Sakharov, A. (1975) *My Country and the World*. New York: Vintage Books.

Schider, K., Tomov, T., Mladenova, M., Mayeya, J. *et al.* (2004) The appropriateness and use of focal group methodology across international mental health communities, *International Review of Psychiatry*, 16(1–2): 24–30.

Sharashidze, N., Naneishvili, G., Silagadze, T., Begiashvili, A., Sulaberidze, B. and Beria, Z. (2004) Georgia mental health country profile, *International Review of Psychiatry*, 16(1–2): 107–16.

Shkolnikov, V., McKee, M. and Leon, D.A. (2001) Changes in life expectancy in Russia in the mid-1990s, *Lancet*, 357(9260): 917–21.

Shorter, E. (1997) *A History of Psychiatry from the Era of the Asylum to the Age of Prozac*. New York: Wiley.

Sjalamov, V. (1995) *Kolyma Tales*. London: Penguin.

Soyfer, V., Gruliow, L. and Gruliow, R. (1997) *Lysenko and the Tragedy of Soviet Science*. Piscataway, NJ: Rutgers University Press.

Stability Pact for South Eastern Europe (2004) *SEE Mental Health Project: Overview of Country Assessment of Mental Health Policy and Legislation in SEE*. Sarajevo: Regional Report, WHO Regional Office for Europe.

Thornicroft, G. and Tansella, M. (1999) *The Mental Health Matrix*. Cambridge: Cambridge University Press.

Tobis, D. (2000) *Moving from Residential Institutions to Community-based Services in Central and Eastern Europe and the Former Soviet Union*. Washington, DC: World Bank.

Tomov, T. (1999) Political abuse of psychiatry in the former Soviet Union, in H. Freeman (ed.) *A Century of Psychiatry*. London: Hardcourt.

Tomov, T. (2001) Mental health reforms in Eastern Europe, *Acta Psychiatrica Scandinavica*, 104 (Suppl. 410): 21–6.

Tomov, T. and Butorin, N. (1997) Attitudes to psychiatric patients: a cross-cultural survey of the psychiatric professions. Paper presented at the WPA Congress, Madrid, 23–8 August.

Tomov, T., Alexandrov, H., Chichek, R. and Ivanov, I. (2003) Leadership in Bulgaria: group relations analysis, in: *State of Society*. Sofia: Open Society Fund, www.osf.bg/sos/.

Tomov, T., Mladenova, M., Lazarova, I., Sotirov, V. and Okoliyski, M. (2004) Bulgaria mental health country profile, *International Review of Psychiatry*, 16(1–2): 93–106.

Townsend, C., Whiteford, H., Baingana, F., Gulbinat, W. *et al.* (2004) The mental health policy template: domains and elements for mental health policy formulation, *International Review of Psychiatry*, 16(1–2): 18–23.

United Nations (2002) *UN Human Development Index 2002*. http://hdp.undp.org.

Varnik, A. (2000) *Depression and Mental Health in Estonia. World Health Organization Report*. Geneva: World Health Organization.

Walt, G. (1994) *Health Policy: An Introduction to Process and Power*. London: Zed Books.

Walt, G., Pavignani, E., Gilson, L. and Bruce, K. (1999) Health sector development: from aid coordination to resource management, *Health Policy and Planning*, 14(3): 207–18.

World Bank (2005) *Dying Too Young. Addressing Premature Mortality and Ill Health Due to Non-communicable Diseases and Injuries in the Russian Federation*. Washington, DC: World Bank.

World Bank (2005) *World Development Indicators 2005*. Washington, DC: World Bank.

World Health Organization (WHO) (2000) *The World Health Report 2000*. Geneva: WHO.

World Health Organization (WHO) (2003) *Mental Health Policy and Service Guidance Package – Organization of Services for Mental Health*. Geneva: WHO.

World Health Organization (WHO) (2005) *Atlas. Mental Health Resources Around the World*. Geneva: WHO.

World Health Organization (2006) *Health For All Database*, January 2006. Geneva: WHO.

chapter eighteen

Global perspective on mental health policy and service development issues: the WHO angle

Michelle Funk, Natalie Drew and Benedetto Saraceno

Over the last few years, several initiatives by the World Health Organization (WHO) have highlighted mental health as a public health problem in need of urgent attention by governments and the international community. In 2001, World Health Day, devoted to mental health, mobilized countries to carry forth the message of 'Stop Exclusion – Dare to Care'. Another milestone in global mental health was the publication of the *World Health Report 2001*. This report made a compelling case for addressing the mental health needs of populations around the world (World Health Organization 2001d). The main messages of the report were that: mental disorders account for a significant burden of disease in all societies; effective interventions are available but are not accessible to the majority of the people who need them; these interventions can be made accessible through changes in policy and legislation, service development, adequate financing and the training of appropriate personnel. The *World Health Report 2001* concluded with a set of ten recommendations that can be adopted by every country in accordance with its needs and resources (see Box 18.1).

Importantly, the WHO Executive Board of January 2002 approved Resolution EB109.R8 (World Health Organization 2002a) on strengthening mental health, which calls on the director general, regional committees and all member states to adopt and implement the recommendations of the *World Health Report* and to increase national cooperation and investments in mental health. The recommendations of this resolution were essentially endorsed by the World

Box 18.1   Recommendations in *The World Health Report 2001*

- Provide treatment in primary care
- Make psychotropic medicines available
- Give care in the community
- Educate the public
- Involve communities, families and consumers
- Establish national policies, programmes and legislation
- Develop human resources
- Link with other sectors
- Monitor community mental health
- Support more research

Health Assembly in Resolution WHA 55.10 (World Health Organization 2002b), reflecting a growing commitment among member states to address the pressing mental health needs of their populations and for the necessity of international support and action in this area.

This chapter outlines the policy and service challenges faced by many countries across the world. It begins with a description of the global burden of mental disorders and their costs in human, social and economic terms as well as the resources that are being invested to address mental health problems. Key policy issues are then highlighted.

Burden of mental disorders

Prevalence of mental disorders

At any given time, 450 million people suffer from some form of mental or brain disorder, including alcohol and substance use disorders. In order of prevalence, 121 million people suffer from depression, 70 million from alcohol-related problems, 50 million suffer from epilepsy, 37 million from Alzheimer's disease and 24 million from schizophrenia (World Health Organization 2001c). Finally, an estimated 815,000 people around the world have committed suicide (World Health Organization 2002c). There is a gender disparity in prevalence rates, notably for depression and substance use disorders, as can be seen in Table 18.1 (World Health Organization 2001e). Many reasons for the higher prevalence of certain mental disorders among women have been put forward, including genetic and biological factors (World Health Organization 2001d). Psychological and social factors also play a part, as the unequal position women hold in society means they experience discrimination in the fields of employment, education and in the exercise of their civil liberties. This, in turn, exposes them to greater stresses and makes them less able to change their stressful environment. The higher prevalence of substance use disorder among men is a consistent finding across the globe, and has been attributed to biological, psychological and psychosocial factors (World Health Organization 2001d). Prevalence rates

Table 18.1 Point prevalence rates of some common mental disorders

Disorder	Point prevalence rates (%)
Unipolar depression	1.9 (for men) 3.2 (for women)
Schizophrenia	0.4
Alzheimer's disease	1–5 5 (for men); 6 (for women) over 60 years
Alcohol use disorders	1.7 (2.8 for men; 0.5 for women)

Source: World Health Report 2001

for this disorder among women are fast increasing in many regions of the world (World Health Organization 2002d).

Global burden of disease

The *World Development Report 1993: Investing in Health* (World Bank 1993) and the development of the disability-adjusted life year for estimating the global burden of disease, including years lost because of disability (Murray and Lopez 1996a, 1996b, 2000) and the *World Health Report 2001*, have all raised awareness of the global burden of mental disorders. According to 2002 estimates, mental and neurological disorders accounted for 12.97 per cent of disability-adjusted life years worldwide. Broken down into regions, the figures are also high: 24.58 per cent in the Americas; 19.52 per cent in Europe; 17.57 per cent in the western Pacific; 11.33 per cent in South-East Asia; 10.80 per cent in the eastern Mediterranean region; and 4.95 per cent in Africa (WHO 2002d). Although the figures are high for all regions, they are comparatively low in developing countries, because of the large burden of communicable, maternal, perinatal and nutritional conditions in these regions.

Mental disorders accounted for 6 of the 20 leading causes of disability worldwide for the 15–44 age group, the most productive section of the population. Unipolar depressive disorders were ranked as the fourth leading cause of disability after lower respiratory infections, perinatal conditions and HIV/AIDs. Mental disorders resulted in more disability than other known public health problems such as ischaemic heart disease and cerebrovascular disease (World Health Organization 2001d). While a greater proportion of the burden is found in developed countries (including those with formerly socialist economies), developing countries are greatly affected and are likely to see a disproportionately large increase in the burden attributable to mental disorders in the coming decades. Although the mental health consequences of major epidemics such as HIV/AIDS have not been studied in detail yet, they are likely to be substantial and will no doubt contribute to the increase in mental health problems in developing countries (World Health Organization 2001d). In the light of this, it becomes increasingly important that countries stop viewing mental health in isolation, but rather as an integral part of the challenge posed by communicable diseases.

Economic and social costs of mental disorders

The economic and social costs of mental disorders fall on societies, governments, people with mental disorders and their carers and families. Given the long-term nature of mental disorders, the most evident economic burden is that of direct treatment costs. For example, the most important contributor to direct costs of depression is hospitalization, accounting for around half of the total in the United Kingdom and three-quarters in the United States (Berto *et al.* 2000).

The indirect costs attributable to mental disorders (from unemployment, increases in absenteeism and decreased productivity) outweigh the direct treatment costs by two to six times in developed market economies (Greenberg *et al.* 1993; Kind and Sorensen 1993), and are likely to account for an even larger proportion of the total costs in developing countries, where the direct treatment costs tend to be low (Chisholm *et al.* 2000). In the United Kingdom, mental health problems were found to be the second most important category of ill health, resulting in 5–6 million working days lost annually (Gabriel and Liimatainen 2000). In the European Union (EU), it is estimated that the cost of mental problems may amount to 3–4 per cent of gross national product (GNP) (Gabriel and Liimatainen 2000).

In most countries, families bear a significant proportion of these economic costs because of the absence of publicly-funded, comprehensive mental health service networks. However, ultimately governments and societies pay a price in terms of reduced national income and increased expenditure on social welfare programmes. Thus, the economic logic for societies and countries is simple: treating and preventing mental disorders is expensive but leaving them unattended can be more so.

In addition to the obvious suffering caused by mental disorders there is a hidden burden of stigma and discrimination, and human rights violations. Rejection, unfair denial of employment opportunities and discrimination in access to services, health insurance and housing are common, as are violations of basic human rights and freedoms, as well as denials of civil, political, economic and social rights, in both institutions and communities. Much of this goes unreported and therefore the burden remains unquantified.

Families and primary care providers also incur social costs, such as the emotional burden of looking after disabled family members, diminished quality of life, social exclusion, stigmatization and loss of future opportunities for self-improvement. The risk of developing a mental disorder is also higher among carers. The end result of high health care costs, lost productivity and social costs is the creation of, or worsening of, poverty.

Global resources for mental health

The WHO survey of mental health resources (World Health Organization 2001a, 2001b) has been a comprehensive and systematic attempt to understand resources for mental health in countries across the world. Although there are a number of methodological limitations to this study which have been described in detail elsewhere (World Health Organization 2001a), project *Atlas* has highlighted the huge gap between the burden of mental disorders and available resources.

Survey results indicated that 40 per cent of countries do not have a mental health policy, ranging from 30 per cent in South-East Asia to 52 per cent in Africa. In Europe, 33 per cent of countries do not have a mental health policy, although some do have a well-developed action plan for mental health. The presence of policy, although an essential part of planning, does not guarantee an effective response to the mental health burden of any particular country. This depends on the comprehensiveness and relevance of the policy as well as its degree of implementation.

Despite the need for legislation and the useful role it can play in protecting and promoting human rights, policy development and implementation, mental health legislation is absent in 25 per cent of countries, covering nearly 31 per cent of the world's population. Of the countries which have mental health legislation, only half (51 per cent) have laws passed after 1990 and 15 per cent of countries have laws that predate the 1960s. In Europe the situation is more positive, with 80 per cent of countries having formulated their legislation after 1990. However, the presence of legislation, even if it has been formulated recently, does not guarantee the protection and promotion of rights of persons with mental disorders. Legislation in many countries is outdated or in many instances takes *away* rights of persons with mental disorders rather than protects their rights. Furthermore, even progressive legislation is of little use if it fails to be implemented effectively, as is the case in many countries.

The findings of *Atlas* provide some indication of the range and often the under-provision of human resources globally. About half the countries of the world have less than 1 psychiatrist and psychiatric nurse per 100,000 population. The medium number of psychiatrists varies from 0.06 per 100,000 population in low income countries to 9 per 100,000 in high income countries. For psychiatric nurses the corresponding figures are 0.16 to 33.5 per 100,000 for low and high income countries respectively (World Health Organization 2001a). Europe has the highest medium number of psychiatrists and psychiatric nurses at 9.0 and 27.5 per 100,000 respectively.

The level of service and treatment resources are also lacking: 37 per cent of countries worldwide do not have community care facilities. This figure is at its highest in the South-East Asian region at 50 per cent, followed by the eastern Mediterranean region, where community care facilities are absent in 45 per cent of countries. In comparison, the European region has a relatively low number of countries without community care facilities, at 26 per cent.

Worldwide, 20 per cent of countries do not have some of the basic psychotropic medicines in primary care settings. In Europe, 22 per cent of countries do not have access to these medicines in primary care. This figure is startlingly high when compared to other regions where the percentage ranges from 21 per cent (eastern Mediterranean region) to 10 per cent (the Americas). Only the African region has a substantially higher percentage of countries without basic psychotropic medicines (29 per cent).

Forty per cent of countries worldwide do not provide treatment for severe mental disorders at primary care level. This figure ranges from 56 per cent of countries in South-East Asia to 35 and 34 per cent in Europe and the Americas respectively. In spite of policy shifts to deinstitutionalization, more than 65 per cent of psychiatric beds in the world are still in mental hospitals. Seventy per cent of countries in Europe have psychiatric beds in mental hospitals, which is higher than both the Americas (47 per cent) and the western Pacific (69 per cent).

These figures are more alarming due to the fact that the level of financial resources being invested to improve mental health is disproportionately low compared with the disability and burden of disease resulting from mental disorders. Twenty-eight per cent of countries do not have a specified mental health budget and of those countries reporting actual mental health expenditure, 36 per cent spend less than 1 per cent of their total health budget on mental health (World Health Organization 2001a). Interestingly, in the European region more than 54 per cent of countries spend more than 5 per cent of their health budget on mental health.

Impact of broader policy issues on the mental health of the population

The mental health of populations and societies is influenced by many macro-social and economic factors, including urbanization, poverty, education and employment among many others. For example, the complex interaction of factors associated with urbanization can increase the risk of developing mental health problems. Urbanization can exacerbate poverty, increase the risk of homelessness and of exposure to environmental adversities such as pollution. It also disrupts established patterns of family life, leading to reduced social support (Desjarlais *et al.* 1995). Poverty is one of the strongest factors affecting mental health. In both market economies and developing countries it is both a cause and effect of mental disorders (Patel 2001). Given the strong linkages between macro-socio, economic factors and mental health, the latter needs to be an important consideration in the implementation of millennium development goals and poverty reduction strategies. Furthermore, government policies impacting on macro-social factors need to be carefully considered for potential negative and unintended effects on mental health before being implemented. Mechanisms should be introduced in order to prevent mental disorders and to monitor the mental health situation that arises in response to policies. Using the case of poverty as an example, government policies aimed at reducing absolute and relative levels of poverty are likely to have a significant positive impact on mental disorders.

Policy and strategic planning

Mental health policy, when well conceptualized, can define a vision for improving mental health and reducing the burden of mental disorders in a population. It allows the expression of an organized and coherent set of values, principles and objectives to achieve the vision and to establish a model for action. Without policy direction, lack of coordination, fragmentation and inefficiencies in the system will weaken the impact of any mental health intervention.

It is not easy to achieve a common vision among stakeholders from diverse backgrounds. Part of the difficulty is that different stakeholders – for example, consumers, family representatives and mental health professionals – interpret the population's mental health needs in different ways. Autonomy may be the most pressing issue for consumers. While families may emphasize the need for adequate information, financial and social support, mental health professionals look towards efficiency and resources, and policy-makers seek cost-effectiveness. However, the process of establishing a vision allows discussion and the sharing of ideas among different stakeholders and helps to negotiate boundaries and define a general image of the future of mental health. This shared vision can provide direction to activities and improve collaboration. The vision adopted will be underpinned by a number of values and principles. If debated and made explicit, values and principles will improve the coherence of strategies adopted to implement the shared vision. Different countries, regions, cultural and social groups within a country have their own values associated with mental health and mental disorders but in essence they should reflect notions of equity, uphold human rights standards and ultimately be reflected in all actions and interventions adopted.

Once the vision, values and principles are defined, a number of objectives, areas for action and strategies can be formulated. Objectives should aim to improve the health of the population, respond to people's expectations and provide financial protection against the cost of ill health (World Health Organization 2001d). A number of strategies simultaneously addressing a number of areas for action need to be identified in order to take these objectives forward. These areas include: financing, legislation and human rights, organization of services, human resources and training, promotion, prevention, treatment and rehabilitation, advocacy, quality improvement, information systems, research and evaluation.

Finally it is essential that policy and planning be based on reliable information about available mental health resources and an epidemiological profile of mental health problems in the country. The information base to guide planning, however, is lacking in many countries and often expert synthesis and interpretation is required of the best available data from local, national, regional and international levels. Currently, around a third of countries have no system for the annual reporting of mental health data, and often data, when available, are not sufficient to guide planning (World Health Organization 2001a).

Key issues for mental health policy and service development

Outlined below are a number of key issues and principles that should guide mental health system reform and inform government action in the area of policy and service development.

Involvement of consumer and family organizations

The mental health system exists for persons with mental disorders and family members and they can – and should – make important contributions to defining what works and how the mental health system can be improved. In addition, families assume a great part of the responsibility for caring for a family member who has a mental disorder, and this is likely to increase with the movement towards deinstitutionalization and community care. Understandably, families' understanding, knowledge and skills can influence greatly the quality of care and support provided to a family member who has a mental disorder. At times, there are notable tensions between the viewpoints of consumer and family groups, some of the most important focusing on involuntary admission and treatment. However, it is imperative that both persons with mental disorders and family members be included in the development of services, in reviewing standards and in the development and implementation of policy and legislation.

Experience demonstrates that the development of consumer and family groups and their active involvement in a number of areas has led to improvements in the quality of services and care provided to persons with mental disorders (World Health Organization 2003d). Consumer and family groups have achieved this through a variety of activities ranging from advocacy to awareness-raising and education, support groups and the development of alternative services.

Financing to support equity, efficiency and reform

Adequate and sustained financing is a critical factor in the creation of a viable mental health system. Financing is not only a major driver of a mental health system but is also a powerful tool with which policy-makers can develop and shape mental health services and their impact.

Although in many countries prepayment-based systems (tax, social insurance, private insurance) have been introduced to protect people from catastrophic financial risk from health care problems, the degree to which they do indeed protect persons with mental health problems depends on whether enough of the prepayment is dedicated to mental disorders. Unfortunately, mental health is often excluded from basic health packages and from health insurance coverage. This results in a significant financial burden on the family, who are sometimes driven to poverty due to the chronic nature of the condition. It also results in a considerable economic burden for the country as a whole.

Indeed, poor work performance and absenteeism due to mental health problems contribute significantly to loss of productivity. Some of the most prevalent and serious mental disorders are often onset in early adulthood when people might be expected to be at their most economically active (Üstün 1999). The financial burden of mental health problems in developed countries is estimated to be between 3 and 4 per cent of GNP and costs national economies several billion dollars a year, both in terms of expenditures incurred and loss of productivity. The average annual costs, including medical, pharmaceutical and disability costs, for employees with depression may be 4.2 times higher than those incurred by a typical beneficiary (Birnbaum *et al.* 1999). However, the inclusion of mental health into prepayment schemes can significantly reduce this financial burden, since the cost of treatment is often completely offset by a reduction in the number of days of absenteeism and productivity lost while at work (World Health Organization 2003a).

Equity and efficiency considerations should be at the forefront when making financing decisions. Financing can be used to address *equity* issues by allocating specific resources to certain disadvantaged population groups or groups at high risk of developing mental disorders and to ensure that persons who meet certain income criteria do not have to pay user fees for services or that they pay in accordance with their incomes. Financing can only address certain aspects of equity however. The stigma and discrimination associated with mental disorders also represent significant barriers to service access, and appropriate measures are required to tackle these problems in order to ensure that people with mental disorders are able to seek and receive the treatment and care that they need.

To enhance *efficiency*, decisions about allocations of resources to different types of services and interventions (hospital-based, community-based, case management, medications etc.) should be based on data about effectiveness and cost-effectiveness and should be closely linked to priorities specified in progressive policy. Financing can also be used, as mentioned above, to *reform* mental heath systems; for example, it can be used to change predominantly psychiatric-focused care to care in the community and general health care settings. Providing financial incentives to community programmes represents one strategy to promote this reform process. In a bonus programme in Texas, for example, mental health agencies received a certain fixed amount for each bed-day reduced and this resulted in relatively rapid deinstitutionalization (World Health Organization 2003b).

Commitment to quality

Quality is a measure of whether services increase the likelihood of desired mental health outcomes and are consistent with current evidence-based practice. A focus on quality helps to ensure that scarce resources are used in an efficient and effective way.

Quality is an essential requirement of any mental health service whether the service is in its infancy, with minimal resources, or well established, with plentiful resources (see Box 18.2). Clearly in settings where human and financial

Box 18.2 Quality standards

A focus on quality helps to ensure that resources are used properly. In most systems, resources are not used optimally. Some systems *overuse* many ineffective services; that is, services do not result in improvement or even cause harm. Other systems *underuse* effective services; that is, systems fail to provide what people need. In either case the lack of a focus on quality results in resources being wasted.

A focus on quality helps to ensure that the latest scientific knowledge and new technologies are used in treatments. In the last decade, major scientific breakthroughs have occurred in medications and treatments for mental disorders. The *World Health Report* (World Health Organization 2001d) documents treatments that work, but also points out that there is a huge gulf between the knowledge base and what is implemented.

A focus on quality helps to build trust in the effectiveness of the system and to overcome barriers to appropriate care at different levels. Satisfactory quality builds societal credibility in mental health treatment. It is the basis for demonstrating that the benefits of treatment for mental disorders outweigh the social costs of having such disorders. Without satisfactory quality funders, the general public and even persons with mental illnesses and their families become disillusioned.

Adapted from World Health Organization (2003c)

resources are lacking, implementing quality standards represents a considerable challenge. Furthermore, access to the latest scientific breakthroughs in mental health treatment is also likely to be limited. Even in such settings, however, quality improvement is crucial, since poor quality services are likely to be ineffective and therefore result in a wastage of already scarce resources. Planners confronted by limited resources therefore need to prioritize in order to make best use of available resources. They may need to decide, for example, whether to provide current service recipients with better services or use the resources to serve more people.

Policy-makers should put in place a number of simple strategies to improve quality. Some of these include building quality standards into policy and legislation, defining professional standards of the mental health workforce and their training, establishing and monitoring services through established standards and accreditation procedures and ensuring the availability of clinical guidelines based on evidence-based practice.

Service organization

In order to deliver a high standard of mental health treatment and care the WHO emphasizes the adoption of an integrated system of service delivery which attempts to comprehensively address the full range of psychosocial needs of people with mental disorders. A number of policy recommendations for service organization have been highlighted in the *World Health Report 2001*, and elaborated upon in the WHO Mental Health Policy and Service Guidance Package. They include:

- shifting care away from large psychiatric hospitals;
- developing community mental health services; and
- integrating mental health care into general health services.

Essentially, ethical and scientific considerations have given impetus to the movement to transfer mental health care from mental hospitals to primary health care, general hospitals and a range of community services in the expectation of enhancing accessibility and acceptability of services, achieving better 'mental' and 'physical' health outcomes and also achieving a better rationalization of resources.

While it is not appropriate to be prescriptive at a global level about the micro-level details of service organization in individual countries, as this will depend on a number of important social, economic and political variables, a number of general recommendations can be made. These are summarized in Figure 18.1 which shows the degree to which different categories of services should be provided and their relative cost. A large part of mental health care can be self-managed and/or managed by informal community mental health services and low-cost resources can be made available in the community to this effect. Where additional expertise and support is needed a more formalized network of

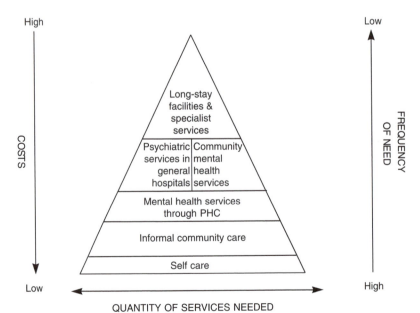

Figure 18.1 WHO-recommended optimal mix of services

Source: Adapted from World Health Organization (2003c)

services is required. In ascending order these include: primary care services, followed by psychiatric services based in general hospitals and formal community mental health services, and lastly by specialist and long-stay mental health services.

However, even if the 'ideal' service organization model as depicted in the diagram is adopted, it would not result in optimal treatment and care for persons with mental disorders unless a number of key principles for organizing services are respected. These include the need to have services and care which promote accessibility, comprehensiveness, effectiveness, continuity and coordination, needs-led care, equity and respect for human rights.

Human resources planning and training

Human resources (HR) are the most valuable assets of a mental health service. In most mental health services, the largest portion of the annual recurrent budget is spent on personnel (Thornicroft and Tansella 1999). A mental health service relies on the skill and motivation of its personnel to promote mental health, prevent disorders and provide care for people with mental disorders.

Yet, there are frequently major difficulties encountered in the planning and training of HR for mental health care. In many countries there are too few trained and available personnel, there are distribution difficulties within a country or region (e.g. too few staff in rural settings or too many staff in large institutional settings), the available personnel are not used appropriately and many staff are unproductive or demoralized.

There are several reasons why HR planning has been so poor, including the lack of an appropriate body responsible for HR planning, long training periods for staff (which mean that decisions to train more staff take time to filter into services), training institutions that are out of touch with service and population needs, the lack of accurate or usable data, the perception by general health authorities that mental health is not a priority, the presence of a significant private sector which can draw professionals away from public sector services, the migration of skilled mental health workers to developed countries (i.e. 'brain drain') and professional attitudes which may hinder some aspects of HR development (Green 1999).

Several courses of action can be taken by countries to address these difficulties. There is a need to develop appropriate policy for HR in mental health to ensure a harmonious fit between the nature and level of knowledge and skills required of mental health workers at different levels of service delivery and service needs. Planning needs to address practical details about the numbers of mental health professionals required at different levels of service delivery and the skill mix and competencies required. Continuing education, training and supervision are fundamental to providing evidence-based care and need to be reviewed periodically and improved, in keeping with the mental health needs of the population. Ongoing education and opportunities for skills development, along with the provision of specialist training, can also act as an incentive to retain individuals who may otherwise be tempted to seek training and employment opportunities abroad. Finally, management strategies need to enhance leadership, motivation, recruitment and the deployment of often scarce personnel.

Conclusions

Mental disorders contribute significantly to the global burden of disease, and are associated with economic and social costs to individuals, families and countries. Reducing this burden is possible given an important evolving information base to guide policy, service development and clinical practice. However, there remains a sizeable gap between what we know in terms of what works and what is actually available in countries. In developed countries, deinstitutionalization has not been accompanied by sufficient provision of community-based residential and occupational facilities. The detection and treatment of mental disorders in primary care settings remains poor and there remain tensions between the competing demands for general versus specialist services. In developing countries, the gross under-provision of resources, personnel and services needs urgent attention. The gap needs to be closed by continued advocacy efforts to raise mental health on the agenda of governments, by continued dissemination of information on effective policies, service development and clinical practice, and the dissemination of international human right standards.

The larger macro-social and economic factors impacting on mental health need to be pursued in this overall effort. Poverty, education and economic development are some of the millennium development goals that, if appropriately addressed, can contribute to reducing the gap. International and multilateral organizations and non-governmental organizations (NGOs) have unique roles to play. These roles necessarily differ according to the specific mandates of organizations and it is not the place of this chapter to elaborate on these. In the end, it will be the political commitment of governments to address mental health problems, the strength of consumer and family movements in countries to ensure that mental health does not disappear from the agenda, the support provided by international and multilateral organizations, NGOs and the international community at large that will ensure continued progress in the area of mental health.

References

Berto, P., D'Ilario, D., Ruffo, P., Di Virgilio, R. and Rizzo, F. (2000) Depression: cost-of-illness studies in the international literature, a review, *The Journal of Mental Health Policy and Economics*, 3(1): 3–10.

Birnbaum, H., Greenberg, P., Barton, M., Kessler, R., Rowland, C. and Williamson, T. (1999) Workplace burden of depression: a case study in social functioning using employer claims data, *Drug Benefits Trends*, 11: 6BH–12BH.

Chisholm, D., Sekar, K., Kumar, K., Saeed, K., James, S., Mubbashar, M. and Murthy, R.S. (2000) Integration of mental health care into primary care: demonstration cost-outcome study in India and Pakistan, *British Journal of Psychiatry*, 176: 581–8.

Desjarlais, R., Eisenberg, L., Good, B. and Kleinman, A. (1995) *World Mental Health: Problems And Priorities In Low-Income Countries.* New York: Oxford University Press.

Gabriel, P. and Liimatainen, M.R. (2000) *Mental Health in the Workplace.* Geneva: International Labour Office.

Green, A. (1999) *An Introduction to Health Planning in Developing Countries,* 2nd edn. Oxford: Oxford University Press.

Greenberg, P.E., Stiglin, L.E., Finkelstein, S.N. and Berndt, E.R. (1993) The economic burden of depression in 1990, *Journal of Clinical Psychiatry,* 54(11): 1–14.

Kind, P. and Sorensen, J. (1993) The costs of depression, *International Clinical Psychopharmacology,* 7: 191–5.

Murray, C.J.L. and Lopez, A.D. (eds) (1996a) *The Global Burden of Disease: A Comprehensive Assessment of Mortality and Disability From Diseases, Injuries and Risk Factors in 1990 and Projected to 2020.* Cambridge, MA: Harvard School of Public Health on behalf of the World Health Organization and the World Bank (Global Burden of Disease and Injury Series, vol. I).

Murray, C.J.L. and Lopez, A.D. (1996b) *Global Health Statistics.* Cambridge, MA: Harvard School of Public Health on behalf of the World Health Organization and the World Bank (Global Burden of Disease and Injury Series, vol. II).

Murray, C.J.L. and Lopez, A.D. (2000) Progress and directions in refining the global burden of disease approach: a response to Williams, *Health Economics,* 9: 69–82.

Patel, V. (2001) Poverty, inequality, and mental health in developing countries, in D. Leon and G. Walt (eds) *Poverty, Inequality and Health: An International Perspective.* Oxford: Oxford University Press.

Thornicroft, G. and Tansella, M. (1999) *The Mental Health Matrix: A Manual to Improve Services.* Cambridge: Cambridge University Press.

Üstün, T.B. (1999) The global burden of mental disorders, *American Journal of Public Health,* 89(9): 1315–18.

World Bank (1993) *World Development Report 1993: Investing in Health.* New York: Oxford University Press for the World Bank.

World Health Organization (2001a) *Atlas: Mental Health Resources in the World 2001.* Geneva: World Health Organization.

World Health Organization (2001b) *Atlas: Country Profiles on Mental Health Resources 2001.* Geneva: World Health Organization.

World Health Organization (2001c) *Mental and Neurological Disorders* (fact sheet No. 265, December). Geneva: World Health Organization.

World Health Organization (2001d) *The World Health Report 2001. Mental Health: New Understanding, New Hope.* Geneva: World Health Organization.

World Health Organization (2001e) *Gender Disparities in Mental Health – Ministerial Round Tables 2001.* Geneva: World Health Organization.

World Health Organization (2002a) *Resolution EB109.R8 – Strengthening Mental Health. One Hundred and Ninth session of the Executive Board.* Geneva: World Health Organization.

World Health Organization (2002b) *Resolution WHA 55.10 – Mental Health: Responding to the Call for Action. Fifty-fifth World Health Assembly.* Geneva: World Health Organization.

World Health Organization (2002c) *World Report on Violence and Health.* Geneva: World Health Organization.

World Health Organization (2002d) *World Health Report 2002. Reducing Risks, Promoting Healthy Life.* Geneva: World Health Organization.

World Health Organization (2003a) *Investing in Mental Health.* Geneva: World Health Organization.

World Health Organization (2003b) *WHO Mental Health Policy and Service Guidance Package: Mental Health Financing.* Geneva: World Health Organization.

World Health Organization (2003c) *WHO Mental Health Policy and Service Guidance Package: Organization of Services for Mental Health.* Geneva: World Health Organization.

World Health Organization (2003d) *WHO Mental Health Policy and Service Guidance Package: Quality Improvement for Mental Health Care.* Geneva: World Health Organization.

Index

Related books from Open University Press

Purchase from www.openup.co.uk or order through your local bookseller

PRIMARY CARE IN THE DRIVER'S SEAT

ORGANIZATIONAL REFORM IN EUROPEAN PRIMARY CARE

Richard Saltman, Ana Rico and Wienke Boerma (eds)

- What is the best way to structure primary care services?
- How can coordination between primary care and other parts of health care systems be improved?
- How should new technologies be integrated into primary care?

There is considerable agreement among national policy makers across Europe that, in principle, primary care should be the linchpin of a well-designed health care system. This agreement, however, does not carry over into the organizational mechanisms best suited to pursuing or achieving this common objective. Across western, central and eastern Europe, primary care is delivered through a wide range of institutional, financial, professional and clinical configurations. This book is a study of the reforms of primary care in Europe as well as their impacts on the broader co-ordination mechanisms within European health care systems. It also provides suggestions for effective strategies for future improvement in health care system reform.

Primary Care in the Driver's Seat is key reading for students studying health policy, health economics, public policy and management, as well as health managers and policy makers.

Contributors
Richard Baker; Sven-Eric Bergman; Wienke Boerma; Mats Brommels; Michael Calnan; Diana Delnoij; Anna Dixon; Carl-Ardy Dubois; Joan Gené Badia; Bernhard Gibis; Stefan Greß; Peter Groenewegen; Jan Heyrman; Jack Hutten; Michael Kidd; Mårten Kvist; Miranda Laurant; Margus Lember; Martin Marshall; Alison McCallum; Toomas Palu; Ana Rico; Ray Robinson; Valentin Rusovich; Richard B. Saltman; Anthony Scott; Rod Sheaff; Igor Svab; Bonnie Sibbald; Hrvoje Tiljak; Andrija Štampar; Michel Wensing.

Contents
List of tables – List of boxes – List of figures – List of contributors – Series editors' introduction – Foreword – Acknowledgements – Part one: Assessing the strategic landscape – Coordination and integration in European primary care – Mapping primary care across Europe – Changing conditions for structural reform in primary care – Drawing the strands together: primary care in perspective – Part two: Changing institutional arrangements – The challenge of coordination: The role of primary care professionals in promoting integration across the interface – The impact of primary care purchasing in Europe: A comparative case study of primary care reform – The evolving public-private mix – Part three: Changing working arrangements – Changing task profiles – Changing professional roles in primary care education – Managing primary care behaviour through payment systems and financial incentives – Part four: Changing quality standards – Improving the quality and performance of primary care – The role of new information and communication technologies in primary care – Index.

2005 280pp
0 335 21365 0 (EAN: 9 780335 213658) Paperback
0 335 21366 9 (EAN: 9 780335 213665) Hardback

HUMAN RESOURCES FOR HEALTH IN EUROPE

Carl-Ardy Dubois, Martin McKee, and Ellen Nolte

Health service human resources are key determinants of health service performance. The human resource is the largest and most expensive input into healthcare, yet it can be the most challenging to develop. This book examines some of the major challenges facing health care professions in Europe and the potential responses to these challenges.

The book analyses how the current regulatory processes and practices related to key aspects of the management of the health professions may facilitate or inhibit the development of effective responses to future challenges facing health care systems in Europe. The authors document how health care systems in Europe are confronting existing challenges in relation to the health workforce and identify the strategies that are likely to be most effective in optimizing the management of health professionals in the future.

Human Resources for Health in Europe is key reading for health policy-makers and postgraduates taking courses in health services management, health policy and health economics. It is also of interest to human resource professionals.

Contributors
Carl Afford, Rita Baeten, James Buchan, Anna Dixon, Carl-Ardy Dubois, Sigrún Gunnarsdóttir, Yves Jorens, Elizabeth Kachur, Karl Krajic, Suzy Lessof, Ann Mahon, Alan Maynard, Martin McKee, Ellen Nolte, Anne Marie Rafferty, Charles Shaw, Bonnie Sibbald, Ruth Young.

Contents
Foreword – Human resources for health in Europe – Analysing trends, opportunities and challenges – Migration of health workers in Europe: policy problem or policy solution? – Changing professional boundaries – Structures and trends in health profession education in Europe – Managing the performance of health professionals – Health care managers as a critical component of the health care workforce – Incentives in health care: the shift in emphasis from the implicit to the explicit – Enhancing working conditions – Reshaping the regulation of the workforce in European health care systems – The challenges of transition in CEE and the NIS of the former USSR – The impact of EU law and policy – Moving forward: building a strategic framework for the development of the health care workforce – Index.

288pp   0 335 21855 5 (Paperback)   0 335 21856 3 (Hardback)

PURCHASING TO IMPROVE HEALTH SYSTEMS PERFORMANCE

Edited by Josep Figueras, Ray Robinson and Elke Jakubowski

Purchasing is championed as key to improving health systems performance. However, despite the central role the purchasing function plays in many health system reforms, there is very little evidence about its development or its real impact on societal objectives. This book addresses this gap and provides:

- A comprehensive account of the theory and practice of purchasing for health services across Europe
- An up-to-date analysis of the evidence on different approaches to purchasing
- Support for policy-makers and practitioners as they formulate purchasing strategies so that they can increase effectiveness and improve performance in their own national context
- An assessment of the intersecting roles of citizens, the government and the providers

Written by leading health policy analysts, this book is essential reading for health policy makers, planners and managers as well as researchers and students in the field of health studies.

Contributors
Toni Ashton, Philip Berman, Michael Borowitz, Helmut Brand, Reinhard Busse, Andrea Donatini, Martin Dlouhy, Antonio Duran, Tamás Evetovits, André P. van den Exter, Josep Figueras, Nick Freemantle, Julian Forder, Péter Gaál, Chris Ham, Brian Hardy, Petr Hava, David Hunter, Danguole Jankauskiene, Maris Jesse, Ninel Kadyrova, Joe Kutzin, John Langenbrunner, Donald W. Light, Hans Maarse, Nicholas Mays, Martin McKee, Eva Orosz, John Øvretveit, Dominique Polton, Alexander S. Preker, Thomas A. Rathwell, Sabine Richard, Ray Robinson, Andrei Rys, Constantino Sakellarides, Sergey Shishkin, Peter C. Smith, Markus Schneider, Francesco Taroni, Marcial Velasco-Garrido, Miriam Wiley.

Contents
*List of tables – List of boxes – List of figures – List of contributors – Series Editors' introduction – Foreword – Acknowledgements – **Part One** – Introduction – Organization of purchasing in Europe – Purchasing to improve health systems – **Part Two** – Theories of purchasing – Role of markets and competition – Purchasers as the public's agent – Purchasing to promote population health – Steering the purchaser: Stewardship and government – Purchasers, providers and contracts – Purchasing for quality of care – Purchasing and paying providers – Responding to purchasing: Provider perspectives – Index.*

320pp   0 335 21367 7 (Paperback)   0 335 21368 5 (Hardback)